ANTIBIOTICS

WHAT EVERYONE NEEDS TO KNOW®

ANTIBIOTICS

WHAT EVERYONE NEEDS TO KNOW®

MARY ELIZABETH WILSON

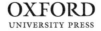

OXFORD
UNIVERSITY PRESS

OXFORD
UNIVERSITY PRESS

Oxford University Press is a department of the University of Oxford. It furthers
the University's objective of excellence in research, scholarship, and education
by publishing worldwide. Oxford is a registered trade mark of Oxford University
Press in the UK and certain other countries.

"What Everyone Needs to Know" is a registered trademark of
Oxford University Press.

Published in the United States of America by Oxford University Press
198 Madison Avenue, New York, NY 10016, United States of America.

Library of Congress Cataloging-in-Publication Data
Names: Wilson, Mary Elizabeth, author.
Title: Antibiotics : what everyone needs to know / Mary Elizabeth Wilson.
Description: New York, NY : Oxford University Press, [2019] |
Series: What everyone needs to know |
Includes bibliographical references and index.
Identifiers: LCCN 2018056947 | ISBN 9780190663407 (paperback : alk. paper) |
ISBN 9780190663414 (hardcover : alk. paper)
Subjects: LCSH: Antibiotics—Popular works.
Classification: LCC RM267.W55 2019 | DDC 615.3/29—dc23
LC record available at https://lccn.loc.gov/2018056947

1 3 5 7 9 8 6 4 2

Paperback printed by Sheridan Books, Inc., United States of America
Hardback printed by Bridgeport National Bindery, Inc., United States of America

To Miriam
Who shares her treasure with me

CONTENTS

2. USE IN HUMANS   43

Deschutes Public Library

Terminal: FE-V5-BEND-04
Date: 04/20/02022 12:33:13 PM

Member: L. S. Lo**********
Membership Number: ********0271

Current Fine: $0.00
On Loan: 13 (0 Overdue)
On Hold: 0 (0 Available to pickup)

Today's Borrowed Items: (5)

35394015835404
Clear the clutter, find happiness : one-mi
nute tips for decluttering and refreshing
your home and yo
                              Due Date: 05/11/2022

35394018169868
The minimalist way : minimalism strategies
 to declutter your life and make room for
joy / Erica Layn
                              Due Date: 05/11/2022

35394018603171
People we meet on vacation / Emily Henry.
                              Due Date: 05/11/2022

35394014488064
Unstuffed : decluttering your home, mind,
& soul / Ruth Soukup.
                              Due Date: 05/11/2022

35394018054102
Antibiotics : what everyone needs to know
/ Mary Elizabeth Wilson.
                              Due Date: 05/11/2022

Please return all items by the due date.
Thank you.
Visit us online at:
www.deschuteslibrary.org

3. CONSEQUENCES OF USE: ADVERSE EVENTS ASSOCIATED WITH USE OF ANTIBIOTICS IN HUMANS 101

4. OTHER USES OF ANTIBIOTICS (NONHUMAN USE)   149

7. INTERVENTIONS TO REDUCE NEED FOR ANTIBIOTICS AND ALTERNATIVES TO ANTIBIOTICS 263

8. PRESERVING ANTIBIOTICS AND DEVELOPING NEW ANTIBACTERIAL TREATMENTS 307

PREFACE

The future of humanity and microbes likely will unfold as episodes of a suspense thriller that could be titled Our Wits Versus Their Genes.

—Joshua Lederberg, winner of the Nobel Prize
for pioneering work on microbial genetics

Why should you read this book?

Antibiotics affect everyone. Most people have taken antibiotics at some point in their lives. But antibiotics can affect even those who have not taken them.

Antibiotics are fundamentally different from other drugs. Antibiotics are a shared resource, a community property. Using them can promote the appearance and sometimes the predominance of bacteria that resist their action. They affect the microbial landscape and biological systems on Earth. They do not disappear when a person takes a dose of penicillin or another antibiotic. Use of antibiotics has had a profound global impact.

A century ago you could die from a cut on your finger. If the break in the skin allowed virulent bacteria, like *Streptococcus*, to enter the body, they could multiply and spread. No available treatment could halt the spread, and a person lived or died depending on whether his or her own immune system could contain the infection. The youngest and the oldest, the most vulnerable, regularly died from what we would consider common infections—but young, healthy individuals also died from serious bacterial infections, like *Staphylococcus* and *Streptococcus*. Women could die from childbirth if disease-causing bacteria entered tissues after they gave birth. Minor injuries or surgical procedures or appendicitis could end in death. Pneumonia, "the old man's friend," often ended in death. During wars and other conflicts, up until World War I, more died from infections than directly from weapons of war.

Bacteria are everywhere—in and on us and animals, in air, in the soil, in water, and in the environment. We live in a sea of microbes. Only a tiny fraction can cause us harm, and many are essential for life as we know it—for each of us personally and for the planet. They are abundant, genetically diverse, resilient, and able to change rapidly. Bacteria make up a large part of life on Earth. We rely on our resident bacteria to help shape our immune systems, to help process our food, to fend off invading bacteria, and for myriad functions that we are just beginning to understand.

Bacteria can also kill us, and antibiotics have saved millions of lives over the decades they have been available. They are currently the best form of treatment for many common and not-so-common infections. They are powerful and potent and can seem magical in their rapid reversal of many infections. They can pull patients back from the brink of death. There is good reason antibiotics were considered miracle drugs when they first became available.

Antibiotics produce immediate as well as long-term consequences. Because of the incredible capacity of microbes to change rapidly through mutation and through horizontal gene transfer and a whole variety of molecular maneuvers, they can evade the effects of antibiotics and facilitate movement of resistance to other bacteria—not necessarily even the same species of bacteria. Exposure to antibiotics (and to antiseptics, disinfectants, and other biocides) thus contributes to the emergence of resistance in bacteria. The wide use of antibiotics has helped shape a microbial world that is composed of many more resistant bacteria than existed before antibiotics were used.

Because antibiotics are relatively cheap, accessible, familiar, and generally safe, they are often used casually, indiscriminately, and thoughtlessly. Antibiotics are used to treat humans, but large quantities are also used in food animals, work animals, pets, and plants. Widespread use of antibiotics ultimately reduces their effectiveness for everyone. This leads to a major challenge: how do we apply these life-saving drugs in ways to save lives and also preserve, for as long as possible, their benefits? Too often we are squandering a precious resource.

Many global organizations, governments, and institutions are awakening to the serious problem of antibiotic resistance and are trying to find ways to reverse this growing menace. This will not be easy. The effort must be global because antibiotic-resistant bacteria and resistance genes move within regions and around the world with the greatest of ease. They are carried by humans, by animals, in food, and in water systems. They contaminate the soil and water in some areas.

Interventions to deal with antibiotic resistance must involve multiple sectors—human and animal health, agriculture, environmental systems, food production, industry, governments, and policymakers. A One Health approach must embrace animal and plant health and the environment as well human health. Urgent needs include provision of infrastructure to provide clean water and sanitary waste disposal to populations that lack them, delivery of effective vaccines, and research into diagnostics, new vaccines, and new antibiotics and other treatment approaches. Stewardship programs can help to improve use and perhaps allow longer use of existing antibiotics, but stewardship alone will not be sufficient. We also need to reduce the incidence of avoidable infections to reduce the need for antibiotics. Three prominent areas include improved access to clean water and sanitary waste disposal, increased use of current vaccines, and interventions to reduce health care–associated infections.

The World Health Organization (WHO) recently (2018) delivered a report that lays out total consumption of antibiotics as described by defined daily doses (DDDs) per 1,000 inhabitants per day in metric tons for 65 countries and areas. The consumption ranges from 4.4 DDDs per 1,000 inhabitants in Burundi to 64.4 DDDs for Mongolia. Even within high- and middle-income countries, use in 2015 varied widely: 9.78 in the Netherlands, 11.49 in Germany, 14.19 in Japan, 17.05 in Canada, 25.92 in France, and 33.85 for Greece. There is also wide variation in antibiotic use by city and region within countries, including the United States. The marked, national variation in use suggests that many countries could achieve good outcomes with substantially reduced consumption of antibiotics.

Globally use of antibiotics can be characterized by excess use in some populations and some sectors and by lack of access in other (low-income) populations. Resistant bacteria and resistance genes also spread more rapidly and widely in areas that lack clean drinking water and sanitary waste disposal. In general, low-income countries have higher burdens of infections and have a greater need for antibiotics than high-income countries.

Why did I write this book?

Many people have had personal experience with taking an antibiotic for an infection and may think of antibiotics narrowly—just another drug taken to treat an illness. This book aims to provide a broader picture of the scope and scale of how antibiotics are used and the global impact they have had and are having on biological systems in individuals and populations and on the environment. Their broad use threatens to undermine their effectiveness. A better understanding of how they work—and their limitations and broad impacts—may promote more thoughtful and informed use. A recent survey suggested that about a third of people in the United States still believe that antibiotics work against viral infections. They often cite personal experience. They had a viral infection, they took an antibiotic, and they got better. The problem with reaching this conclusion is that if they had a viral infection and did not take an antibiotic, they would also get better—in the same period of time.

This book provides a broad view of antibiotics—where they come from, how they were discovered, how they work, and how they are used in people, food animals, pets, plants, and aquaculture. The book examines in detail the consequences of their use, including adverse drug reactions, impact on the microbiota, and especially the development and spread of resistant bacteria and resistance genes. The consequences of antibiotic-resistant bacteria are already apparent. People are dying today from infections that cannot be treated with the available antibiotics and from consequences of taking antibiotics (e.g., *Clostridioides difficile* colitis). Many interventions ranging from simple (like handwashing) to difficult and expensive can be undertaken to markedly reduce the burden from infections and the need for antibiotics. We should focus on these at the same time we support research and development of better diagnostics, new vaccines, new antibiotics, and other forms of treatment that do not involve antibiotics.

After new antibiotics are developed and approved by the US Food and Drug Administration (FDA) for use (a long, expensive, and uncertain process), they often follow a typical course over time as more and more bacteria find ways to resist them. Antibiotics will continue to play a role in the treatment of infections, but we should not focus all of our research efforts into just finding more antibiotics of the traditional sort. Most antibiotics available today are crude instruments for eliminating bacteria causing an infection or illness because they also destroy many beneficial bacteria along with the disease-causing bacteria. We do not fully understand the consequences of disrupting the microbiota. We need better and more precise tools. Ideally we should hit the target bacteria and leave the others unscathed.

An evolution of thinking about bacteria resident on and within our bodies has come from a better understanding of the microbiome and appreciation of the many services our microbiota provides throughout life. We are learning that our microbiota are a treasure to be maintained and nourished. We are learning this as many residents in many high-income countries are being found to harbor impoverished microbiota. Efforts are underway to create banks to save bacteria that are at risk of being eliminated from human populations. New approaches are looking at ways to work with and harness beneficial microbes rather than using a search-and-destroy strategy. The microbes have a remarkable capacity to adapt to our interventions. We must use our wits to survive.

In this book, I have sought to convey a perspective on antibiotics that stretches from history into the future; that demonstrates how antibiotics are a precious, misused, fragile, and imperfect resource; that respects the subtlety and complexity of human interaction with our microbial surround; and that provides practical information and a clear-eyed view of the challenges evoked by this fascinating topic, antibiotics.

ACKNOWLEDGMENTS

I elected to pursue postgraduate medical training in Boston, home of many towering figures in the discipline of infectious diseases. These included Max Finland at Boston City Hospital, who pioneered in studies of penicillin in the United States and called attention to potential problems with antibiotic resistance as early as 1946. From the start, he was critical of indiscriminate use of antibiotics. In 1975 he wrote about antibiotics in animal feed and salmonellosis in animals and humans. Other leaders such as Edward Kass and Louis Weinstein also recognized early on the potential problems with overuse and misuse of antibiotics and were articulate in conveying this message. Weinstein, blunt and direct, was an outspoken critic of the misuse of broad-spectrum antibiotics. For many years I attended regular teaching rounds in Boston with Edward Kass, Louis Weinstein, Morton Swartz, Arnold Weinberg, Robert Moellering, and other leaders in the field. My thinking about antibiotics was shaped by masters in the field, individuals who were participants from the beginning of the antibiotic era and who helped define the modern discipline of infectious diseases.

My internal medicine and infectious diseases training was done at Beth Israel Hospital in Boston in the Harvard program. Our weekly rounds included the infectious diseases team from Brigham and Women's Hospital where Thomas O'Brien, a global leader in the study of antibiotic resistance, had a laboratory. He joined and contributed to our conferences. During the second year of my infectious diseases fellowship, I spent 3 months in Haiti working at the Albert Schweitzer Hospital. Although only a few hours' flight, it was a world away from Boston. Common medical problems were malaria, tuberculosis, intestinal parasites, tetanus, and typhoid fever, along with the familiar infections like streptococcal and staphylococcal infections. Here I was surprised to learn that about 90% of the *Staphylococcus aureus* isolates were sensitive to penicillin. In contrast, in Boston at that time about 90% of the *S. aureus* isolates were resistant to penicillin. On reflection, it made sense. The staphylococcal bacteria carried by residents in a largely rural area near Deschapelles, Haiti, had limited exposure to antibiotics and were more like naïve bacteria seen in the preantibiotic era.

I did not choose to do my postmedical school training in Boston because of prior awareness of the depth of knowledge to be found there in infectious diseases and antibiotics, but I fortuitously landed in that rich environment. I am humbled when I think of the masters who informed my experience in infectious diseases and thinking about antibiotics and resistance. They were among the best in the world.

After my fellowship, I took a clinical position in infectious diseases at Mount Auburn Hospital, a Harvard community teaching hospital in Cambridge. Dr. John Moses, head of infectious diseases, strongly favored prudent use of antibiotics. Long before antibiotic stewardship programs became common (or required), he had instituted careful scrutiny of use of newer and broader-spectrum antibiotics. This involved many discussions with residents in training and clinicians about choices of antibiotics and resulted in more restrained and more appropriate use of antibiotics than occurred in most hospital settings. It also helped to inform my philosophy about antibiotics and their use.

In 2006 I was invited to be a member of the Pew National Commission on Industrial Farm Animal Production. One key area we examined was the use of antibiotics in food animals. Work with the commission entailed visits to concentrated animal feeding operations where we viewed chickens, pigs, and cattle being raised in massive numbers—the mass production of biomass for food. This also provided an education about the extensive use of antibiotics, including for growth promotion, in animals. We learned about another kind of resistance—reluctance on the part of some in the agricultural sector to eliminating use of antibiotics for growth promotion. Our thoughtful chair, John Carlin (former governor of Kansas), and other members, including Robert Martin and Robert Lawrence, helped to assemble and present our recommendations, which included stopping use of antibiotics for growth promotion.

Many others have shaped my thinking. I have great respect and admiration for the work by long-time colleague Stuart Levy, at Tufts in Boston, who has made a career studying antibiotic resistance and has worked for decades to engage the global community and research laboratories in the study of resistance. He has also been an advocate for ways to limit its spread and started the Alliance for the Prudent Use of Antibiotics.

Other colleagues whose impressive work related to antibiotics has helped to inform the world and shape my thinking include Ramanan Laxminarayan, founder and director of the Center for Disease Dynamics, Economics and Policy, whose knowledgeable staff and partners have been relentless in bringing data and analysis related to antibiotic use, access, and resistance to the attention of the world through talks, publications, and freely available materials on the center website. His database is global and includes animal as well as human use. He has raised attention to the issues on a global stage.

Other friends and colleagues are providing essential elements and contributions that can inform policy and action. These include Marc Mendelson, Keith Klugman, Steve

Zinner, and Heiman Wertheim. Dame Sally Davies, chief medical officer for England and chief medical advisor to the UK
government, has been enormously influential in the United
Kingdom and globally. Jeremy Farrar, head of the Wellcome
Trust, has provided financial and intellectual support, creating
broad awareness and seeking solutions to problems related to
antimicrobial resistance.

The Microbial Threats Forum at the National Academies in
its early years was chaired by Joshua Lederberg and Margaret
(Peggy) Hamburg. Members and leaders in the Microbial
Threats Forum at the National Academies in recent years have
continued to bring visibility to issues related to antibiotic resistance. These include James Hughes (who codirects the Emory
Antibiotic Resistance Center), Lonnie King, Keiji Fukuda,
and Peter Sands. John Rex, now the chief medical officer and
expert-in-residence at the Wellcome Trust, has been working
tirelessly across sectors to identify solutions to antimicrobial
resistance.

David Relman and Martin Blaser have done key research
related to the microbiome and the roles of resident microbiota
and have brought wide visibility to the science in these areas.
My work in travel medicine neatly reinforced my interest in
emerging infections and the global movement of pathogens,
especially the role of travelers in acquiring and moving resistant bacteria and resistance genes.

I thank Jaime Sepulveda, executive director of Global
Health Sciences at the University of California San Francisco,
who understands big issues related to global health and has
given me the flexibility to work on this book.

I thank Chad Zimmerman at Oxford University Press for
suggesting that I consider writing this book. Fortunately, he
convinced me that it should not take a long time to write it, so
I agreed to take on the project. It did take a long time. I learned

much in the process of composing this book, but its content emerges from decades of experience in the clinical arena and thinking about the issues.

Finally, I thank my dearest friend and loving husband, Harvey Fineberg, who has been steadfast in his support, honest in his feedback, and always creative in his ideas.

ANTIBIOTICS

WHAT EVERYONE NEEDS TO KNOW®

1

ORIGIN AND FUNCTION

What is an antibiotic?

The word "antibiotic" comes from the terms "anti," meaning "against" or "opposing," and "bios," meaning "life," and refers to a substance that works against bacterial life. Originally the term was used to describe substances, such as penicillin or streptomycin, produced by or derived from other living organisms, like bacteria or fungi, with the capacity to destroy or stop the growth of bacteria. But over time the term "antibiotic" has come to be used more broadly by most people to refer to all medicines that are used against bacteria causing infections. Today many drugs used to treat bacterial infections are semisynthetic or synthetic molecules made in the laboratory, but in general usage they are all called antibiotics. Many other substances, such as vinegar, chlorine, alcohol, and metals (e.g., copper), have antibacterial activity, but they are not referred to as antibiotics.

What is the difference between an antibiotic and an antimicrobial?

The term "antibiotic" usually refers to substances active against bacteria, whereas the term "antimicrobial" refers to all substances active against all microscopic (too small to see with the naked eye) organisms—or microbes—that cause human infections. All antibiotics are antimicrobials; not all antimicrobials are antibiotics.

Many classes of organisms cause human infections. In addition to bacteria that cause strep (streptococcal) and staph (staphylococcal) infections and tuberculosis, other microorganisms include viruses, like influenza, measles, and HIV; protozoa; and fungi. See Table 1.1 for examples of infections of each type. It is relevant to know which one is causing an infection because the treatment is often completely different depending on the cause. Today the broader term "antimicrobial" is often used to describe penicillin and other antibiotics. Another term, "anti-infectives," is also sometimes used to refer to drugs that have been developed to treat any kind of infection, whether bacterial, viral, fungal, helminth (worms), or protozoan in origin. Helminths (worms) are not included in the table because many helminths that infect humans can be seen with the naked eye. Helminths include the parasites that cause schistosomiasis, filariasis, and worm infections of the intestinal tract (like tapeworms, hookworms, and ascaris). Helminths can range in size from microscopic to worms like tapeworms that can reach meters in length.

The term "germ" is a general, informal term that is sometimes used in the popular literature to describe microorganisms that cause disease, especially bacteria and viruses. (For example, a doctor might say, "We know there's a germ that's causing this, but we're still figuring out what.") Only a tiny fraction of bacteria that exist on Earth have the capacity to cause infection or disease in humans (or plants or animals).

Other terms are sometimes used to describe drugs that have focused activity or specific targets. For example, an antiviral drug works against viruses, an antiparasitic drug against parasites, an antiprotozoal drug against protozoan parasites, and an antifungal drug against fungi. The mechanisms of action of these drugs are typically different from antibiotics,

Table 1.1 Types of Microorganisms and Examples of Infections They Cause

	Clinical Syndrome/Tissues Infected
Bacteria	
Staphylococcus aureus	Skin infection, abscess, bacteremia, endocarditis, wound infection, bone infection
Streptococcus pyogenes	Tonsillitis, sore throat, skin and soft tissue infection, scarlet fever
Streptococcus pneumoniae	Pneumonia, meningitis, ear infection, sinus infection
Enterococcus faecalis, Enterococcus faecium	Endocarditis, urinary tract infection, peritonitis
Clostridium (Clostridioides) difficile	Infection of bowel, diarrhea
Escherichia coli	Urinary tract infection, bacteremia, gastrointestinal infections
Klebsiella pneumoniae	Pneumonia, bacteremia, hospital-acquired infections
Neisseria gonorrhoeae	Gonorrhea, urethritis, cervicitis
Neisseria meningitidis	Meningitis
Vibrio cholerae	Cholera, severe diarrhea
Yersinia pestis	Plague, pneumonia, meningitis, bubo
Haemophilus influenzae	Respiratory infections, otitis, meningitis
Mycobacterium tuberculosis	Tuberculosis, lung infection, extrapulmonary infection
Viruses	
Influenza	Flu, pneumonia, bronchitis
Respiratory syncytial virus (RSV)	Upper respiratory infection, pneumonia
Rotavirus	Diarrhea
HIV	AIDS, leads to immune compromise and opportunistic infections
Varicella zoster	Chickenpox, pneumonia, shingles
Herpes simplex	Cold sores, genital herpes, encephalitis (rare)
Middle East Respiratory syndrome virus (MERS)	Pneumonia
Rubeola virus	Measles, fever, skin rash, pneumonia

(continued)

Table 1.1 Continued

	Clinical Syndrome/Tissues Infected
Protozoa	
Plasmodium species	Malaria
Giardia duodenalis	Diarrhea
Entamoeba histolytica	Amebiasis, dysentery, liver abscess
Toxoplasma gondii	Toxoplasmosis, lymphadenopathy
Fungi	
Candida albicans	Vaginitis, yeast infection of throat
Histoplasma capsulatum	Pneumonia
Coccidioides immitis	Pneumonia, meningitis, "valley fever"
Aspergillus fumigatus	Allergic bronchopulmonary infection, lung and other infections in immunocompromised patients
Cryptococcus neoformans	Meningitis in immune compromised
Pneumocystis jirovecii	Pneumonia in immune compromised

reflecting the different biologies of these other classes of microorganisms.

In other instances, terms describing the drugs may indicate activity against specific infections, such as an antimalarial drug, an agent that works against malaria; an antituberculous drug, which works against tuberculosis; and an antistaphylococcal drug, which treats staph infections.

Antibiotics are sometimes described by their mechanism of action or structure. Antibiotics are described in various classes or families (Table 1.2 lists the main classes of antibiotics). A parent drug, like penicillin, which is defined as a beta-lactam antibiotic because of a certain part of its structure, has spawned multiple generations of penicillins and related drugs, sometimes identified as third- and fourth-generation drugs. The most recently developed cephalosporins, for example, are considered fifth-generation drugs. The beta-lactam antibiotic classes have been spectacularly successful. In addition to

Table 1.2 Classes of Antibiotics

Class	Examples
Sulfonamides	Sulfamethoxazole
Beta-lactams	Penicillin, ampicillin, cephalosporins, carbapenems (e.g., meropenem)
Chloramphenicol	Chloramphenicol (now rarely used in the United States)
Tetracyclines	Doxycycline, minocycline, tigecycline
Aminoglycosides	Streptomycin, gentamicin, tobramycin
Macrolides	Erythromycin, azithromycin
Glycopeptides	Vancomycin, teicoplanin
Quinolones	Nalidixic acid, ciprofloxacin, moxifloxacin
Streptogramins	Synercid (combination of dalfopristin A and quinupristin B)
Oxazolidinones	Linezolid, tedizolid (formerly torezolid)
Lipopeptides	Daptomycin
Polyketides	Rifampin
Diarylquinolines	Bedaquiline

the penicillins, other classes of beta-lactam antibiotics include the cephalosporins, the carbapenems (e.g., imipenem and meropenem), and monobactams (e.g., aztreonam). Table 1.3 lists several classes of antibiotics and the multiple generations of drugs that have followed based on the same molecule.

In many instances the initial antibiotic in a class was based on a naturally occurring substance, often from a soil bacterium or fungus that was observed to have antibacterial

Table 1.3 Generations of Antibiotics Approved for Use in the United States

Cephalosporins	Quinolones	Tetracyclines
Cephalothin	Nalidixic acid	Oxytetracycline
Cefuroxime	Ciprofloxacin	Doxycycline
Ceftazidime	Levofloxacin	Tigecycline
Cefepime	Moxifloxacin	Eravacycline
Ceftaroline		

properties. Chemists have subsequently been able to alter the structure or add or change portions to create semisynthetic drugs with different, and typically more desirable, characteristics—or a broader or different antibacterial spectrum of activity, fewer side effects, etc. Thus, many general classes of antibiotics contain both natural and semisynthetic antibiotics. Some antibiotics, like the quinolones, are completely synthetic.

Antibiotics are sometimes described in terms of the classes of bacteria that they kill. A broad distinction is made between Gram-negative and Gram-positive bacteria. This refers to the staining characteristics of the bacteria when visualized under the microscope. How they stain reflects fundamental differences in their cell walls or bacterial cell envelopes. Another broad grouping of bacteria is by the growth conditions that the bacteria require. Some bacteria cannot grow in the presence of oxygen—so-called anaerobes. Some bacteria require oxygen for growth; others do not require it but can tolerate it. Still others are killed by the presence of oxygen. Anaerobes play an important role in many infections, including many mixed infections involving bacteria from the intestine. Examples are a ruptured appendix or perforated bowel when a mix of bacteria spill into the abdominal cavity. Many antibiotics have little or poor activity against anaerobes, so it is relevant to know which antibiotics are active against anaerobes when making decisions about the choice of antibiotics.

Antibiotics are also sometimes described by the way they affect bacteria. Do they kill them outright or do they just slow their growth? The killers are called "cidal" or bactericidal antibiotics, and those that slow growth are "bacteriostatic."

Antibiotics may also be described by their toxic effects, for example, nephrotoxic (toxic to kidneys), ototoxic (toxic to ears, or more specifically, affecting hearing or balance), allergenic (frequently causing allergic reactions), neurotoxic (toxic to the nervous system), hepatotoxic (toxic to the liver), and so forth.

How do antibiotics work?

Antibiotics kill, disable, or slow the growth of the targeted harmful bacteria that cause disease. Sound simple? Consider the challenges to creating a safe and effective antibiotic. The antibiotic must reach the bacteria, which may be found in a remote part of the body, such as in a sinus, a kidney, or the brain—so it must diffuse through tissues. It has to kill or disable the target bacteria without causing severe damage to the human cells. Although one might prefer to kill harmful bacteria, slowing the growth may be sufficient to allow the person's immune system time to clear the infection. Sometimes the rapid killing of bacteria can release toxins that can cause tissue damage or other problems. In fact, antibiotics alone may not be able to cure an infection. They work in concert with the body's immune system. They may reduce the number of disease-producing bacteria or slow their growth so that the body's own immune defenses can finish the job.

Antibiotics use multiple mechanisms to kill or disable bacterial cells. Antibiotics have many different targets in the bacterial cell and work through multiple different pathways. The common antibiotics, penicillins and cephalosporins, target biosynthesis of the cell wall of the bacteria. If the wall is weakened, bacteria will be split apart by changes in osmotic pressure. One of the newer antibiotics, daptomycin, disrupts the integrity of another part of the bacterial cell, the cell membrane, which normally is a barrier to leakage of ions and small molecules in and out of the bacterial cell. Uncontrolled leakage may be lethal to the bacterial cells. To survive, grow, and divide, bacteria must also make thousands of proteins. Many antibiotics, such as tetracyclines, erythromycins, and aminoglycosides, block protein biosynthesis by the bacterial cell, another approach that can lead to death of the bacterial cell. Yet another approach is to interfere with DNA replication or the transcription of DNA into RNA. The fluoroquinolones and rifampin block information transfer to lead to bacterial cell death. Another major mechanism is to inhibit folate synthesis, essential for survival.

Sulfonamide antibiotics act as competitive inhibitors in a key step in folate synthesis.

What is the difference between broad- and narrow-spectrum antibiotics?

Different antibiotics target different kinds of disease-causing bacteria. Some antibiotics have a very specific narrow range of bacteria they can kill and are known as narrow-spectrum antibiotics; others can kill a wide range of bacteria and are known as broad-spectrum antibiotics. As a general rule, one would like to use the narrowest-spectrum antibiotic that will hit the bacteria targeted.

But there can be benefits to using an antibiotic active against a wide range of bacteria if one does not know which particular type of bacteria is causing an illness, particularly early in the course of infection before results from diagnostic tests are available that may pinpoint a specific cause of illness.

Another situation that may prompt use of a broad-spectrum antibiotic is an infection that involves multiple types of bacteria, known as polymicrobial infection. This occurs most often when there is a leak of bacteria from the intestines, as occurs with a perforation (e.g., from an injury, like a gunshot wound), a problem known as diverticulitis, or acute appendicitis, which may lead to rupture of the appendix. The intestine is filled with trillions of bacteria that help perform normal body functions, but if they spill into the peritoneal cavity, the normally sterile area around them, they can cause severe, acute illness that can ultimately be fatal. Antibiotics are often used along with a surgical procedure that may be needed to repair damaged tissue, remove an inflamed appendix, drain an abscess, etc. Antibiotics may be administered in combination to provide broader range of coverage, or better activity against a specific bacterial target, if one drug has marginal activity, or to prevent emergence of resistant forms. Some combinations are also synergistic—meaning the combination provides enhanced activity against the target bacteria and is better than either alone. Some combinations of drugs can also be antagonistic. For example, the combination of a drug that works only on actively replicating bacteria with one that slows the growth of bacteria may be less effective than either one alone. These may work at cross-purposes and reduce the effectiveness of treatment.

Even though antibiotics may not damage the human cells of the body, they have impact on a key constituent of the human body. All antibiotics have an effect on the normal resident bacteria living in and on the human host, even though they are not the target of the antibiotic. So there is always a collateral effect—or potential damage—from the use of antibiotics.

Antibiotics are a crude tool; they kill or disable a wide range of normal resident bacteria (sometimes called "off-target killing") along with the harmful bacteria. So far, we do not have antibiotics that can target only the harmful bacteria and leave all the others unscathed. Antibiotics vary greatly in their impact on our resident bacteria. In general, the broad-spectrum antibiotics have a greater impact on our resident bacteria than the narrow-spectrum antibiotics, and a longer duration of treatment will have greater impact on the resident bacteria. Bacteria live in communities with multiple species inhabiting each part of the body. Antibiotics given for whatever reason may upset the composition of the community and potentially alter the way it functions. Disruption of the normal community of bacteria, which provide competition to invaders, may make it more likely that bacteria or yeast that are harmful can thrive. The term "colonization resistance" is sometimes used to describe the benefit from normal healthy bacteria that can resist the invasion and colonization by bacteria or other microbes that do not normally inhabit a particular body site, such as the gut, vagina, or mouth.

Bacteria have developed a range of ingenious ways to survive that have nothing to do with the usual resistance to antibiotics. Some bacteria can survive extreme environmental conditions (extremophiles) of heat, cold, acidity, or other conditions that would kill human cells and most other bacteria. Some bacteria that cause disease have survival mechanisms not related to a specific antibiotic but that have developed over eons as ways to stay alive, especially under adverse conditions when proper nutrients or other essential conditions for survival may be lacking. Some bacteria, such as *Clostridia*, form spores, a sort of armored shell that protects them from conditions that would be lethal for most bacteria. Others produce capsules that surround the bacteria, making it more difficult for the human immune system to attack them. The bacteria that cause tuberculosis, *Mycobacterium tuberculosis*, a long-time companion of humans, can form into a tubercle, a latent or suspended stage during which the bacteria do not actively reproduce. Because antibiotics generally work only when the bacteria are metabolically active and replicating, drugs may not be able to quickly kill these inactive forms. Swarms of bacteria may be walled off by the body, by the creation of what we call an abscess that has a wall that encloses an inner collection of pus. Sequestered behind the wall of the abscess, the bacteria may be protected from the antibiotic. Even if the unshielded bacteria would ordinarily be killed by antibiotics, the drugs may be unable to reach them, so they are functionally resistant. Bacteria create biofilms, privileged sites for survival. Many devices used in the modern hospital setting provide favored places for biofilms— prosthetic joints, indwelling urinary catheters, intravenous lines used to deliver drugs, etc. These provide special niches where bacteria can thrive, unreachable by usual host immune defenses and antibiotics.

Why do we have so many different antibiotics?

We have hundreds of different forms of antibiotics, but they fall into about 15 major classes. The period of 1940 to 1960, sometimes known as the golden age of antibiotic discovery, is when most of the major classes of antibiotics still used today were discovered. Two important synthetic antibiotic classes, the fluoroquinolones and oxazolidinones, have been developed since 1960. Although 30 new antibiotics were approved by the US Food and Drug Administration (FDA) between 1983 and 1992, only 7 new antibiotics were approved between 2003 and 2012, many based on molecules already known. In short, the pipeline was reduced to a trickle.

The reasons we have so many antibiotics fall into several big categories: the range and diversity of bacteria and infections they cause and the diversity of human hosts; the location of the infection within the body; the quest to find safer, more effective antibiotics that work for everyone and all infections; and the ongoing constant evolution of bacteria and resistance to antibiotics.

Infections are caused by a wide range of distinct and different bacteria that affect different parts of the body. Many antibiotics target only a few or may be able to penetrate only certain tissues or parts of the body. Over the years there has been a search to find antibiotics that work against all infections, even those that are obscure, and in all types of patients—all ages and in those with underlying problems like kidney or liver problems. Because of massive global travel and trade, unusual infections that may have originated in a remote part of the world may now be seen anywhere.

There is also a desire to make antibiotics that are safer and less likely to cause allergic reactions or damage the kidneys and other organs—to reduce antibiotic-related adverse events. One also wants to create formulations with different attributes (e.g., broader or different spectrum of activity, longer half-life, easier route of administration). Some people are allergic to common antibiotics, like penicillin, so it is especially useful to have alternative drugs to use. Many drugs, including many antibiotics, are not safe to take during pregnancy because they can cross the placenta and potentially damage the developing fetus. Some pass into breast milk and can be harmful for a breastfeeding infant. This is another reason having multiple choices is helpful. Patients who have kidney disease may be unable to take certain antibiotics because normally kidneys excrete the excess drug or the breakdown product of the drug. The drug may accumulate to toxic levels if used in someone with failing kidneys. Other drugs are broken down by the liver and so cannot be taken safely by someone with liver disease. So for multiple reasons relating to the quirks and differences among humans, it is useful to have multiple choices. In the future, it may be possible to predict with more precision than currently possible which individuals are likely to have a bad reaction to a specific drug or to develop toxic levels so that we can choose an appropriate alternative at the outset of treatment. Today we may have a general idea about the probability that someone will have a specific adverse reaction to a drug (based on studies in large populations), but we usually do not have the tools to identify which patient is likely to have an adverse reaction so that it can be avoided in that individual.

We have a growing older population and more individuals who are immunocompromised, diabetic, or on dialysis or who have other conditions that place them at risk for infections and for adverse events related to antibiotics. Ideally one wants a menu with multiple choices of antibiotics to treat diverse infections and patients. Medical care is also evolving, with more individuals having surgery for placement of artificial hips and knees and prosthetic devices. Antibiotics play an important role in preventing infections when artificial material is placed in the human body.

Although many factors contribute to the need and desire for new antibiotics, overwhelmingly the most important reason for the need for additional antibiotics is development of resistance to them. With use, antibiotics are, in a sense, used up. The antibiotics do not become resistant, but the bacteria do. Bacteria are alive and respond to the presence of antibiotics. They are just trying to survive—and the fittest do. Antibiotics are unique among drugs in that using them leads to them to become less effective. Although there may be exceptions, in general, the more they are used, the more resistance in bacteria appears, leading to reduced effectiveness. Every antibiotic that has ever been developed and released has followed the familiar path of increasing resistance of bacteria to it over time (see chapter 5 on antibiotic resistance). To some extent, this means antibiotics have a limited lifespan against some infections. In contrast to drugs that are developed to treat high blood pressure, for example, which continue to work the same way decade after decade, for antibiotics the landscape changes. They often lose value over time. The use of antibiotics and response to their use is a dynamic process.

So reasons for having a robust supply of a range of different antibiotics include the need to have antibiotics that actually work against the whole wide range of bacteria that cause human infections. Bacteria become resistant when exposed repeatedly to antibiotics, in a dynamic dance, with humans always trying to stay a step ahead with a drug that will work against the bacteria causing today's infection. And then the specific choice must be tailored to the specific person and the current circumstances.

Do antibiotics work against viruses?

Antibiotics do not work against viruses—even though a substantial proportion of all antibiotics consumed are taken for viral infections, especially viral respiratory infections (prescribed and consumed on the mistaken impression that they will work). Occasionally viral infections are complicated by bacterial infections, such as the case of viral influenza infection followed by bacterial pneumococcal pneumonia. But this is the exception.

Individuals request antibiotics for viral upper respiratory infections because they think they might work and because the individuals often are unaware of possible harm. Busy clinicians prescribe antibiotics for viral respiratory infections because patients request them; prescribing antibiotics takes less time than explaining why they are unnecessary and un-likely to work. Also, clinicians usually do not have a rapid, point-of-care diagnostic test that can confirm without a doubt that a viral infection and not a bacterial infection is causing the illness. Studies show that outcomes are the same with and without antibiotics for viral upper respiratory infections. But adverse events are common after a course of antibiotics. Overall, it is estimated that up to 40% of prescribed antibiotics are unnecessary.

We do have antimicrobial (antiviral) agents that work against some respiratory viruses, which means the old adage that nothing can be done for a viral infection except chicken soup, honey and lemon, or whatever your grandmother ad-vised you to use is no longer true. We have drugs that work against many strains of influenza, a major cause of respira-tory infections. But most upper respiratory infections—and some of the lower respiratory tract infections—are caused by a whole range of respiratory viruses, such as rhinoviruses, adenoviruses, respiratory syncytial viruses, and others, for which we do not have antiviral agents for routine use. We do have highly effective specific antiviral drugs for treating a few other viruses, such as HIV, varicella, and herpes viruses.

Why do people confuse bacteria and viruses?

Confusion abounds about bacteria and viruses, the two most common types of microbes to cause human infections. Symptoms caused by bacterial and viral infections can be sim-ilar. Both can cause fever. The term "germ" is commonly used to refer to both, in part because the common name of an infec-tion does little to convey whether it is caused by a virus or bac-terium. Additionally, many infections were named before the distinction between bacteria and viruses was known; bacteria were identified long before the much smaller viruses were recognized. For example, the terms "tularemia," "plague," and "influenza" do not make clear the type of microbe involved in causing the infection. To cause more confusion, plague is caused by *Yersinia pestis*, a bacterium with a name that is totally unlike "plague." This confusion is exacerbated when the term "plague" is colloquially used by the media and general public to refer to any awful outbreak. Tuberculosis was sometimes called the "White Plague" to distinguish it from the "Black Plague" that killed millions during the Middle Ages. Early in the HIV epidemic, the infection was sometimes called the "gay plague." The bacteria *Haemophilus influenzae* cause serious infections, such as meningitis and pneumonia—so much so that a vaccine was developed and infants are now routinely immunized (in most countries) with the Hib (*Haemophilus influenzae* type b) vaccine. But influenza is caused by the influenza virus, an infection sometimes referred to as "the flu." But the term "flu" is also used more generally to refer to any disease that causes aches and fever. Sometimes illnesses are called "stomach flu" when diarrhea or gastrointestinal symptoms are common. This almost certainly is not caused by the influenza virus, which targets the respiratory tract and commonly causes fever, aches, and cough and respiratory symptoms.

How were antibiotics discovered?

When asked about the discovery of antibiotics, most people will cite the story of the young scientist, Alexander Fleming, whose agar plate became contaminated with a fungus that had floated in the air. The fungus fell on an agar plate in the laboratory and was able to flourish, producing a fluffy white patch of growth. The observant scientist noted a clear zone around the fungus where bacteria, like staph, which he was studying at the time, were killed or unable to grow. He surmised that something that diffused from the fungus (he called it "mould juice") was preventing bacteria from growing. Alexander Fleming shared the Nobel Prize for Physiology or Medicine in 1945 with Howard Florey and Ernst Boris Chain for the discovery of penicillin.

The basic elements of this part of the story are correct, but the broader history of antibiotics is much richer, much longer, and more interesting—involving war, conflict, soil, brilliant observations and blind alleys, and many disciplines (Gaynes 2017). (Apocryphal tales of applying moldy bread to infected wounds in ancient Egypt or using moldy soybean curd to treat boils in ancient China add some intrigue to this history, unquestionably.) In terms of documented history, the origins of antibiotics are attributed at least in part to the work of Louis Pasteur, the French scientist well known for his many scientific contributions, including the recognition that heat could kill microbes, which led to use of pasteurization in the wine industry, and later in milk. Pasteur (1822–1895) observed in the 1870s that some bacteria inhibit other bacteria—or in other words, that bacteria or other microbes produce substances that affect the growth of other bacterial populations.

One of Pasteur's contemporaries, the German Paul Ehrlich (1854–1915), used aniline dyes, discovered in the 1850s, to stain blood cells, other body tissues, and bacteria. Ehrlich's efforts facilitated his observation that organic chemicals had different reactions to various cells or cell parts. This in turn allowed him to develop methods (some of them still used today) to see morphological/structural characteristics of cells in order to identify different types of cells (e.g., different types of white blood cells) and bacteria, including the bacteria identified by Robert Koch in the 1880s as the cause of tuberculosis. Ehrlich surmised that the staining of cells must be the result of a chemical reaction and that molecules of a chemical must bind to cell receptors—what he called a "key-lock principle." From there he sought to find a chemical that could kill pathogenic (disease-causing) microbes like bacteria (or tumor cells) without damaging normal tissues. In theory, the chemical (or "magic bullet," as he described it) would go straight to the target organism or cell, bind to it, and not damage others.

At that time syphilis was a major scourge—and it remains with us today. This sexually transmitted infection manifested with multiple stages of infection, each with different but characteristic signs and symptoms. Without treatment, infection could last a lifetime. Late-stage syphilis led to dementia and ultimately death. Mental institutions were filled with patients with the diagnosis of *dementia paralyticus*, or late-stage syphilis. Although many treatment approaches had been tried over centuries, the substance mercury (rubbed on the skin, given by injection, taken by mouth, or vaporized) was the mainstay of treatment, but it was toxic and not usually effective. A common saying at the time was "a night with Venus and a lifetime with mercury." The cause of syphilis, a spirochete (a type of bacteria) called *Treponema pallidum,* had just been discovered in 1905. A blood test to diagnose syphilis was developed in 1906 and was refined over the subsequent decades. Researchers could not grow the spirochetes in the laboratory the way they could grow staph and strep, but they could infect rabbits and some other animals with the spirochete, an important advance. This allowed them to test various treatments. In 1913 a Japanese scientist working at Rockefeller University demonstrated spirochetes in the brain of a person with progressive paralysis and thus linked the late-stage neurologic disease to syphilis.

Compound number 606, a chemical screened in Ehrlich's laboratory, was active against spirochetes found in other animals (fowl), so Ehrlich decided to test it in rabbits infected with the spirochete that causes syphilis in humans. Compound 606 was highly effective against the spirochetes in the rabbit model, so Ehrlich then tested it in humans. He named the drug salvarsan (chemical name: arsphenamine). The first clinical trial of the drug was carried out in 1909 and involved 50 patients with late-stage syphilis. Salvarsan had a beneficial effect, as was announced at a scientific conference in 1910. A huge demand for the drug ensued, and a chemical company, Hoechst Chemical Works, manufactured the drug on a large scale and distributed 65,000 doses free of charge. Unfortunately, the drug was not easy to prepare or to administer to patients, and many serious adverse events were reported from the drug. Ehrlich's lab continued to screen other related compounds and found another one that was more easily manufactured and administered; they named it neosalvarsan. Its use was not without controversy, mostly moral: Some individuals and groups voiced concern about the breakdown in sexual inhibitions if sexually transmitted infections could be treated.

Salvarsan/neosalvarsan was the best agent for treating syphilis in the early 1900s, but failure and relapse were common among individuals treated with it. Better options were needed, but use of this chemical nonetheless proved the concept that injections or infusions of drugs could potentially modify the course of bacterial infections—an enormous breakthrough in understanding infectious diseases. The leading causes of death in the early 20th century were infectious diseases, many of them bacterial.

Amid recognition that salvarsan/neosalvarsan did not produce reliable or long-lasting remissions in syphilis, another German researcher, Julius Wagner-Jauregg, took a totally different approach. In 1917 he injected nine patients suffering from progressive paralysis (syphilis) with malaria parasites; he based this approach on past observations that patients with syphilis who developed a high fever or suffered serious illness unrelated to the syphilis would sometimes actually show improvement in the syphilis symptoms. Six of the nine patients injected with malaria parasites showed extensive remission. Wagner-Jauregg expanded his testing and in 1920 reported his results to the German Psychiatric Society in Hamburg. Use of malaria as a treatment for syphilis gained wide acceptance and became a mode of treatment in other parts of Europe, North America, South America, South Africa, and Japan.

For his discovery of the therapeutic value of malaria inoculation in the treatment of syphilic dementia, Wagner-Jauregg was awarded the Nobel Prize for Physiology or Medicine in 1927. It was also an early example of one microbe being used to alter or eliminate another but by a very different mechanism than by the use of antibiotics.

The compound sulfanilamide was prepared in 1908 by the Austrian chemist Paul Joseph Gelmo (1879–1961) for his doctoral dissertation and patented in 1909; it was used as a constituent of azosulfonamide dyes. Perhaps inspired by Ehrlich's earlier work with dye components, the German scientist Gerhard Domagk (1895–1964) worked with two chemists decades later to test how such compounds might be active against microbes. In 1931 they found a compound that had some activity against streptococci in mice; they modified its structure and produced a compound with dramatic antimicrobial activity in mice, particularly against streptococci (the cause of scarlet fever, rheumatic fever, strep throat, and other serious infections in humans). They named it prontosil rubrum (for its red color), or prontosil. One hundred percent of the mice injected with live streptococci that received doses of the prontosil survived. Domagk continued to investigate the drug over the next 3 years and published results in a 1935 paper entitled "Streptococcus Experiment." During the time he was studying the drug, his 6-year-old daughter developed a severe streptococcal infection in her arm after a minor injury from an unsterile needle. This was an infection that could be fatal and was sometimes treated with amputation to try to save the person's life. Domagk gave his daughter large doses of the drug, and she was cured.

The drug was found to be active against many bacteria that caused common infections. French scientists at the Pasteur Institute showed that prontosil was actually what was called a "prodrug," the precursor to the actual active agent. Subsequent work on sulfonamides produced a large number of derivatives, some of which are still in wide use today, sometimes in combination with other drugs to extend their activity. Prontosil and other sulfonamides gained rapid and wide use. Within a year of publication of Domagk's paper, studies with the drugs had been done in three European centers.

In 1939 Gerhard Domagk was named as a recipient of the Nobel Prize for his discovery of the antibacterial effect of prontosil, but Nazi leaders in Germany prevented him from accepting it. After the war ended, he traveled to Stockholm in 1947 to receive his medal (but no money).

Sulfonamides were cheap to produce and linked easily to other molecules, so this discovery set off the development and production of many related compounds. Sulfonamides were first used in the United States by a physician at Columbia University in 1935. Researchers at Johns Hopkins University also did pioneering work with sulfonamides and published a report in 1937 describing the treatment of 19 patients. Others showed that it could be used to treat gonorrhea. By 1941 a paper was published in the United States with results of more than 1,000 patients with various infections. One sad note was that an attempt in 1937 in the United States to produce a raspberry-flavored version in liquid form that would be easy for children to take (sulfonamide elixir) ended up causing more than 100 deaths because the liquid used to dissolve the sulfanilamide was toxic (see chapter 1, How are antibiotics made?). By the 1940s massive amounts of the sulfonamides were being produced and used, including extensively in World War II. Soldiers were given packets of sulfa powder and told to put powder in wounds if injured. Sulfa was also used to treat meningitis, and deaths from meningitis fell from 39.2% during World War I to 3% during World War II. Back in the United States, it was used to treat puerperal fever, the infection following childbirth that was often fatal (an infection often caused by streptococci). One Swedish researcher, Nanna Svartz (1890–1986), combined it with salicylate (similar to aspirin) and used it to treat rheumatoid arthritis and ulcerative colitis (a type of inflammatory bowel disease). A form of that combination is still in use today.

The sulfonamide era lasted only a few years—some characterize it as 1937 to 1942. As early as 1938 researchers were aware that sulfonamides worked against some infections but not against many others. It had a narrow spectrum of activity, but it found wide use because it was the only agent available. As sulfonamide drugs were used more frequently, researchers also learned about their toxic side effects and allergic reactions, sometimes severe. Some chemical modifications to the sulfonamides achieved better activity against bacteria and reduction of their adverse effects, but they still were far from ideal. Even more ominous was the early appearance and dissemination of bacteria that resisted sulfonamides' action. In all, the long-term contribution of sulfonamides was a demonstration that a substance taken by mouth or injected could influence the course of an infection—and in some instances save lives.

While some investigators in the 1920s and 1930s continued to look for agents based on dyes and poisons, others looked to the natural world. Selman Waksman (1888–1973), born in Russia, came to the United States in 1910, enrolled at Rutgers University, and was appointed a research assistant in soil bacteriology in 1915. (Even today, soil bacteria provide a rich resource for understanding the interactions among biological life, as they rank among the most abundant and diverse group of organisms on Earth.) Waksman began to work with actinomycetes in 1915, observing that many soil microbes (fungi and bacteria) had the capacity to inhibit the growth of other microbes. He and his team systematically screened soil to try to find microbes that would produce chemical substances that would inhibit or destroy pathogenic organisms—including microbes that can cause human disease (Waksman 1940). He coined the term "antibiotic" in 1942, which at the time he meant as a reference to chemicals from living organisms. (As noted in an earlier section the term now has a broader meaning, but some purists prefer to use the term as it was originally defined.) He and his colleagues identified a streptomycin-producing organism, *Streptomyces griseus*, in September 1943 from farmland soil near their laboratory. Once the streptomycin's properties were discovered, the substance was submitted to clinical trials with partners at the Mayo Clinic, and its remarkable properties were revealed. It worked against the bacteria that caused tuberculosis and also against many other Gram-negative bacteria that caused severe infections, such as typhoid fever, cholera, tularemia, and plague, and the bacteria that caused common urinary tract infections. Waksman received the Nobel Prize in 1952 for "ingenious systematic and successful study of the soil microbes that have led to the discovery of streptomycin." In his Nobel Lecture delivered on December 12, 1952, he noted how the subsequent introduction of para-aminosalicylic acid (PAS) and isoniazid (two other drugs used to treat tuberculosis) foretold "the conquest of the 'Great White Plague,' undreamt of less than 10 years ago." Alas, today we face tuberculosis that is resistant to all three drugs, plus others. The Great White Plague is still with us and globally kills more than a million people each year.

As noted earlier, the name most associated with the discovery of antibiotics is Alexander Fleming, sometimes also called the "penicillin man." If chance favors the prepared mind, Fleming's was prepared. Fleming (1881–1955) was born on a Scottish farm and later moved to London where he studied medicine. He joined the research department at St. Mary's Hospital and became a professor of bacteriology.

In September 1928, at a time when he was studying staphylococci in his laboratory, he returned from vacation and found one petri dish/agar plate contaminated with a fungus, which he later identified as *Penicillium notatum*. He also observed a clear zone around the fungus, an indication that the bacteria, like staphylococci, were unable to grow in that zone. He surmised that the fungus was producing a substance that diffused into the agar. He carried out additional studies with the fungus and the "mould broth filtrates," or "mold juice," which he named "penicillin" after the name of the fungus. He found that it was active against staphylococcus, streptococcus, and some other bacteria that commonly caused infections but not against the bacteria that caused typhoid fever. In a paper published the following year (1929) in the *British Journal of Experimental Pathology*, he laid out his key findings (Fleming 1929). The substance secreted by the fungus was active against bacteria that caused infections producing pus, like staph and strep, but not against some other bacteria; it was not toxic to animals; and it did not interfere with the function of white blood cells (which are an important body defense in fighting infection).

He did not envision this substance as a magic bullet that could be used to treat systemic infections and that would ultimately save millions of lives. He and his laboratory assistants did some work to prepare crude extracts, but he and his collaborators lacked the knowledge of chemistry to purify and produce this substance. They tried to concentrate it but found it was easily destroyed. In 1940 he wrote in the *Pharmaceutical Journal*, "We have used it in the laboratory for over 10 years as a method of differential culture. It was used in a few cases as local antiseptic, but although it gave reasonably good results the trouble of making it seemed not worthwhile" (Fleming 1940). After receiving the Nobel Prize in 1945 he wrote, "When I saw changes on my culture plate as the result of the mould contaminant, I had not the slightest suspicion that I was at the beginning of something extraordinary" (Fleming 1945).

Other scientists and a team effort were necessary to rescue Fleming's observation from obscurity and continue the story of discovery and realization. Fleming made a key observation and published it, but it took a team of researchers with other skills to purify, stabilize, and produce this magic substance from mold—and to scale up production of this life-saving substance.

Howard Florey (1898–1968), an Australian, attended Oxford as a Rhodes Scholar and spent most of his life in the United Kingdom, becoming Oxford's chair of pathology in 1935. His team picked up and continued research on penicillin in 1939, purifying the substance from *Penicillium* and producing enough to begin studies in animals and then in humans. In March 1940, penicillin-receiving mice infected with streptococci bacteria survived. The results were published in August 1940 in *The Lancet*, which set off increased demand to both extract and purify penicillin for broader use and study (Chain 1940). The Oxford team had to process up to 500 liters per week, using whatever containers they could find—milk churns, biscuit tins, pie dishes, bedpans—to hold the liquid cultures. They later developed stackable ceramic containers that replaced the initial containers for fermentation. Shortages related to war activities markedly limited their resources, but the Oxford laboratory was turned into a penicillin production space. Women dubbed the "penicillin girls" were paid 2 pounds per week to help to "farm" the *Penicillium* in order to produce a few milligrams of penicillin per week. The process used to purify the substance was excruciatingly inefficient, and its activity also had to be tested. The full sequence—grow, extract, purify, and test activity—had to precede any trials in humans.

The first human trials began in 1941 (Abraham 1941). The first patient, a 43-year-old man with life-threatening infection, showed dramatic improvement after receiving the penicillin, but when supplies of the substance were quickly exhausted, the infection relapsed and the man died. In the early days, penicillin was in such short supply that they collected urine from patients who had received the precious drug to extract penicillin that had been excreted for reuse in other patients.

In 1941 the UK pharmaceutical companies were engaged in producing drugs for the war activities and had little capacity to take on industrial production of penicillin. Massive scale-up was needed. Florey and colleagues traveled to the United States and had a series of meetings aimed at generating interest from the US pharmaceutical industry in producing penicillin on a large scale. Through their meetings, aided by Florey's connections and credibility from previous time spent in the United States, they were able to find experts in fermentation and *Penicillium* mold. The Department of Agriculture's

Northern Regional Research Laboratory in Peoria, Illinois, undertook the program to scale up production, led by Robert Coghill, chief of fermentation. One of his scientists found that they could increase the yield of the cultures by using corn-steep liquor, a by-product of the corn wet-milling process. It was cheap, available in large quantities, and remarkably effective. They produced penicillin in massive, deep fermentation tanks. The teams found multiple innovations to increase yield and make the production more efficient. After searching far and wide in soil and elsewhere for better penicillin-producing strains of *Penicillium*, the one they identified as the best was from a moldy cantaloupe from a Peoria fruit market. They were able to create an even more productive mutant organism by treating the *Penicillium* with X-rays and ultraviolet (UV) radiation.

Production of penicillin in the United States started in 1942. Major pharmaceutical companies were told they would be serving the national (read: war) interest if they began penicillin production. It was given high priority for federal funds. Multiple companies participated—Merck, Squibb, Lilly, and Pfizer. The initial penicillin produced was stockpiled for use by the military. Supplies were also sent to designated investigators in multiple centers in the United States. The drug was shown to be effective against streptococcal, staphylococcal, and gonococcal infections. By 1944 it had also been shown to be effective in treating syphilis—and previous approaches for treating syphilis with malaria therapy and toxic chemicals were quickly abandoned. Civilian use was initially rationed because of the limited supplies in the early 1940s. Troops received priority for treatment. Because it was in short supply in the early years, it was sometimes used in combination with another drug, probenecid, which inhibited the excretion of the penicillin and so could prolong its action.

By 1944 US production had increased dramatically, increasing from 21 billion units in 1943 to 1,663 billion units in 1944 and to more than 6.8 trillion in 1945. Restrictions on penicillin use in the United States were removed in March 1945. In the United Kingdom, penicillin became available by prescription to the general public in June 1946. In 1945 Alexander Fleming, Ernst Chain, and Howard Florey received the Nobel Prize for the discovery of penicillin and its curative effects in various infectious diseases.

The production and scale-up of work with penicillin was a remarkable achievement—hastened by significant investment of resources resulting from the need to ramp up production rapidly because of the war. A period of great optimism and discovery followed with the identification of multiple other antibiotics. Infections that were previously fatal—meningitis, pneumonia, bacterial endocarditis (infection of the heart valves), and tuberculosis—could be cured, sometimes with a few doses of an antibiotic.

From the earliest days, Fleming and others warned about the risk of bacteria becoming resistant to antibiotics—but to most this seemed like a distant or unlikely threat.

Where do antibiotics come from?

The period between about 1940 and 1960 is considered the golden age of antibiotic discovery. During this period most of the classes of antibiotics that we use today were introduced—penicillins, cephalosporins, aminoglycosides, chloramphenicol, tetracyclines, macrolides (such as erythromycin), and glycopeptides (such as vancomycin). From there, medicinal chemists created generations of semisynthetic antibiotics based on these original discoveries. A fully synthetic antibiotic class, fluoroquinolone (e.g., ciprofloxacin), was introduced in 1960 and many other quinolone antibiotics have followed since then.

These early antibiotics came from soil, microbes in the environment, and chemicals that could be synthesized in the laboratory. The search today for new antibiotics includes looking for natural molecules that may inhibit the growth of bacteria.

New tools available to scientists today allow them to tinker with existing molecules or to create new substances with desirable characteristics; nothing is off limits. Plants have been the source of drugs like artemisinin and quinine, used to treat malaria. The vast biodiversity could potentially hold other biological treasures that could be used to treat infections and improve health. Plants and wild animals are also affected by infections, and some may have evolved protective approaches that could be useful to humans. Komodo dragons and marine animals have been studied as possible sources of compounds with valuable properties.

What follows is a short overview of the origins of several classes of antibiotics:

Cephalosporins are beta-lactam antibiotics originally derived from the fungus *Acremonium chrysogenum*. The fungus that yielded the first cephalosporin was found in the sea in Sardinia by an Italian pharmacologist in 1945. The cephalosporin drugs were not marketed until 1964. Many semisynthetic derivatives have followed. Some are derived from *Streptomyces* spp.

Yale microbiologist, Paul Burkholder, discovered a microorganism in 1947 in a field in Caracas, Venezuela, that inhibited both Gram-negative and Gram-positive organisms. It was later named *Streptomyces venezuelae* after the country where it had been found. The antibiotic it produced was named chloramphenicol. It was subsequently synthesized and the drug has been widely used globally and is on the World Health Organization (WHO) list of essential medicines. It has many desirable characteristics (relatively broad spectrum, good absorption when taken by mouth, good central nervous system penetration, cheap) but occasional severe side effects that have limited its use.

Aureomycin (later known as chlortetracycline) was produced from an organism later named *Streptomyces aureofaciens*.

A soil botanist isolated it from soil on the campus of the University of Missouri. It produced a yellow substance (hence its name from aureus, meaning golden) with antibiotic activity. It was the first tetracycline and was first isolated in 1944. A soil bacterium, *Streptomyces rimosus*, isolated near the Pfizer laboratories, yielded oxytetracycline. It was patented in 1949 and available commercially starting in 1950. An American chemist determined its chemical structure, which enabled mass production of the drug, sold under the trade name of Terramycin. A derivative of oxytetracycline, doxycycline, was developed in the pharmaceutical laboratories at Pfizer and remains in wide use today.

The organism that yielded vancomycin was isolated in 1953 by a scientist working at Eli Lilly from a soil sample from the interior jungles of Borneo. The organism is now known as *Amycolatopsis orientalis*. The drug was given the generic name of vancomycin after "vanquish" because of its antibacterial effects.

The aminoglycoside kanamycin came from *Streptomyces kanamiyceticus*, isolated in Japan in 1957. Gentamicin, another aminoglycoside, was found to be produced by bacteria of the genus *Micromonospora* in 1963 by scientists at Schering Corporation.

Polymyxins came from spore-forming soil bacteria, *Bacillus* (*Paenibacillus*) *polymyxa*, first identified in 1940; colistin was isolated from *Bacillus polymyxa* var. *colistinus* in 1949 in Japan. There are five polymyxins: polymyxin A, B, C, D, and E. Only two, polymyxin B and polymyxin E (colistin), are in wide use. They were initially thought to be too toxic for systemic use but have returned to clinical use as "last resort antibiotics" because of widespread resistance of bacteria to other antibiotics. They are often used topically, including in animals. Colistin is administered as a prodrug, colistimethate sodium, thought to be less toxic than its parent.

Erythromycin was isolated from a strain of *Streptomyces erythreus* (now known as *Saccharopolyspora erythraea*) and became available in 1952. Various salts and esters of erythromycin were later developed that are less likely to be inactivated by stomach acid. Chemical synthesis was successful in 1981. Multiple semisynthetic antibiotics related to erythromycin have followed including azithromycin and clarithromycin.

Lincomycin was isolated from a strain of *Streptomyces lincolnensis* in the Upjohn Research Laboratories in 1963. Researchers chemically modified the antibiotic to improve it and created the superior antibiotic clindamycin, which is still widely used.

After discovering azomycin, a substance from a *Streptomyces* species that was weakly active against *Trichomonas*, chemists at Rhone-Poulenc Research Laboratories synthesized similar agents and discovered a drug that was later found to be active against many anaerobic bacteria (important in many infections related to the gastrointestinal tract), as well as *Giardia*, amebae, and *Trichomonas vaginalis*. The drug was metronidazole, which has found wide use globally (and is also on the WHO list of essential medicines).

After substances with antibacterial activity are found in nature, they must be purified, characterized, analyzed, and assessed for safety. The structure of the substance is determined. If the agent has potential commercial value, then the means must be developed for scale-up and production.

Discovery of the initial structure of an antibiotic may be the most exciting step, but it's hardly the last. After the structure of an antibiotic is determined, it can then be manipulated in ways that may broaden its spectrum of activity, reduce toxicity, or change excretion or metabolism by the body or other characteristics. For example, we now have dozens of different penicillins. To reach to this point, researchers started with the substance Fleming first observed, which itself took more than a decade to purify. From there the chemical structure of penicillin was first proposed by Edward Abraham in 1942 and confirmed by Dorothy Hodgkin at Oxford in 1946. A chemist at MIT later completed the first synthesis of penicillin, making it possible to attach other molecules to the structure and create new forms of penicillin. Ampicillin was created through this approach in 1961. A related drug, amoxicillin, still used widely today, was also developed at Beecham in 1971.

Synthetic antibiotics can come from what is called *rational design*. Rather than through trial and error—or looking for a needle in the haystack by culturing soil and other natural substances all over the world—scientists can now identify a specific receptor or enzyme or part of a bacterial pathogen and try to design an antibiotic in the laboratory to carry out a specific task. Nature provides many examples of approaches to take, but some antibiotics, like the quinolones, are created in the laboratory.

Although many collaborators are always involved, most of the antibiotics discovered/designed/developed between 1929 and 2000 came from the United States. The United Kingdom, European countries including Italy and Germany, and Japan have also had active research programs in antibiotic development.

How are antibiotics made?

Antibiotics licensed in the United States today are made in modern manufacturing sites. Control is stringent and the FDA has extensive oversight. The raw materials used to manufacture antibiotics may come from many sources, many of them outside of the United States.

The main regulatory standard for ensuring high quality and consistency is the CGMP, the Current Good Manufacturing Practice regulations for human pharmaceuticals. These are enforced by the FDA. Adherence to these regulations is necessary to ensure the identity, strength, quality, and purity of drugs. Manufacturers of medications must control manufacturing operations. Aspects covered include management systems, quality of raw materials, detecting and investigating deviations in quality, and maintaining reliable testing laboratories. This is intended to prevent contamination and poor-quality products. The CGMP regulations are minimum standards that must be maintained by the drug manufacturer. The FDA inspects pharmaceutical manufacturing facilities globally, including those that manufacture active ingredients. If a manufacturer distributes a drug that fails to meet certain standards, for example, by having too little or too much active ingredient, the company can recall the product voluntarily. If a company does not recall a substandard drug, the FDA can send a warning to the public and can also seize the drug. Violations can include problems with sanitation or cleanliness of the facility or faulty equipment. Before a pharmaceutical company can submit an application for a new drug approval, it must meet the CGMP regulations.

Although adverse events and side effects with use of antibiotics remain common, the manufacturing process is highly regulated. All of this strict regulation is born of historical cases that illustrate what happens when regulations aren't in place. One example is the sulfanilamide event, the history of which led to the passage of the 1938 Federal Food, Drug, and Cosmetic Act. Sulfanilamide was an organic compound that had been shown to work against some infections in the mid-1930s in Europe. It was dissolved in diethylene glycol, a solvent, by a pharmaceutical company in the United States and sold in elixir form. Diethylene glycol is poisonous to humans and other mammals, and reports of its toxicity had been published in medical journals; this was either not widely known nor well heeded. In 1937 a pharmacist mixed the drug with the solvent, added raspberry flavoring, and marketed it; no animal or other premarketing testing was required at the time. More than 100 people in 15 states died after taking the elixir, many of them children with sore throats and other minor ailments. The resulting Food, Drug, and Cosmetic Act increased the FDA's authority to regulate drugs, though prescriptions for antibiotics in the US were not required until 1951. The pharmacist and chemist who created the preparation committed suicide while awaiting trial.

Are new antibiotics created in the laboratory or discovered in nature?

Historically many antibiotics have been based on substances found in nature. The quest to find natural substances that have antibacterial activity continues, but much of the drug discovery and development today involves the creation of new molecules that may have desirable characteristics.

One potentially valuable resource for natural products is the National Cancer Institute's program for Natural Product Discovery, started years ago as a resource for cancer drug discovery. The Natural Products Branch now has a global collection of extracts from more than 230,000 sources. About 161,000 are plant based, about 41,000 marine based, and about 30,000 microbial based. The goal at the institute is to create a library with about a million semipure natural product samples that can be screened for antimicrobial activity—and other desired activities.

What happens after a compound with antibacterial activity is discovered? How does it come to be used to treat infections?

The development and approval of a new antibiotic is a long, arduous, and expensive process. Decades can pass between identification of a molecule of interest and its use in the clinical setting. Most candidates do not survive the rigorous process. Only a tiny fraction of potential candidates are actually approved for clinical use by the FDA. On average it takes 12 to

15 years to complete the process for drugs that are successful—and can cost up to half a billion dollars or more to complete the process. If 5,000 compounds are tested, perhaps 5 will make it into clinical trials, and 1 might ultimately be approved.

When a candidate of interest is discovered, initial testing is done in the laboratory and in animals to assess its safety and biological activity. Drugs that survive the preclinical testing are tested in a small number of volunteers—initially (typically) 20 to 100 healthy adults—to establish safety and dosage. Investigators also assess how the drug is metabolized and excreted. Those drugs that perform well in this phase are next tested to assess the drug's effectiveness and to continue to look for side effects. The drug may be compared with a similar drug or a placebo—an inactive agent. This phase may include hundreds of patients. Those that show favorable results in this phase move to the next phase of testing, which typically includes thousands of patients. If the drug performs well, the pharmaceutical company may apply for FDA approval. The company completes what is called a New Drug Application (NDA), which may include tens or hundreds of thousands of pages of material for the FDA for review. This NDA includes all of the background information about clinical trials, including efficacy and side effects, the structure of the molecule, what ingredients are included in the drug, how the drug is handled by the human body, and how the drug is manufactured, processed, and packaged. Adverse events and side effects of antibiotics that are identified in early trials are listed in detail when drugs are approved by the FDA. Even if a drug is approved and marketed, postmarketing safety monitoring and surveillance continues.

Some drugs are approved the first time they are reviewed. Many are not. Some are never approved. Sometimes the FDA requires more information or additional clinical studies to be completed before it will reconsider whether a drug should be approved.

The list of drugs that are approved for use varies by country. Some drugs that are FDA approved in the United States are not approved for use in other countries. The reverse is also true. When drugs are approved, the approval includes the specific indications for which the drug is to be used. For example, a drug may be approved for treating specific bacteria (e.g., *Staphylococcus, Streptococcus, Escherichia coli*) or types of infections (e.g., community-acquired pneumonia, complicated urinary tract infections, and meningitis). Common restrictions or warnings on the recommended use of drugs include age (e.g., not recommended for children younger than 2 years or not recommended for those older than 60 years), pregnancy, underlying diseases like renal or liver disease, coadministration of other drugs, and type or body site of infection.

Some of these indications are limited because the drug has not been tested in a particular group, for example, young children or the elderly. In other instances, certain groups are excluded because of increased risk for adverse events. Physicians can prescribe a drug for indications other than those that are approved, but this is considered "off label" use of the antibiotic.

Many examples exist of antibiotics that were approved by the FDA for use for specific indications but then recommendations for use were changed. Based on postmarketing safety data, unexpected adverse events may come to light. Clinical trials done before FDA approval typically include a few to several thousand participants. Rare side effects that occur only 1 to 2 times per 100,000 patients or even less frequently are not likely to be identified during the clinical trials. Only when a drug is released and used widely in a larger population—tens of thousands or millions—will these rare events be observed. If these are serious, for example, those causing severe disease, disability, or death, changes in the way the drug is prescribed will need to be made. If it is possible to identify those at risk for the severe adverse event by age, underlying disease, or another cofactor like simultaneous use of another drug, it may be possible to warn doctors to avoid the drug in specific situations. If the serious event is idiosyncratic—totally unpredictable and coming out of the blue—the drug may be withdrawn from the market or its use restricted. That decision will be based in part on the seriousness of the type of infection being treated and the availability of other drugs for treating that same infection. The decision could vary, for example, if the treatment was for a fatal infection for which no other treatment was available versus a mild self-limited infection for which many other options were available for treatment.

In some instances, the FDA will require a so-called black-box warning to alert clinicians to a particular risk or danger from using a drug. Usually these have the effect of restricting or reducing the use of the drug. In some instances, FDA approval is withdrawn. In other instances, restrictions on the use of a drug and negative publicity about the drug have so eroded confidence in the drug and its use that pharmaceutical companies have voluntarily withdrawn the drug from the market. One example is telithromycin, a semisynthetic oral macrolide antibiotic that was approved for treatment of community-acquired pneumonia of mild to moderate severity. It was developed by a French pharmaceutical company and approved by the European Commission in 2001. The FDA approved the drug in 2004. Within a couple of years reports of severe drug-induced liver injury and deaths were published and received wide visibility in the medical community. The FDA revised the label to remove some of the initial indications for the drug and added a black-box warning. In the United States, Sanofi-Aventis withdrew the drug from active sales.

Tigecycline, a tetracycline derivative, was approved by the FDA in 2005 and marketed by the pharmaceutical company Pfizer. Subsequent studies found that patients treated with tigecycline had an increased risk of death compared to other treatments for the same kinds of infections. This was seen most clearly in patients with hospital-acquired pneumonia. The FDA required the addition of a black-box warning in 2010.

A frequently used class of antibiotics, the fluoroquinolones, has continued to generate new warnings. The fluoroquinolones have been approved for use for more than 40 years in the United States and are widely used for many types of infections. They have many benefits: They can be taken orally, are generally inexpensive, and have broad activity against many Gram-positive and Gram-negative bacteria. Currently FDA-approved fluoroquinolones include levofloxacin, ciprofloxacin, moxifloxacin, ofloxacin, gemifloxacin, and delafloxacin. They are available in more than 60 generic versions.

Other FDA-approved quinolones have been removed from use in the United States after postmarketing surveillance identified unrecognized problems. Temafloxacin was approved in the United States in 1992 and was withdrawn shortly after because of reports of severe allergic reactions and hemolytic anemia, causing at least three deaths. Grepafloxacin was withdrawn from the global market in 1999 because of adverse cardiac events. In the United States the FDA in 1999 advised doctors to limit prescriptions of trovafloxacin because it had been associated with severe liver failure and death. It was later withdrawn from the market. Yet another quinolone, gatifloxacin, introduced in 1999 was withdrawn from the market in 2006 because of reports of severe hyperglycemia (high blood sugar) and hypoglycemia (low blood sugar). It is still available as an ophthalmic solution.

The fluoroquinolones provide an illustrative example of the ongoing refinement of recommendations for use and warnings about new adverse events decades after initial FDA approval. In 2008 the FDA added a black-box warning for increased risk of tendinitis and tendon rupture (although this had been listed for many years as a potential adverse event). In 2011 the FDA added risk of worsening symptoms of myasthenia gravis to the black-box warning. Risk of the potential for irreversible peripheral neuropathy (e.g., serious nerve damage) was added in 2013. In 2016 the FDA required enhanced warnings about disabling and potentially permanent side effects involving tendons, muscles, joints, nerves, and the central nervous system and restricted use for certain uncomplicated infections, observing that "the risk of the serious side effects generally outweighed the benefits for patients with acute bacterial sinusitis, acute bacterial exacerbation of chronic bronchitis, and uncomplicated urinary tract infections" (FDA 2016). They concluded that fluoroquinolones should be reserved for treating patients with infections for which no good alternative treatment options were available.

In July 2018 the FDA required labeling changes for all fluoroquinolones to strengthen warnings about risks of mental health side effects and low blood sugar levels. The new warning about mental health is to be listed separately from other central nervous system side effects and to be consistent across all fluoroquinolones. Warnings specifically mention disturbances in attention, disorientation, agitation, nervousness, memory impairment, and delirium. All fluoroquinolones are now also required to explicitly mention the potential for risk of coma with hypoglycemia (low blood sugar).

Although the FDA offers recommendations, warnings, and information, the prescribing habits of clinicians and preferences of patients can be slow to change. As long as a drug is FDA approved, clinicians can prescribe it, sometimes for indications that are not listed in the FDA approval.

In the United States fluoroquinolones are the third most commonly prescribed antibiotic class in adults, with an estimated 115 prescriptions per 1,000 persons annually.

Are the same antibiotics used all over the world?

The common classes of antibiotics are generally available throughout the world, although they may have different names, come in different strengths, and have different appearances. The same antibiotics may be licensed or approved for different indications in other countries. Many of the newer and very expensive antibiotics may be unavailable or difficult to obtain in low- and middle-income countries. Many large pharmaceutical companies distribute antibiotics globally. India is now a major producer and exporter of antibiotics. One example is faropenem, an oral penem (similar to carbapenems) antibiotic, approved for use in Japan and India. It is manufactured in India, and its use in India has increased 154% since it was approved in 2010. It has not been approved by the FDA.

A major difference among countries and regions is where and how antibiotics are obtained. In the United States we are accustomed to obtaining a prescription for any antibiotic we use, with a possible exception being topical ointments. Globally this is not true. In many countries antibiotics are sold without a prescription. They may be sold at local markets or by roadside vendors. Licensed health providers, including doctors, nurses, and pharmacists, are in short supply in many low-income countries. Drugs may be provided or dispensed by village health workers with little knowledge of the indications or side effects from antibiotics. A study that tried to estimate the global extent of the non-prescription supply of antibiotics in community pharmacies around the world estimated that 62% of antibiotics were given without a prescription (Auta 2018). Most often they were given without a prescription to patients with symptoms of urinary tract infections and upper respiratory infections. The most commonly used antibiotics for these symptoms were fluoroquinolones and penicillins.

Another study that estimated by country the percentages of antibiotics obtained without a prescription found wide variation: 46% in Brazil, 25% in Peru, 36% in China, 18% in India, 3% in northern Europe, and 100% in Nigeria and Sudan.

As has been documented repeatedly, even in places that require a prescription, many antibiotics are prescribed when none is needed—and the duration, dose, or drug prescribed may be wrong or suboptimal.

Another problem today is that many antibiotics for humans, animals, and plants are available over the internet. Antibiotics that are not licensed for sale in the United States can be obtained over the internet. Antibiotics that require a prescription for use in the United States can also be obtained over the internet. Quality may be an issue for these drugs.

How common are substandard and falsified antibiotics?

Globally the selling of falsified and substandard drugs is a major problem (NASEM 2013). Substandard and falsified products also include vaccines and diagnostic tests. Although these falsified and substandard products have been found in every region of the world, the problem is most severe in low- and middle-income countries, particularly in countries where regulation is lax. The problem affects both generic and name-brand products and exists for any product that has a market. The problem with antimalarial drugs has received much attention, but antibiotics are also among the many drugs that may be substandard or falsified. The WHO has a Global Surveillance and Monitoring System for substandard and falsified medical products that provides regulatory authorities with an interconnected network. It is especially useful to countries that lack strong regulatory oversight (WHO 2017). Among the substandard and falsified products identified by the WHO surveillance system between 2013 and 2017, the two most common types of drugs were malaria medicines (almost 20%) and antibiotics (about 17%)—but the list includes everything from contraceptives and heart and diabetes medicines to pain medicines and cancer treatments.

Substandard drugs are officially defined as "authorized medical products that fail to meet either their quality standards or specification or both" and may result from poor manufacturing, shipping, or storage conditions. It also describes drugs sold after the expiration date.

Substandard drugs may have been transported under conditions that allowed deterioration of the product. They may have the wrong amount of the active ingredient. They may not dissolve properly when taken by mouth (technical term is "dissolution delay") so the active medicine in the pill may not be absorbed. They may be contaminated with toxic substances, like lead or other products that should never be ingested. They may not be sterile and may be heavily contaminated with bacteria, fungi, or other microbes that could cause illness. Drugs that are substandard include all types of formulations (pills, liquid medicines, injectable). Falsified products are those that deliberately or fraudulently misrepresent their identity, composition, or source.

The potential adverse consequences of substandard and falsified antibiotics are many. People can die or have serious complications or prolongation of illness from an infection that is not treated with the right amount of an active drug. Receiving low doses of an antibiotic in a substandard or falsified drug can contribute to the development of resistance in bacteria. Contaminants in these drugs can cause illness, allergic reactions, or even death.

A recent study done in Malawi highlighted some of the problems with medications. Research team members (covert shoppers) (Chikowe 2018) posed as patients or guardians of patients and visited private pharmacies and medicine stores in Blantyre, Malawi, and requested amoxicillin, saying they wanted the medication for the flu or a cold. Researchers then analyzed the tablets, in duplicate: one tablet was analyzed locally using a new tool, a paper analytic device, and another tablet from the same sample was analyzed via high-performance liquid chromatography in a research laboratory in the United States.

In all they visited 56 shops and were able to obtain amoxicillin samples from 42 of them; 95% of sellers sold the amoxicillin without a prescription, even though in Malawi antibiotics are supposed to be regulated as prescription only. The analysis found that all samples contained amoxicillin. This was successfully verified with the paper analytic device locally and confirmed in the high-tech laboratory. The amount of active drug was also correct. Almost all samples had been repackaged and only a third had expiration dates displayed.

Many approaches have been developed to try to identify falsified and substandard drugs, including use of spectroscopy and chemical analyses. These take expertise and resources—and suspicion of a problem. Many of the producers of falsified drugs are extremely sophisticated in being able to reproduce pills and packaging that look like the original product. There is a huge market and trade in falsified drugs. Pharmaceuticals are big business, with the global sales of medicines being greater than $1 trillion. Substandard drugs may be cheaper to produce but there is no intent to deceive. Falsified products are deliberately designed to deceive.

The Pharmaceutical Security Research Institute reported that in 2015 Asia had the highest incidence of drug crime cases among the WHO world regions. More than 3,000 cases were reported; many defective products were transported across national borders. The WHO estimates that globally about 10.5% of medicines are substandard or falsified. A recent study that estimated the prevalence of poor-quality essential medicines in low- and middle-income countries found that the overall prevalence was 13.6% and was highest in Africa, where almost 19% of drugs were poor quality (Ozawa 2018). They estimated that 12.4% of antibiotics were substandard or falsified. Dr. Joel Breman, who has studied falsified and substandard drugs, wrote in July 2018 that approximately 122,000 African children under 5 die each year as a result of being treated with fake antimalaria drugs.

What is the WHO model list of essential medicines?

Since 1977, the WHO has published a model list of essential medicines, defined as those that "satisfy the priority health care needs of the population." The list is revised every 2 years in consultation with an expert committee. The WHO also encourages each country to develop its own list taking into account local priorities. The initial list 40 years ago included 208 medicines; the most recent update in 2017 listed more than 300.

Medicines are removed and others added with each revision. The document lists medicines, formulations (e.g., powder for oral liquid, solid oral form, powder for injection, oral liquid, tablet), and first- and second-choice indications for the antibiotic. In 2017 the WHO committee developed three categories for antibiotics: Access, Watch, and Reserve (see chapter 8 on preserving antibiotics).

In addition to antibiotics, the list includes drugs to treat other kinds of infections (e.g., antiviral, antimalarial, antileprosy, anti-HIV, antituberculosis, and antifungal medicines), as well as medicines for reproductive health, cardiovascular disease, diabetes, pain, cancer, and other medical problems. There is a separate list of essential medicines for children that was first published in 2007.

2

USE IN HUMANS

How are antibiotics administered? What are the routes
of administration besides by mouth and by injection? What
determines how they should be given?

How an antibiotic is administered depends on the type and
location of the infection and the characteristics of the antibiotic. Some antibiotics are too toxic to be taken internally and
are used only for surface infections of the skin or on superficial
tissues, like the conjunctivae (surface lining) of the eyes. This
was true of some of the earliest antibiotics that were discovered. Most infections affect tissues or organs deep in the body,
like the lungs or kidneys, and the antibiotics must reach the
bacteria causing the infection to be effective. Typically the antibiotic must reach the bloodstream, which will then carry the
antibiotic to other tissues and organs.

For treating most common infections the antibiotic is taken
by mouth as a pill, a capsule, or sometimes a liquid. Infants
and young children are unable to swallow pills so liquid or
gel forms are often used for them. Taken orally, an effective
drug must survive the stomach acid and digestive enzymes
in a form that is still active. It must dissolve or change to a
form that can be absorbed into the bloodstream so that it can
reach infected tissues. It cannot be so irritating that it damages
the lining of the stomach or small bowel—or provokes nausea,

vomiting, or diarrhea in the recipient. The location within the gastrointestinal tract where the drug is absorbed—and the amount that is absorbed—will vary by drug. If a drug can potentially be destroyed by stomach acid or irritate the stomach lining, the drug may be made with a protective coating (enteric coat) to allow it to pass through the stomach before dissolving. A few drugs are nonabsorbable so their antibiotic activity can continue throughout the course of the gastrointestinal tract. Clinicians can take advantage of this feature and use these antibiotics for their effect on the bowel bacteria, but this accounts for a small minority of drugs. The goal for most oral antibiotics is for them to be rapidly and completely absorbed into the bloodstream and then to reach various tissues.

Different hurdles exist for antibiotics that are given by injection—typically either injected into a vein (usually a superficial vein in the arm or back of the hand where there are generally visible, accessible veins) or injected into a muscle. The antibiotic liquid cannot be irritating to the tissues, cause local bleeding or inflammation, or cause red blood cells to break down. This means it cannot be too acidic or too alkaline. Drugs infused directly into a vein cannot contain substances that are toxic to the heart or that could affect heart rhythm—for example, those containing high amounts of potassium. When drugs are given as an injection into the muscle, there is a limit to the volume that can be injected at one time. When given through a vein, the drug can be diluted in fluid, like saline (salt water) or a glucose (sugar water) solution, and dripped in over a period of time, even many hours in some instances.

One advantage of administering an antibiotic by injection is the reliability of the drug reaching the bloodstream. Some individuals, like infants, can't swallow pills. But any drug that requires repeated injections will not appeal to patients. Over many decades more alternatives to injections and intravenous antibiotics have become available.

Antibiotics can be altered by chemists to change some of their characteristics. For example, the originally produced penicillin (besides containing impurities) was destroyed by acid in the stomach. Ultimately a pill form was made that could survive stomach acid. For injectable penicillin, chemists added a local anesthetic, procaine (like novocaine used by dentists), to penicillin to reduce the pain at the injection site. Procaine penicillin has been used since 1948. With procaine penicillin, peak blood levels of penicillin are reached about 2 hours after injection and some of the drug persists in the body for 24 hours. Another common preparation involves mixing penicillin with the local anesthetic benzathine. This slows the absorption of penicillin from the muscle. Benzathine penicillin became available in 1950. After an injection of this formulation, penicillin can still be detected in low levels 14 days after an injection. Regular penicillin would have to be given as an injection every 6 hours to achieve persistent levels of activity. Regular penicillin is eliminated by the kidneys with more than 70% of the dose passed in the urine within 6 hours, mainly as the active drug. This is why in the early days when penicillin was in short supply, urine was sometimes saved and taken to a laboratory where the penicillin could be recovered and reused in another patient.

Different forms of an antibiotic, like the penicillin examples just described, are needed because different types of infections require different levels of an antibiotic and lengths of treatment. Specially prepared formulations may be used to treat infections in specific locations, such as superficial infections of the skin, of the outer part of the ear and ear canal (but not middle ear infections), and of the conjunctivae of the eyes. Only certain antibiotics that are made in fluids or ointments that are not damaging to the delicate cornea and structures of the eye can be used to treat eye infections. Putting the antibiotic in ointments can help provide longer contact. Most antibiotics do not readily penetrate intact skin but can be absorbed through broken skin or through mucous membranes, such as the conjunctivae (eyes), vagina, rectum, and mouth.

In some instances, antibiotics are injected directly into tissues close to the site of infection, for example, into the belly (intraperitoneally) to treat peritoneal infection or into the area around the spinal column (intrathecally) to treat meningitis when drugs that penetrate the blood-brain barrier are unavailable.

Delivering drugs by aerosol (spray) has been tried for treating lung infections, but this approach is not common. Recently the US Food and Drug Administration (FDA) approved an antibiotic (amikacin) that can be inhaled to treat a specific type of lung infection (*Mycobacterium avium* complex) that is often difficult to treat. The treatment is delivered through a nebulizer.

Are pills as effective as injections?

In some cultures injections are viewed as more effective than pills. Injections are perceived as "strong" and pills as "weak." Some patients even request *une piqure*, or a shot, and think they have been shortchanged by a health provider who fails to deliver an injection. If it hurts, it must work, right? But injections are not always more effective; some antibiotic pills are more effective than some antibiotics given by injection. It depends on the specific antibiotic, its form, and the amount used.

Some antibiotics are available in both pill and injectable form; some are made only as pills and others only as injectable forms. The properties of the specific antibiotic will determine whether it can be absorbed from the gastrointestinal tract if taken by mouth. Chemists have become expert at modifying molecules to create the desired properties in a drug.

Because infants and young children—and sometimes others—may be unable to swallow pills or capsules, some antibiotics commonly used in infants and young children have been prepared in liquid formulations, and with flavors like cherry and strawberry that make them appealing. These have to be carefully tested to make certain the altered form is still absorbed.

Injectable antibiotics can be given as injections into the muscle or tissues or delivered directly as a liquid into a vein (blood vessel). There are several advantages to infusing the drug directly into the vein. With many antibiotics one can deliver a much larger dose of the antibiotic, perhaps 20 to 30 times or more, directly into the vein than in pill form or injection into muscle. The delivery is fast and certain. In contrast, pills taken by mouth might be vomited or not be absorbed. It takes longer for antibiotics in pills to start to work against bacteria. The patient may forget to take pills or decide not to take them. For severe infections or if the person is unable to take oral antibiotics (e.g., is unconscious or vomiting), antibiotics are usually given by injection. A needle or small plastic catheter may be inserted into a vein and taped in place so that repeated doses of an antibiotic in a fluid can be given without requiring a new needle puncture of the skin for each dose. This way the drug is delivered directly into the bloodstream. Giving a drug by injection into the muscle is fast and reliable but also painful, and most people are not eager to receive repeated injections. Also, the amount of drug given per injection is limited. The disadvantages of intravenous antibiotics are the discomfort of an intravenous line, the need for regular medical attention (though in recent years there has been more use of outpatient and even home intravenous treatment, so intravenous therapy does not always require being in a hospital as it did in the past), and the occasional complications like clotting of the vein and infection related to the presence of the foreign material (needle or catheter) that are risks from intravenous lines.

Pills or capsules, on the other hand, are convenient and portable. They can be taken anywhere—at home, at work, on the road—and only require the person to remember to take them. Some must be taken with food to avoid stomach upset or to improve absorption; others must be taken on an empty stomach for optimal absorption. Some may interact with specific foods or other medications—like antacids, milk, iron pills, and bismuth subsalicylate (Pepto-Bismol®). The main reasons they may not work as well as injections is that the levels of the antibiotic in the bloodstream from drugs in pills and capsules are generally lower than from injected drugs—and people forget to take them or decide to stop taking them. Many oral antibiotics must be taken three or four times daily, which is difficult to do consistently—especially if one is feeling better.

Many of the newer antibiotics have been designed with more favorable characteristics, for example, better absorption so good blood levels can be achieved after a single dose and altered molecules so that they remain active longer. Some need to be taken only once daily—a big improvement over the antibiotics that required multiple doses every day. With some of the newer drugs a single dose may deliver several days of action against bacteria.

There have also been improvements in the drugs given by injection so that some of them last longer—also an advantage. Antibiotics are a foreign substance that the body typically breaks down and eliminates, in one way or another. Some of the older chemicals used to treat infection, like mercury and molecules related to arsenic, could accumulate in the body to toxic levels and cause side effects, but antibiotics used today are typically eliminated within hours to days.

For treating some infections there are clear advantages to having a drug that stays around for a long time. The patient does not have to keep taking doses of the drug. However, there are also downsides. A long duration of treatment is unnecessary for many infections. Ideally one wants an antibiotic to be present only as long as necessary to treat an infection. If a person turns out to be allergic to a drug, continued presence of the antibiotic can prolong the stimulus for the allergic reaction.

Where does the antibiotic go in the body? Does it reach all
organs and tissues? What is its fate? Does any part of the
antibiotic leave the body in urine or feces?

What happens to an antibiotic after it is swallowed or injected depends on the specific drug. The general sequence for all drugs is absorption, distribution in the body, binding to certain cells and tissues, biotransformation, and finally elimination. The amount of antibiotic that reaches various organs and tissues varies. Some drugs penetrate into white blood cells more readily than others and so may be especially useful in killing bacteria that have found a way to survive inside cells. One part of the body that is notoriously difficult to reach is the brain and the lining of the brain (meninges, which become infected and inflamed in meningitis) because of what is known as the blood-brain barrier. The barrier is able to keep some drugs from freely entering that space, which is important to know when a person has an infection of that space. There has been extensive manipulation of many antibiotics to try to craft ones that work well under specific circumstances and for special infections like meningitis. What if the infection has spread into bone? We need antibiotics that will penetrate bone in high enough concentrations that they can reach and clear the bacteria.

When considering antibiotics, one can think of the body as having multiple compartments, even though, of course, they are all linked and connected through many visible and not-so-obvious pathways. In choosing an antibiotic to treat an infection, it is useful to know the type of bacteria causing the infection, the characteristics of that particular strain (e.g., which antibiotics are active against it in the laboratory), and the location of the infection in the body. Even if the same species of bacteria are involved, a different antibiotic might be chosen to treat an infection in the bone than one in the brain. In an ideal world, treatment for each infection would be customized based on knowing the specific bacterial strain and location of infection in the body. In the real world, clinicians often make decisions based on fragments of information and best guesses. Today, however, scans that give clear images of many parts of the body, as well as other tests, provide details that were not available in past decades.

Detailed studies are done on any substance that might be used as an antibiotic in humans. If a substance is shown to kill or inhibit growth of bacteria, that is only a first step. Initial studies are done in animals or on cells in the laboratory to learn if the drug damages tissues or cells. Does it affect the normal functioning of the body? Can drug levels be achieved that are high enough to kill bacteria in an animal (first) or person without causing harm to the person? Studies called pharmacokinetic studies are done to assess how rapidly the drug is absorbed and enters the bloodstream. One measure that is determined is the half-life of the drug or the time it takes for the level of the drug in the plasma (bloodstream) to reach half of its original peak concentration. This value will influence how often doses of the antibiotic will have to be given. In animals and then in humans detailed tests are done to learn other characteristics.

Some antibiotics taken by a pregnant woman can reach the developing fetus, potentially causing damage to the fetus during vulnerable stages of development. Every new drug that is being considered is analyzed for its capacity to cross the placenta and reach tissues in the fetus. It is always important to know if a woman might be pregnant when choosing an antibiotic. Some antibiotics can be safe to use during pregnancy. Many are not. Some antibiotics have a different effect depending on the stage of the pregnancy and the age of the fetus. For example, the tetracycline antibiotics can affect development of bones and teeth in the fetus.

Antibiotics are typically broken down (biotransformed) by the body, whether they are taken by mouth or given by injection. The byproducts of the metabolism (breakdown) may also have activity against the bacteria. Sometimes these byproducts are more active than the parent compound. Many of the enzyme systems involved in the biotransformation of drugs are located in the liver. The cytochrome P450 system includes multiple enzymes that are responsible for the biotransformation (metabolism) of drugs and toxins. These enzymes can be induced (increased or turned on) or inhibited (slowed down or stopped) by some drugs, including some antibiotics. An individual's genetics may determine in part how an antibiotic is metabolized—and the levels of the drug. Antibiotics can be eliminated from the body unchanged in the urine. The kidneys are the most important location for elimination of the antibiotic or its metabolites (the byproducts that result when the drug is broken down). This means that if a person has kidney failure, the drug or its byproducts can accumulate and, in some instances, be toxic. For antibiotics that are biotransformed primarily by the liver, the dosage may have to be adjusted if a person has liver disease, such as cirrhosis, that affects liver function.

What happens with antibiotics after they leave the body?

Some of the byproducts of antibiotics are formed in the liver when the antibiotic-containing blood passes through the liver; they end up in the bile and are then excreted through the intestine, where they are eliminated with the feces. This means that residues of antibiotics (and sometimes unchanged antibiotics) end up in wastewater, sewage treatment plants, or wherever human waste is processed or discharged. In lower-income countries where toilets are unavailable and open defecation (depositing feces on the ground) is common, untreated human waste (urine and feces) can end up in streams, rivers, lakes, and surface waters. In Delhi, India, for example, only 56% of human sewage is appropriately treated (Peal 2015). Our environment—soil, water, and air—is loaded with bacteria, and these antibiotic residues from waste that reach soil and water can affect some of those bacteria as well.

An estimate from a recent UN report is that up to 80% of antibiotics are excreted without being broken down through human urine and feces. For example, with amoxicillin, a commonly used, well-absorbed oral antibiotic, well over half (58% to 68%) is eliminated in unchanged form in the urine within 6 hours of taking an oral dose.

In many countries human waste goes into sewage systems and is treated. Animal waste plus antibiotics and their byproducts become part of manure, which may be spread on fields to fertilize crops and can affect soil bacteria. Runoff can enter local streams and surface water.

Most animal waste from agricultural facilities is not treated and can contaminate streams, rivers, and estuaries. A study by Zhu and colleagues (Zhu 2017) examined sediments from 18 estuaries that spanned over 4,000 km of eastern coastal China. They found that residues of all the major classes of antibiotics were widespread. Antibiotics are not "used up" when they go into a person or an animal and can still act on bacteria even after they leave the body. In the United States most human waste (but not animal waste) is treated in facilities where harmful bacteria and residues of drugs are mostly eliminated, however, some antibiotic resistant microbes can survive processing even in advanced wastewater treatment plants (LaPara 2011).

Why are antibiotics that are not absorbed used?

Usually antibiotics are taken by mouth as a way to deliver the drug into tissues throughout the body. But some antibiotics are not absorbed from the stomach or intestine and are used specifically to treat bacteria in the gut. When taken by mouth, they pass through the body staying within the gastrointestinal (GI) tract and are eliminated with the feces. Why are they used this way? As the antibiotic passes through the intestine, it can kill bacteria it comes into contact with. How many are killed depends on how broad its activity (how broad-spectrum the antibiotic) is. Clinicians sometimes intentionally use an antibiotic that is not absorbed (like oral vancomycin) to treat an infection that is localized to the GI tract (like *Clostridioides difficile*). They also have used this approach to eliminate bacteria from the bowel in preparation for bowel surgery when the bowel wall will be cut and there is risk that bowel bacteria could contaminate the wound. Antibiotics that are not absorbed from the GI tract, such as polymyxin and gentamicin, may be used for this purpose. Bowel bacteria can leak out of the bowel and into the bloodstream in individuals whose immune systems are severely compromised—and nonabsorbable drugs have been used in some instances to try to reduce the abundance of bacteria that might leak from the bowel and cause infection. Vancomycin and gentamicin are also used to treat infections in other parts of the body, but in those instances, the drugs must be given by injection because the drug will not reach bacteria outside the gut if it is taken by mouth. In contrast, an antibiotic named rifaximin was developed specifically to treat infections of the bowel. It is poorly absorbed and so acts only on the gut. It is sometimes used to treat travelers' diarrhea and is also active against *C. difficile*. Another drug rifamycin SV, just FDA approved in 2018, is formulated to be minimally absorbed so that the drug is delivered to the distal small bowel and colon. It is indicated for some cases of travelers' diarrhea. In contrast to ciprofloxacin, it was not associated with acquisition of multidrug resistant bacteria (Steffen 2018).

How does one decide which antibiotic to use?

Ideally the clinician knows what type of bacteria is causing the infection, for example, *Staphylococcus*, *Streptococcus*, or *Escherichia coli*. Under the best of circumstances, the person's bacteria causing the infection are cultured in the laboratory (often grown on an agar plate where colonies of bacteria can be seen without a microscope) so that the patient's own strain can be tested. Traditionally the testing was done by spreading a layer of fluid containing the bacteria on a large agar plate, dropping discs impregnated with known amounts of multiple different antibiotics on the agar plate, and carefully spacing them so that the discs were not too close together. The agar plate with the film of bacteria and discs were incubated overnight, and the bacteria were allowed to grow to the point that they became visible. The antibiotics within the discs would diffuse into the agar around them. Bacteria that were resistant to a particular antibiotic would grow right up to the disc (see Figure 2.1). Those that were sensitive could not grow in the

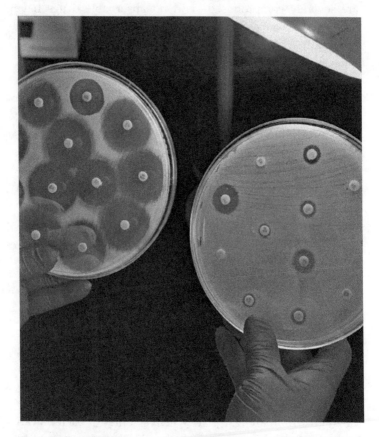

Figure 2.1 Testing for antibiotic resistance. Clear zones where bacterial growth is inhibited around the antibiotic discs indicate sensitive (susceptible) bacteria.

Centers for Disease Control and Prevention (CDC). Atlanta, GA.

presence of the antibiotic, so a visible clear zone would be present around that particular antibiotic disc. By examining the agar plate and measuring the size of the clear zone, typically in millimeters (or noting its absence), the microbiologist could report that the patient's bacteria were sensitive (or likely to respond) to certain antibiotics or resistant (unlikely to respond) to others. Many of the systems for testing bacteria for susceptibility to antibiotics are now automated and give detailed information on a printout or computer screen, but the basic idea is the same—checking to see if that patient's particular strain of bacteria will grow in the presence of an antibiotic in an amount (determined after extensive testing in the laboratory and linking this with clinical outcomes) that can be achieved in the human body.

Often decisions about the choice of an antibiotic are made without having the patient's own strain of bacteria. Sometimes antibiotics need to be started before the laboratory results are available. In those cases, if the clinician knows that the particular type of infection is usually caused by staph or another disease-causing bacterium, an antibiotic choice is made based on probabilities of antibiotic susceptibility profiles from recent experience—in that patient, that clinic, that hospital, or that geographic region, or in the published literature.

Many other factors go into the choice of antibiotic to treat an infection in a particular patient. Some minor, superficial infections may not need an antibiotic at all. So the first question is always: is the patient likely to benefit from an antibiotic? If yes, which antibiotics are likely to work for that particular infection given its cause and location? Is there a pill form that is likely to work? Can the patient take pills? Does the patient have allergies that would make it necessary to avoid some antibiotics? Does the patient have kidney or liver disease that would make it unwise to use certain drugs or that would require readjusting the usual dose? Antibiotics also vary greatly in cost, with many of the newer drugs being much more expensive. Can the patient afford the drug? Unfortunately, sometimes when patients learn the price of a drug, they may decide to skip filling the prescription—and may be embarrassed to tell their doctor what has happened.

When the type or types of bacteria causing the infection are unknown, the clinician must make an educated guess about which bacteria are likely involved and which antibiotics are most likely to work. Does one choose an antibiotic that is active against a relatively narrow group of bacteria (narrow-spectrum drug), or does one go with a broad-spectrum drug or even a combination of drugs to cover more types of bacteria? That decision will depend in part on how sick the patient is. In a patient with septic shock (a potentially fatal type of infection) or severe illness in whom the use of an ineffective drug could lead to death within a few hours, broader antibiotic coverage is often chosen initially—and sometimes drugs with more potential side effects. In some types of infections multiple different bacteria are involved and a single antibiotic may not cover all of them. These are so-called polymicrobial infections. Examples include appendicitis or perforation of the bowel and leakage of bowel bacteria into the peritoneal cavity. Many pieces of information need to be integrated into the decision making about use of an antibiotic.

A major hurdle in medical decision making is insufficient information at the time the clinical situation requires making a choice. A huge gap in our medical tool kit is lack of point-of-care or bedside diagnostic tests that would allow rapid confirmation of the cause of an illness. Is the illness caused by or complicated by an infection? Is the infection caused by bacteria that are likely to respond to antibiotics or by a virus that will not? Which antibiotics are likely to work for this person's infection? Are the benefits of an antibiotic likely to outweigh the risks associated with the antibiotic? Using antibiotics when they have no benefit means squandering a precious resource.

What information about each antibiotic is available to the pharmacist, the health provider, and the patient?

For every antibiotic that is approved for use in the United States, the FDA document titled "full prescribing information," or FPI, is created. In a standard format, it supplies detailed information about the drug based on data presented to the FDA in the New Drug Application at the time of the request for drug approval. These FPI documents have detailed information and may run 25 pages or longer. There is a shorter version called "highlights of prescribing information" that includes a summary of the key points and most of the practical information the health provider needs to know to prescribe the drug. Table 2.1 displays the categories of information provided in the FPI. This includes the types of infections that can be treated with it. After an antibiotic is approved, if a pharmaceutical company wants to change the content of the FPI, for example, to add new indications for the use of the drug or to highlight new adverse events that have been recognized, these changes must be approved by the FDA. If the FDA recognizes new problems with an antibiotic after it has been approved, it may require the pharmaceutical company to make changes to the FPI document describing the drug. Health providers typically review this information carefully before prescribing an antibiotic to make certain a specific drug is a good choice for a particular patient.

Patients who fill prescriptions for antibiotics (and other drugs) are also given background about the specific drug. This always includes categories about common uses, how to take the drug, cautions, and possible side effects. Sometimes these are written in a question-and-answer format to make the content more easily understandable. Patients are urged to contact their health care provider or pharmacist if they are concerned about possible side effects. Information sheets given to patients also include an 800 number for the FDA that they can call if they want to report possible side effects from the drug.

Table 2.1 Full Prescribing Information Provided for Drugs

Section	Comment
Boxed warning (also known as black-box warning)	Included only if FDA has required special warning about use of the drug, side effects, other
Indications and usage	Lists medical conditions and types of infections for which the drug is indicated, for example, community-acquired pneumonia, acute bacterial skin infection
Dosage and administration	Amount of drug to be given and route of administration; may vary by type of infection. May include separate tables for adult and pediatric patients. Gives recommended duration of treatment
Dosage forms and strengths	Describes pills, capsules, oral suspension, injectable, or other forms and amount of drug in each
Contraindications	Lists situations when the antibiotic should not be used. Examples include known hypersensitivity to drug, history of liver disease
Warnings and precautions	Describes events that have followed use of the drug, such as hypersensitivity reactions, liver toxicity, heart rhythm change, tooth discoloration, *C. difficile* diarrhea. Also describes action to be taken for each adverse event, such as discontinue drug immediately, evaluate, or contact provider
Adverse reactions	Lists most common adverse reactions and the percentage of patients who developed these during clinical trials, for example, diarrhea (5%–14%), nausea (3%–18%), vomiting (2%–7%). For drugs approved several years ago it includes experience with adverse reactions after the drug was marketed. Lists abnormalities in laboratory results related to the drug
Drug interactions	Lists known interactions with other specific drugs and their consequences, such as increased risk of bleeding, increased risk of liver damage, or risk of damaging hearing

Table 2.1 Continued

Section	Comment
Use in specific populations	May indicate certain patients who should not receive the drug, such as infants or young children, pregnant women, nursing mothers, older individuals
Drug abuse and dependence	Indicates potential for drug causing dependence. This has not been described for any antibiotics
Overdosage	Potential for adverse events in the event of overdose
Description (dosage forms, ingredients, pharmacological or therapeutic class, and other relevant information)	Gives chemical name and displays chemical structure. Lists other ingredients found in the tablets
Clinical pharmacology (mechanism of action, pharmacodynamics, pharmacokinetics, microbiology)	Describes how the drug works, how much is absorbed if taken as pill, how long it stays in the body, and how it is cleared from the body. Describes which bacteria can be killed by it and which ones are resistant to it
Nonclinical toxicology (carcinogenesis, mutagenesis, impairment of fertility, animal toxicology, and/or pharmacology)	Describes whether the drug can cause cancer or mutations or decrease sperm counts. Usually results are from animal studies
Clinical studies	Describes the outcomes when the drug was used to treat infections in people
How supplied/ storage and handling	Size of vials or bottles; appearance of pills, for example, yellow, diamond shaped, film-coated tablet
Patient counseling information	Describes common side effects and how to take pills, for example, with or without food and possible interference if taken with antacids, multivitamins, other pills

How long does it take for an antibiotic to work? Why are
some antibiotics given as a single dose and others prescribed
for weeks or longer?

Improvement in some infections can be dramatic and rapid.
High fever from an infection may drop within hours in response to an antibiotic, but it depends on the type of bacteria
and the location within the body. In typhoid fever, fortunately
no longer a common infection in the United States, fever drops
slowly, often in a stepwise fashion—a little lower each day
until it is gone. Clinical response in most infections is faster.
Some infections can be treated with one or a few doses of an
antibiotic—like gonorrhea or a bladder infection. Infections
that are in bone or that involve the heart valves (endocarditis)
can take weeks to cure. Bacteria that are enclosed in an abscess cavity may not respond even to high doses or prolonged
antibiotic courses because the bacteria are walled off and
antibiotics may not reach the bacteria or be active in the pus in
an abscess cavity.

When a patient does not respond as expected to antibiotic treatment, several possibilities exist. Maybe the bacteria
causing the infection are resistant to the antibiotic. Maybe the
antibiotic cannot reach the bacteria because they are walled
off or protected by foreign material, like a catheter. Or maybe
the initial diagnosis was wrong and the fever or the symptoms
were caused by something else.

A successful resolution to an infection usually requires
participation from the human host and the human immune system, which includes white blood cells known as
phagocytes that help to enclose bacteria and other small cells
and particles. They are found throughout the body; they en-
gulf and kill bacteria and are essential for fighting infection.
Each person normally has billions of them. The antibiotic
alone may not be able to completely clear the bacteria that are
causing the problem. When foreign material is present, such as
an artificial (prosthetic) knee or hip, a graft in a blood vessel,
mesh placed in a hernia repair, or an artificial heart valve or

other artificial material, the bacteria may be able to survive by clinging to the artificial material or some of the debris (old clot, sutures, etc.) in a biofilm where they can evade the immune response and action of the antibiotic. Sometimes treatment can be successful with a very long course of antibiotics, and sometimes the foreign material must be removed to clear the infection.

Treatment of tuberculosis, another bacterial infection, may take 6 months to a year or more to cure. It is always treated with multiple antibiotics because treatment with one or two drugs often leads to the development of resistant forms of infection.

What determines the right dose of an antibiotic?

Antibiotics that are used in humans have been selected because they can kill bacteria in the body at levels that are not toxic to human tissues and organs. Many other substances have potent antibacterial activity but may also damage human tissues at doses that kill the bacteria. More than 100 years ago Paul Ehrlich put forth the idea of an agent that attaches to or attacks only the disease-causing bacteria that infect a person and does not affect any of the other cells in the human body, but this does not yet exist in routine practice.

Antibiotics vary as to their safety at doses that are effective in treating infections in humans. This has been defined as the therapeutic index or the therapeutic ratio. Scientists determine how much of the drug is required to have the desired effect in 50% of cases (efficacious dose in 50%, or ED50) and the dose that will cause adverse effects in 50% of cases (toxic dose in 50%, or TD50). The therapeutic index is determined by dividing the TD50 by the ED50. The higher the therapeutic index or number is, the safer the drug. One would prefer to use drugs with a high therapeutic index, which means a wide margin of safety. This allows more flexibility in increasing the dose if an infection is especially hard to treat because it is in a difficult-to-reach part of the body or if the bacteria are only marginally sensitive to the antibiotic.

A few drugs that are commonly used today have a narrow therapeutic window, meaning the toxic dose is not much higher than the therapeutic dose—the dose that is likely to be effective. When these drugs are used to treat infections, the clinician will carefully calculate the exact dose of the drug to be administered, taking into account the weight of the patient, kidney function, liver function (if relevant for that specific drug), and the patient's age to estimate the initial dose. Some of the body systems that metabolize drugs become less effective in older people, and lowering the dose may be necessary. After the drug has been started (usually after a few doses to allow equilibration of the drug in the body), the level of the drug in the blood will be measured. The range of safe levels has been determined by multiple previous studies, so the clinician can then compare the level in a particular patient with the desired range and can increase or decrease the dose as needed. Depending on the duration of treatment needed, the levels may have to be measured more than once. For most antibiotics, there is no need to measure levels because there is a wide range of safe levels.

The human body is a dynamic system and many factors can influence levels, including genetics, other drugs, and changes in kidney function over time. A class of drugs called aminoglycosides, still commonly used today because they often work against infections for which few or no other treatments are available, has a narrow therapeutic window and can cause kidney damage and deafness. Even if they can effectively treat an infection, a patient can potentially end up with severe side effects, which can be irreversible. Vancomycin is another commonly used antibiotic (to treat staph and enterococcal infections) that has a relatively narrow therapeutic window and can be toxic to the kidneys when levels are high.

The type and location of infection will also influence the dose of an antibiotic. Infections in the brain and lining of the brain, like meningitis, typically require high doses of an antibiotic because the antibiotics may penetrate poorly. Other hard-to-treat infections that may require high doses and a long duration of treatment are infections of the heart valves (endocarditis) and infections of bone (osteomyelitis).

There are other reasons for high doses of antibiotic. A patient's bacteria may be only marginally sensitive to a particular antibiotic that is otherwise a good choice for the infection because of its safety, tissue penetration, and other characteristics. If the antibiotic dose can be safely boosted, it may be increased to target the specific strain of bacteria.

Can one overdose on an antibiotic?

Most oral antibiotics used today have a wide therapeutic window, so if someone takes extra doses, there are likely to be few consequences, at least in older children and adults. Some antimalaria drugs, such as chloroquine and quinine, used to prevent and treat malaria can be toxic in young children. Some antibiotics given by injection, as noted earlier, can have adverse consequences if levels are high. Some antibiotics like penicillin given intravenously at high doses can cause seizures, but this is not an "overdose" as we would traditionally think of it.

Does an antibiotic have any effect other than against the bacteria being treated?

Antibiotics are typically given to treat a specific infection, and the clinician will try to give a drug that is the best match for the bacteria causing the infection—but the antibiotics don't just affect the bacteria causing the infection. They also kill some of the normal resident bacteria. Taking an antibiotic can have a profound effect on the bacteria in many parts of the body, but especially in the gut or the gastrointestinal tract, where the largest number of bacteria reside.

Currently available antibiotics are not programmed to selectively eliminate the bacteria causing the infection and nothing else. They are a blunt instrument and will kill sensitive bacteria that they reach, wherever they are in the body. This means there is a lot of collateral damage to resident bacteria or off-target killing.

Bacteria that cause disease (known as pathogens) are often closely related to many of the trillions of bacteria that live in and on us. So treating an infection—say, using penicillin to treat a strep infection of the throat—may cause mass casualties among other bacteria that live in the throat, in the gut, and elsewhere in the body. The intended target may be the Group A *Streptococcus* in the throat that is making a person sick, but antibiotics, so impressive and elegant in many ways, kill any bacteria in their path that are sensitive to them. Group A *Streptococcus* is a bad actor and has traits (virulence factors like toxin production) that allow it to cause severe disease and death (streptococcal sepsis, streptococcal skin infections, streptococcal pneumonia and meningitis, scarlet fever, rheumatic fever, etc.). But there are many other types of streptococci that are part of our resident bacteria (mouth, throat, gut, skin) and may be killed by an antibiotic. Those bacteria that are resistant to the antibiotic survive—and may in fact flourish because some of their bacterial competition for space and food (nutrients) has been killed off.

One of the severe consequences of using antibiotics is the selection of resistant bacteria. Resistance in bacteria is a major and serious global problem, but the consequences of antibiotic exposure on the body's bacterial residents goes far beyond promoting the survival of bacteria resistant to the antibiotic. At the time of birth infants begin to acquire their resident bacteria—starting with passage through the birth canal and later swallowing colostrum and breast milk. Each individual develops a unique collection of populations of bacteria. The bacteria in the gut are most abundant, but all body surfaces and mucous membranes like the mouth, conjunctivae, and vagina are inhabited by resident bacteria. Each person carries a unique constellation of bacteria—like a microbial fingerprint—that can remain remarkably constant over time, if there are no disturbances. The bacteria that live between the toes show a different composition than those that live on the elbow or behind the ear. Those in the mouth and throat differ from those in the stomach. Different parts of the intestine have different kinds of bacteria. The bacteria in the vagina and rectum are different. In an individual the bacteria show a certain constancy over time—but many factors can affect them, such as age, sex, diet, illness, activities and exposures, travel, drugs, and pregnancy. Our knowledge about the constellation of bacteria (and yeast, viruses, and other microorganisms) that live on and in us is still at a rudimentary level.

We know enough to understand that our microbiota are fundamental to our health and well-being. The microbiota influence immunity, hormones, and other chemicals and may contribute to allergic, inflammatory, neoplastic, metabolic, and other diseases. These microbial communities are complex and may be shared among human populations. See a more detailed discussion in the section on microbiomes.

How long does the effect of an antibiotic last?

This question should be broken into two parts. The first part is, how long does the antibiotic (the drug) stay in the body or in any of the tissues? The second is, how long does the effect of the antibiotic on the resident bacteria last?

The length of time the antibiotic persists in the body is highly variable and depends on the specific antibiotic. With most antibiotics the peak amount or level of the drug will be reached shortly after the drug is consumed or injected—minutes to hours—and then the levels fall off as the body transforms or breaks down the drug and eliminates it. The antibiotic may be active in treating the infection only when the levels are relatively high even though small amounts of the drug may persist for days or longer in some tissues or cells.

If a drug causes an adverse reaction, this can be brief and completely reversible or longer lasting and occasionally irreversible. An adverse reaction to a drug can start after a person has stopped taking a drug and can persist even after a drug is completely gone from the system.

The most profoundly important effect and one that potentially affects the larger community is the impact of the antibiotic on the person's resident bacteria. In the early days of antibiotic therapy most of the attention was on the magical nature of these substances that could miraculously bring people back from the brink of death. In the early years of their use, even in the 1940s, it became apparent that the bacteria that were the intended target of the antibiotics could develop resistance to the antibiotics. It was also learned early on that resistant bacteria could spread from one person to another. There was less awareness of the abundance and importance of the normal resident bacteria—the microbiota—that can help to keep us healthy.

An individual taking an antibiotic can potentially have consequences beyond the individual. Antibiotics affect biological systems. Bacteria are alive, mutable, and shared among humans and animals. Bacteria selected because of exposure to antibiotics in one individual may be shared with others and cause future infections in others near and far. Unlike most other drugs, use of antibiotics potentially affects the community and the future. The impact of taking antibiotics can be long lasting.

Why are some infections, such as tuberculosis, always treated with multiple different antibiotics taken simultaneously?

Two or more antibiotics are used at the same time under several circumstances. A combination of drugs will cover more bacteria than one, so if one is uncertain of the cause or is treating a polymicrobial infection (an infection that involves many different bacteria), one may use two or more antibiotics. For some especially difficult-to-treat infections, a combination may be synergistic, providing better antibacterial activity than either could provide alone. In endocarditis, an infection of one or more of the heart valves that was always fatal in the pre-antibiotic era, the infecting bacteria are lodged in nodular, ir-regular growths, called vegetations, on the heart valves—the delicate cusps or leaflets. The colonies of bacteria are relatively protected by fibrin and other material and can be difficult to reach with an antibiotic, even though the infection is often caused by a type of streptococci that live in the mouth and are very sensitive to many antibiotics. The infection is also bathed by the blood, but the valve leaflets do not have a good blood supply. To overcome the barriers to curing this otherwise le-thal infection, one typically uses high doses of antibiotics, usually given intravenously for many weeks. In this setting, a second antibiotic may be given to help ensure the killing of all of the bacteria, even though the type of bacteria may be sensitive in the laboratory to low doses of the primary antibi-otic used. Infection is more common on valves that have been scarred or damaged by other diseases (or abnormalities pre-sent from birth); infection of the heart valve can cause further damage to the delicate leaflets, sometimes leading to ulcera-tion, destruction, or abscesses at the base of the valve. Surgery is sometimes necessary to replace or repair a damaged or leaky valve or to help clear the infection if antibiotics alone are not working well.

Tuberculosis is a bacterial infection (caused by a type of bacteria called mycobacteria) that is often slow to develop and is slow to be cured, at least with the drugs we have today. Streptomycin was the first antibiotic shown to be active against tuberculosis in the 1940s by Waksman, but the initial joyful opti-mism was quickly tempered when patients, after experiencing early improvement, then relapsed. Other drugs were added (para-amino salicylic acid or PAS and isoniazid in the 1940s and additional drugs later). For active tuberculosis, what is considered a "short" course of treatment is a 6-month regimen typically involving four drugs. Multiple drugs are taken at the same time to prevent the appearance and proliferation of drug-resistant bacteria. Tuberculosis (TB) remains a major problem today. Two potent factors have made control extraordinarily difficult: the HIV pandemic and drug resistance. Infection with HIV makes individuals especially susceptible to TB and its progression to active infection. A quarter to a third of the global population is infected with the bacillus (*Mycobacterium tuberculosis*) that causes TB, but most have inactive (latent) TB and have no symptoms and usually do not know that they are infected. Becoming infected with HIV markedly increases the risk that TB will become active and disseminate in the body and potentially become contagious and spread to others. Many deaths in HIV-infected individuals are from TB that was unrecognized and untreated. In general, people who have in-active (latent) TB have about a 10% risk of developing active TB over their lifetimes. In HIV-infected individuals, the risk can be as high as 10% per year. The problem of drug-resistant TB is discussed in chapter 5 on resistance.

Does one always have to take the entire course of prescribed antibiotics?

This is a hot-button issue getting lots of attention. It was prompted by a 2017 article in a British journal suggesting that often antibiotics can be stopped when the patient is feeling better. The traditional teaching, which is repeated in many official documents and found on websites, is that one must always take every last pill as prescribed. That traditional recommendation is receiving more scrutiny as we think about ways to safely reduce antibiotic use.

A first question we should ask is, do we know how long to treat a particular infection—be it a kidney infection, pneumonia, or ear infection? In most instances, there have not been good studies to determine exactly how long antibiotics are needed. Typically studies are done on a population of people, and the characteristics of the participants may not match the age, severity, and other features of the current individual seeking treatment. The prescribed courses are estimates of what is needed to cure that particular infection. Many courses of antibiotics are prescribed for 1 week, 10 days, or 2 weeks—but never 9, 11, or 13 days. Published studies for many kinds of infections provide general estimates of whether a longer or shorter course may be necessary but are sometimes rigid or dogmatic about duration without good evidence to support it.

Recent studies assessed whether a shorter course would work in treating ear infections in young children and found that the shorter course was not as effective long ones (Hoberman 2016]. In contrast, recent studies on sinusitis found that there was usually no benefit to taking courses longer than 5 days (Chow 2012).

Studies in hospitalized patients have found that it is possible to give shorter courses of intravenous antibiotics to treat pneumonia than traditionally used and still achieve similar results. Studies comparing traditionally used longer versus shorter courses for other infections, such as skin and soft tissue, kidney, and intraabdominal infections have also found shorter courses give good outcomes. A motivation behind some recent studies is to assess whether shorter courses can be effective because there is a strong desire to eliminate unnecessary antibiotic use without losing the benefits of treatment.

In some serious infections, such as endocarditis, meningitis, joint infection, and osteomyelitis (infection of the bone), we do not want to run the risk of undertreating an infection because incomplete or failed treatment could lead to tissue damage and potential serious long-term consequences. We are more willing to accept occasional failures or relapses for infections that are less serious.

Infections of the kidney may take longer to clear than infections of the bladder (cystitis), which may be superficial and cured with one or a few doses of antibiotic, even though both are diagnosed by finding white blood cells and bacteria in the urine. Often the available diagnostic tests do not clearly show the exact body site of infection within the urinary tract.

In the absence of ideal diagnostic tests, various markers are used to provide clues as to whether an infection is coming under control. These include white blood cell count, fever, redness or tenderness of a wound, and the patient's symptoms. Antibiotics work along with the body's immune system. Typically it is unnecessary to kill every last bacterium involved in causing an infection. If one reduces the bacteria to a low number, the body's own immune defenses may be able to mop up the remaining disease-causing microbes.

This again portrays the deficiencies in our diagnostic capabilities. What if we had a simple diagnostic test that would tell us when the infection had been cured in a particular person? Right now, we base decisions about individuals on population data—for example, the outcomes of infection for 200 patients treated with antibiotic X, Y, or Z for a defined duration. It is likely there is spectrum of durations needed to cure individuals in a population. Most might be cured in 4 days; a few might take 15 days. By default, we may prescribe 14 days for all. Better diagnostic tools would allow for more precise treatment of individuals and likely reduction in overall antibiotic use.

In the meantime, we should study shorter courses of antibiotics for common infections to see if they work as well as traditional or standard courses. In instances where we know shorter courses work, we should use them.

Can one take leftover antibiotics for a new infection? Or give it to a family member or friend?

In general, an antibiotic is matched to a specific infection (cause and location) and person. In selected instances, a person may need to take another course of antibiotics for the same or a similar infection and the leftover antibiotic may be appropriate to use, if not beyond the expiration date. One should never give one's antibiotic to a friend or family member. It may be the wrong drug or the wrong dose for that person, one may be allergic to it, a woman may be pregnant, or one may be taking other drugs that adversely interact with it. Or the person may not even need an antibiotic. In general, the antibiotic should be taken only by the person for whom it was prescribed—and for that specific infection.

What should one do with leftover antibiotics?

Several options are available. Some local pharmacies are willing to accept and appropriately dispose of unused or expired drugs including antibiotics, or they have envelopes that can be used for shipping them for incineration. Some have medication disposal boxes where drugs can be dropped during business hours. In the community there may also be other authorized permanent collection sites in hospitals, clinics, and police departments. The Drug Enforcement Administration (DEA) periodically hosts national drug take-back events where temporary collection sites are set up for the safe disposal of prescription drugs. It took back almost a million pounds of drugs during the May National Prescription Drug Take-Back Day.

Containers of leftover antibiotics should not be thrown unchanged into the trash where a child may find them or someone else may retrieve them. If they are discarded in the trash, it is recommended that they be mixed with soil, cat litter, coffee grounds, or another unpalatable substance and sealed in a plastic bag or other container and then discarded.

It is interesting that people are often told not to flush unused pills down the toilet, yet unchanged antibiotic molecules and active metabolites of antibiotics are excreted into the urine—and guess where most of that goes!

Is it dangerous to take expired antibiotics?

Two questions to answer are, will they still work, and do they become toxic? Antibiotics do not turn to inactive dust or become toxic when the expiration date is reached. In 1979 a law was passed requiring drug manufacturers to stamp an expiration date on their products—so every antibiotic that you receive (in the United States) will have an expiration date on the bottle, the packet, or sometimes stamped on individual pills. Pharmacists cannot dispense a drug after the expiration date, and hospitals must discard drugs that have passed the expiration date. These expiration dates are not necessarily based on detailed studies of each antibiotic (Diven 2015).

A study done by the military many years ago found that most drugs (they were not just looking at antibiotics) retained high levels of activity long after the expiration date. Drugs vary in how stable they are, especially under conditions of high heat and/or humidity. They may lose potency (strength) with time, but many retain a high level of the original activity—but the drug manufacturer cannot confirm that full activity will remain longer than the expiration date.

The two main concerns with a drug over time are loss of potency (active ingredient in the drug loses some of its strength) and potential breakdown of ingredients into forms that could be toxic. Decades ago a form of tetracycline was manufactured in a way that could permit expired drug to become toxic, but that process is no longer used.

Before medications are licensed, they are tested for stability under different conditions of heat and humidity and each is given an expiration date, typically 12 to 60 months after the drug is produced. The duration may vary depending on the specific medication and formulation of the medication (tablet vs. capsule vs. liquid suspension vs. injectable form). In general, solutions and suspensions are less stable than pills and capsules. Some medications, however, are extremely stable and remain fully active long after the expiration date (Lyon 2006). The expiration date simply indicates the time for which the pharmaceutical company has proved that the drug is safe and effective (for which it will still contain the amount of active ingredient listed on the label). It is somewhat of a misnomer, however. The antibiotic activity does not disappear on that date, but its guarantee by the drug company does.

The US military maintains large stockpiles of medications (and vaccines and other materials). This vast, valuable stockpile includes medications that reached their expiration dates in the 1980s. Instead of discarding every medication once it reaches its expiration date (at a cost of millions of dollars), the US military started a program, the Shelf Life Extension Program (SLEP), that involved testing the stability of drugs that were due to expire. The US Department of Defense/FDA SLEP studies showed that 2,650 of 3,005 lots of 122 products stored in their original containers remained stable an average of 66 months after the expiration date. For some drugs the expiration date was extended by more than 20 years. They also found that for every dollar spent in testing the activity of stockpiled drugs, they saved $13 to $94 in what it would cost to acquire new ones. The list of drugs tested included many antibiotics. Some of these and the number of months extended included ampicillin capsules (49 months), tetracycline capsules (50 months), ciprofloxacin tablets (55 months), and cephalexin capsules (57 months). These drugs were in their original containers and stored under ideal conditions, and not in a steamy bathroom in a small container that had been opened—so these numbers should not be taken as the times one can safely save and use these antibiotics from a home medicine cabinet.

In a small study unrelated to military stockpiles, researchers studied a collection of eight medications (no antibiotics included) stored in their original containers that had expired 28 to 40 years (that is correct—*years*) earlier. These were discovered in a forgotten back closet of a retail pharmacy and studied by a researcher who specializes in analyzing chemicals. They found that 12 of the 14 drug compounds in them were present in at least 90% of the amount listed on the label. Three of the drug compounds were present in amounts greater than 110% of the amount listed on label. Aspirin, however, retained less than 5% of its potency (strength). Today the FDA considers acceptable amounts of active drug that fall between 90% and 110% of the amount listed on the label as "reasonable variation."

Because it is illegal for pharmacists to dispense and for hospitals, nursing homes, and other facilities to administer expired drugs, billions of dollars' worth of drugs that still have activity are probably being discarded. Some groups and individuals have called for more active testing of drugs past expiration to reduce the waste and cost to the health care system. Any such effort would probably have to be led by the FDA because pharmaceutical companies have no incentives to have patients take expired medications rather than buy new ones.

In the meantime, consumers in the United States are reasonably well protected against being given expired drugs. Drug labels from pharmacists may also have "beyond use," "do not use after," or "discard after" dates, sometimes required by a state board of pharmacy. After an original container from the manufacturer is opened (and pills dispensed into a small bottle or other container), the original expiration date is not considered reliable because the change in storage could affect the stability of the drug. The "use by" dates are typically 1 year after the drug is dispensed and would never be later than the expiration date for the drug. Increasingly drugs, including many antibiotics, are being dispensed in individual pill or capsule packages that include the name of the drug and the expiration date. Generic drugs are usually repacked into small bottles. The "use by" date may come long before the original expiration date (which may be unknown to the consumer).

As of 2018, 38 US states had passed laws that provide for unused prescription drugs to be donated and redispensed. The details vary by state, but several features are common to all. They include only prescription drugs in unopened, sealed, and tamper-proof packaging with visible expiration dates, usually at least 6 months later than the donation.

See also the section on substandard and falsified drugs in chapter 1.

When are antibiotics used to prevent infections (in contrast to treating an established infection)?

The main reason for giving antibiotics to people is to treat an infection, but a substantial portion of antibiotics are also given to prevent infections. This is called antibiotic prophylaxis. These preventive antibiotics can be given to an individual, a group, or a specific high-risk population. The range of infections for which prophylaxis is given is broad. Sometimes it is given to prevent a specific bacterial infection, like Group A *Streptococcus*. Other times it is given to protect a vulnerable part of the body, such as an artificial heart valve, or a vulnerable patient, such as someone undergoing bone marrow transplantation or a surgical or other procedure.

In the early days after penicillin was discovered, when enthusiasm about its benefits exceeded knowledge about its consequences, it was added to many products, such as throat lozenges, toothpaste, and lipstick, even though by 1947 an outbreak of staph infections that did not respond to penicillin had been reported. Starting in 1951, however, a prescription for penicillin was required in the United States, which provided more control over its wide and indiscriminate use. It seems hard to believe now that in the early years after antibiotics were developed pharmaceutical companies did not have to show that the drugs were effective in treating (or preventing) a particular infection for them to be FDA approved. That requirement came decades later.

The early decades after antibiotics were first marketed were marked by an expanding number of preventive applications. Subsequently studies were done to try to define which procedures might benefit from preventive use of antibiotics and which drug, dose, and duration gave the greatest benefit while also weighing the risks from antibiotics. In general, over the years there has been a movement to give shorter preventive courses of antibiotics for many surgical procedures, often a single dose. Studies have also found that the timing of the antibiotic dose relative to the start (incision) time of surgery can also affect how well it will work. If given too soon, its activity will be gone before the surgical operation starts. Over the years, there has been a huge expansion in the number of surgical procedures for which preventive antibiotics are recommended. One major area is in the placement of artificial or prosthetic joints, most often the hips or knees. Even though this is considered "clean surgery," the presence of artificial material makes it more difficult for the body's immune system to eliminate even small numbers of bacteria that can survive in the local environment created by the prosthetic device. Even bacteria that normally do not invade tissues or cause serious infections, like resident bacteria that live on the skin (*Staphylococcus epidermidis* and others), can survive in the protective environment of artificial material, causing low-grade infection. Once an infection has developed in an artificial joint, it can be difficult or impossible to clear the infection with antibiotics alone, so the stakes are high and surgeons are eager to take steps to avoid infection of such a joint. Manufacturers have also played a role in selecting materials for the joints that are less likely to predispose to infections, and sometimes during the surgery materials or cements are used that are impregnated with antibacterial substances, like antibiotics or metals with antibacterial activity.

How are antibiotics used to prevent infections in surgery?

Surgery is often classified as "dirty" or "clean." The former refers to procedures that involve cutting or manipulating a tissue in a part of the body where bacteria normally are present in large numbers, such as the bowel, or when an infection is already present. An example of a clean surgery would be removal of the thyroid gland. Risks of infection after surgery are vastly different depending on the type of surgery.

In the United States in 2006 approximately 80 million surgical procedures were performed (46 million at inpatient facilities and 32 million at ambulatory settings). Between 2006 and 2009, almost 2% of surgical patients in hospitals experienced a wound infection during their hospital stay. This underestimates the overall rate because about half of surgical wound infections only become apparent after the patient is discharged. These complications of surgery generate enormous costs that can exceed $90,000 per infection, especially if the infection involves a prosthetic joint or bacteria that are resistant to multiple antibiotics. In general, rates of surgical site infections are much higher in most low- and middle-income countries than they are in the United States.

With an aging population that desires to remain active, prosthetic (artificial) joint surgery, such as knee and hip replacement, is likely to increase. In 2011 about 1.2 million prosthetic joint surgeries were performed in the United States, with knee surgery accounting for more than half, followed by hip procedures (Berrios-Torres 2017). The annual rate of knee replacements in the United States doubled between 2000 and 2015. Shoulder, elbow, and ankle replacements are much less common. These joint surgeries are projected to increase to 3.8 million procedures per year by 2030. Globally more than a million total hip replacements are done each year. Currently the infection rate is just over 2%, but this is projected to increase to over 6% by 2030 because patients who are at higher risk for infections are expected to have surgery. Factors such as diabetes and obesity, for example, can increase the risk for infections.

Antibiotics are now routinely used prior to many surgical procedures. The antibiotic is injected, typically intravenously, so that it is present in tissues and serum at the time the surgeon makes the surgical incision. In addition to joint replacements,

surgical procedures where antibiotics have been shown to reduce rates of infection and are routinely used include hip fracture surgery, heart pacemaker implantation, spinal surgery,
transrectal prostate biopsy, removal of the uterus, appendec-
tomy, and surgery involving the bowel (colon and rectum).

Another common surgical procedure is cesarean section.
Globally the number of cesarean section births has nearly
doubled in the past 15 years, reaching almost 30 million or 21%
of live births in 2015. Of the approximately 4 million babies
born annually in the United States, about a third are delivered
by cesarean section. Infectious complications are 5 to 10 times
more frequent after cesarean section than after vaginal delivery and preventive antibiotics are generally given, usually a
single dose of the antibiotic cefazolin in the United States. For
cesarean section procedures, it is recommended that the antibiotic be given before the skin incision is made. Obese women
are at higher risk for post–cesarean procedure infection. In 2014
about a quarter of women giving birth in the United States had
a body mass index (calculated based on weight and height) of
greater than 29.9, which is considered obese. A recent study
found that giving a single dose of intravenous azithromycin to
women undergoing a cesarean procedure (along with routine
preventive antibiotics) reduced the rate of infections occurring
within 6 weeks of delivery from 12% to 6% (Tita 2016). The
antibiotic azithromycin concentrates in the myometrium (the
muscle of the uterus) and stays there and in fat, which may
help explain its benefit in this situation.

In what other settings are antibiotics used to prevent infections (antibiotic prophylaxis)?

Group B *Streptococcus*

In the United States the antibiotic ampicillin is given routinely to pregnant women who test positive (vaginal and
rectal cultures) for carrying a particular bacterium, Group B

Streptococcus. This bacterium is related to the better-known Group A *Streptococcus* that is the cause of strep throat, scarlet fever, and other serious infections. Group B *Streptococcus*, which is present in the vagina in about 10% to 30% of healthy women, can be transferred to the infant during labor and delivery. Infants who become infected can develop meningitis, which can be fatal. Giving ampicillin during labor prevents transmission to the infant. Use of ampicillin around the time of labor and delivery has dramatically reduced the number of infants with Group B streptococcal infections in the United States. Giving antibiotics during labor reduces the risk that the infant will develop Group B *Streptococcus* disease from about 1 in 100 to 1 in 4,000—or a 20-fold reduction in risk. The downside is more administration of antibiotics to healthy women.

Cancer chemotherapy

Antibiotic treatment is also an integral and essential part of cancer chemotherapy and management. After patients receive intense chemotherapy, their white blood cells (the cells that help protect against infection) may fall to dangerously low levels, putting them at high risk for bacterial infections that can kill them. Use of antibiotics is a standard part of some protocols for chemotherapy.

Use in dental procedures

The healthy mouth is alive with billions of bacteria. During and/or after dental procedures, especially procedures that cause local bleeding, like dental extractions, dental implants, root canals, and oral surgical procedures, the dentist may prescribe antibiotics. With these procedures, bacteria often enter the bloodstream. Individuals who have an artificial heart valve or a scarred heart valve or other prosthetic material (such as an artificial joint) may be at increased risk for developing an infection with mouth bacteria at one of these sites. In the past, there were detailed guidelines about the use of preventive antibiotics and a long list of circumstances when they were recommended for dental work, including many patients who had a heart murmur. Over the years the list of indications for preventive antibiotics for dental procedures has shrunk markedly.

Most recently the American Heart Association and European Society for Cardiology recommended preventive antibiotics in patients who have heart conditions associated with the highest risk of adverse outcome if infective endocarditis occurs. The UK National Institute for Health and Care Excellence advises against routine antibiotic prophylaxis to prevent endocarditis.

Meningococcal meningitis

The bacteria *Neisseria meningitidis* (meningococcus) can cause outbreaks of meningitis, which can be rapidly fatal. Fortunately these outbreaks are now much less common in the United States than in the past. These often occur in young people living in crowded conditions (like colleges or camps). Close contacts of those infected (like household contacts or roommates) are at increased risk of also developing meningitis. Giving close contacts a brief course of a preventive antibiotic (that is active against the target strain) can almost eliminate secondary cases among contacts. We now have good meningococcal vaccines, so the problem is less common than in the prevaccine era; however, vaccines are not active against all strains of meningococci and not everyone has been vaccinated. This means that there is still sometimes a role for use of preventive antibiotics in some outbreaks.

In the past, close contacts of patients with *Haemophilus influenzae* meningitis were sometimes given antibiotic prophylaxis to prevent infection. With the wide use of the Hib (*Haemophilus influenzae* type b) vaccine, *H. influenzae* meningitis has virtually disappeared, so this is no longer a reason for its use.

Group A *Streptococcus* and rheumatic fever

Rheumatic fever, an illness that follows infection with Group A *Streptococcus*, is characterized by joint pain, skin rash, and inflammation of the heart. Repeated infections can severely damage heart valves. It is recommended that people who have had a bout of rheumatic fever should remain on penicillin (or another drug if they are allergic to penicillin) for life to reduce the likelihood of repeat infections that may cause more damage to the heart valves. Rheumatic fever has been largely eliminated in North America and other high-income countries because of good access to diagnoses of strep infections and treatment with antibiotics, though there still are occasional clusters of infections. Globally it remains a problem. In 2015 an estimated 33.4 million people suffered from rheumatic heart disease and more than 300,000 died from it.

Another infection caused by Group A *Streptococcus*, erysipelas, manifests as an acute infection of the skin, which becomes red, hot, and tender to touch. High fever and elevated white blood cell count are common. Common sites for these infections are the face and leg. It can sometimes affect the arm in women with lymphedema (swelling) after mastectomy. It can be recurrent and in that setting preventive treatment with penicillin may be recommended.

In 2017, in response to an outbreak of invasive Group A streptococcal infections caused by one strain of streptococcus that seemed to be circulating in the homeless population in Anchorage, Alaska, leading to more than 40 hospitalizations, a decision was made by public health authorities to give a single dose of azithromycin to 391 homeless people they were able to reach at six sites for homeless services. Rates of infections and hospitalization dropped rapidly (Mosites 2018).

Other

A more controversial use of preventive antibiotics is prescribing a tetracycline (doxycycline) for men having sex with men to prevent sexually transmitted infections. Although one study showed it could decrease new infections, it could also contribute to the development and spread of resistant infections.

In the past, some clinicians advocated taking preventive antibiotics during international travel to reduce the likelihood of developing what is called travelers' diarrhea. Subsequent studies found that carrying a few doses of an antibiotic that would likely be active against many of the bacteria that cause travelers' diarrhea and using it in case diarrhea developed was also a good option. Recent studies and increasing global resistance among many bacteria have led to a shift in recommendations. Now antibiotic use is discouraged for mild and moderate diarrhea and reserved for severe infections that are likely to be caused by bacteria. Travelers are an important conduit in the global movement of bacteria, including those with resistance genes.

Women with recurrent urinary tract infections are sometimes prescribed "preventive" treatment, but in general this approach has not been effective and is associated with increasing resistance of bacteria cultured.

A major observation is that preventive use of antibiotics also contributes to the total volume of antibiotics administered and can help to select resistant bacteria. As more bacteria become resistant to antibiotics, preventive use may likewise become less effective. See chapters 5 and 6.

The best current estimates are that more than half of the tons of antibiotics used on Earth are given to animals. Antibiotics used in animals may be used to promote growth, to prevent infection, or to treat a specific infection. See section chapter 4, other uses of antibiotics (non-human use).

When are antibiotics used to treat entire populations in mass treatment campaigns?

Mass drug treatment campaigns are not new. Typically these programs involve giving everyone in a village, a community, or an area a medication, taken by mouth as a pill or liquid or given by injection. Mass vaccination campaigns have also been used in some areas in an attempt to vaccinate large numbers of individuals as efficiently as possible. They are sometimes used in response to outbreaks, such as those caused by yellow fever, measles, diphtheria, or polio or other diseases for which vaccines exist. Other times they are used to try to obtain wide coverage of a population. Mass treatment campaigns have often been used to try to eliminate a specific infection from a population.

Probably the most widely used over many decades are in attempts to control transmission of malaria in tropical and subtropical areas. Drugs used over the decades have included a long list of antimalarial drugs—proguanil, pyrimethamine, chloroquine, amodiaquine, sulfadoxine, and sometimes a combination of two or more. In some instances use of drugs was combined with spraying DDT or other insecticides or with other interventions, like bednets. In some countries in the past, when most malaria parasites were still sensitive to chloroquine, the drug was combined with table salt (used for cooking and seasoning food) and distributed as "chloroquinized salt" for daily use. A range of approaches for mass treatment of malaria have been tried at various times in African, Asian, and South American countries. These interventions were often followed by a decrease in cases and then a reappearance of infections unless control measures were sustained. Long-term benefit was most often seen on small islands and highland areas. The massive and wide use of antimalarials in some of these campaigns probably contributed to the increase in resistance of the malaria parasite to antimalarials, now a serious global problem. Most drugs regularly used to treat the malaria parasite do not have antibacterial activity and so are unlikely to contribute to the development of antibiotic resistance. There are two exceptions. Tetracyclines and sulfadoxine and other sulfonamides have been used to treat malaria and are also used to treat bacterial infections. Some of the general principles about mass treatment and impact on bacteria and parasite populations are relevant.

Drugs used in mass treatment campaigns must have a good safety profile. One potential problem with mass drug treatment programs is the administration of drug to people who may be allergic or have other reasons (such as being pregnant) they should not receive a drug. Many drugs are unsafe to use during pregnancy. For some drugs studies have never been done to show whether or not they are safe to use in pregnant women.

Today targeted mass drug administration programs are actively being used to try to eliminate five different diseases that are so-called neglected tropical diseases. These infections are present in poor, often rural populations, often in tropical regions, and cause chronic disease and disfigurement and prevent people from working and functioning normally. The five that are targeted by a global network are lymphatic filariasis, schistosomiasis, onchocerciasis, soil-transmitted helminths (like hookworm and ascaris), and trachoma. Safe and effective treatments are available for all. Drug companies have donated billions of dollars' worth of drugs to be distributed through programs that focus on populations most affected by these diseases. These drugs include the antibiotic azithromycin from Pfizer and the antiparasitic drugs ivermectin from Merck, albendazole from GlaxoSmithKline, and mebendazole from Johnson and Johnson. Eisai has contributed diethylcarbamazine (DEC), and praziquantel is available free through a donation from Merck Serono to the World Health Organization (WHO).

All of these infections except trachoma are worm (helminth) infections. Trachoma is caused by a strain of *Chlamydia trachomatis* that infects the eyes and is spread from person to person. It is often spread by direct contact, flies, or shared towels or other items in areas with poor hygiene and poor access to handwashing. It causes acute infection of the eyes that can become chronic and can be associated with scarring and ultimately can lead to blindness. Because it is a bacterial infection, it can be treated with antibiotics and can be cured. Many different agents, both topical (applied directly to the eyes) and systemic (taken by mouth and reaching tissues throughout the body), have been tried over decades, and several are effective. An antibiotic that is highly effective is the well-known macrolide antibiotic azithromycin. Because its activity lasts for days, it is effective when given as a single dose. Its other virtues are that it can be used in children as young as 6 months of age and is safe to use in pregnancy, which means women of childbearing age do not have to be excluded from treatment or tested for pregnancy before being treated. The drug is well tolerated. The pharmaceutical company Pfizer has donated the drug, making it available for mass treatment programs in low-income countries. More than 600 million doses of azithromycin have been distributed—85 million in 2016 alone.

Trachoma is not the only chlamydial infection in humans. Other related infections caused by *Chlamydiae* are the serotypes of *Chlamydia trachomatis* that cause genital infections in women and men; *Chlamydophila pneumoniae*, a cause of pneumonia; and *Chlamydia psittaci*, which infects birds and can also cause pneumonia (psittacosis) in humans.

Another bacterial infection that has been targeted for mass treatment campaigns is yaws, an infection that many people have never heard of. Yaws is a chronic infection caused by a bacterium (*Treponema pallidum* subspecies *pertenue*) genetically closely related to syphilis. It is transmitted by direct contact with contagious skin lesions (bumps and ulcers of skin) of an infected person. It can cause a chronic, disfiguring, painful infection. It primarily affects children in rural tropical areas where high humidity and poverty and poor hygiene make it easy for transmission from person to person to occur.

Decades ago, penicillin treatment given by injection was used widely to eliminate yaws from entire populations. This effort was promoted by the WHO and the United Nations Children's Fund from 1952 to 1964 in an attempt to eliminate the disease in 46 countries. Although these mass drug treatment campaigns did not succeed in eliminating yaws, they did reduce the number of active cases in the world by 95%. The main reason they did not succeed was because of the presence of latent yaws, infection that did not cause obvious signs or symptoms at the time of treatment. Today yaws persists in at least 13 countries in Africa, Southeast Asia, and the Western Pacific region. It remains endemic in countries home to 89 million people.

The availability of new drug strategies has renewed interest in trying to eliminate yaws. The current approach supported by the WHO includes mass administration of azithromycin followed by targeted treatment of people who have been missed or have persistent infection. Recently a study assessed how well this worked by doing follow-up evaluation 42 months after mass treatment (Mitja 2018). On an island in Papua New Guinea with a population of about 16,000, mass treatment with azithromycin reached 84% of the population and reduced the percentage of people with active yaws from almost 2 in 100 to only 1 in 1,000. However, they observed that by 2.5 years after the mass treatment, they started to see an increase in infections. Many of the newly identified active cases were in residents who missed being treated when the mass therapy was given. The researchers concluded that to be effective in eliminating yaws, the mass treatment programs would have to reach at least 90% of the population—a goal difficult to achieve—and that a second or third round of the antibiotic might also be necessary.

They also identified another worrisome finding. Some of the newly recognized active cases during late follow-up were studied in detail, and bacteria causing yaws were found to have mutations in their ribosomal RNA genes that made them resistant to azithromycin. Several of those with resistance had contact with each other, suggesting that the resistant bacteria were able to spread from person to person. This means that any mass treatment campaigns will need to be accompanied by clinical surveillance and laboratory support to detect drug resistance, and those with resistant bacteria treated with an alternative, effective drug before resistance spreads. These are sobering findings. This again underscores the complexities and consequences of antibiotic treatments in biological systems. Mass antibiotic treatment campaigns can select for resistance among the targeted bacteria (*Treponema pallidum* subspecies *pertenue* in this case), as well as among the normal resident bacteria in the host.

What are the consequences of mass treatment with antibiotics?

Several years ago investigators noticed that childhood deaths seemed to drop after they carried out mass treatment for trachoma with azithromycin in Ethiopia. Could azithromycin be saving lives of young children in poor areas? This led them to conduct a massive study in more than 1,500 communities (almost 200,000 children) in Malawi, Niger, and Tanzania. Clusters of healthy children 1 month to 5 years of age were randomly assigned to receive one dose of azithromycin or placebo (dummy pill) every 6 months for 2 years. The investigators counted the rates of death in the children who had received antibiotics and compared them with those in the children who had received placebo pills. The results were published in 2018 (Keenan NEJM 2018). They found that deaths were 13.5% lower in communities that received azithromycin than in those that received placebo. The benefit varied by country, ranging from 3.4% lower in Tanzania to 18.1% lower in Niger. Niger is a country with one of the highest child death rates in the world (about 90 children out of every 1,000 die before 5 years of age). The greatest benefit by age was seen in those aged 1 to 5 months, where azithromycin prevented almost a quarter of the deaths. This is also the age group with the highest rate of death in general. Researchers were unable to determine whether any serious adverse event was caused by azithromycin. The study was not set up to investigate how the drug decreased deaths in children. The authors' hypothesis was that the antibiotic may have reduced respiratory infections, diarrhea, and malaria—major killers in these tropical, low-income populations. Azithromycin is active against many bacteria that cause respiratory infections and diarrhea and has been shown in earlier studies to even have some activity against malaria parasites, especially when used with another drug. It has slow but potent activity against the *Plasmodium falciparum* apicoplast, an organelle essential for the malaria parasite's survival.

The results of this study have generated excitement and intense debate. Is it ethical not to provide a well-tolerated, relatively inexpensive intervention today that could save millions of lives in poor countries? It has been estimated that 15,000 children die each day, many from preventable diarrhea and pneumonia, and most of them in low-income countries. At the same time, should one use a treatment that will contribute to the development of antibiotic resistance that will affect future generations—and may make many infections, not just those in childhood and not just those in poor countries, untreatable with these antibiotics in the future? Azithromycin is already widely used today to treat many different kinds of infections and is one of the few remaining options for treating the sexually transmitted infection gonorrhea. Does one save lives today or save effective treatment for the future? One must also ask, if azithromycin is routinely administered to children in low-income countries, how long will it remain effective? Provision of clean water, sanitary facilities, and good nutrition would likely do as much good as or more good than providing widespread antibiotics—but providing clean water and sanitary facilities takes a lot longer to put in place and is expensive. The difference in results by country studied suggested that the lower the current childhood mortality is in the country, the less the benefit from the antibiotic.

Azithromycin cannot be a long-term solution, but many argue in favor of using this intervention as a stopgap measure to save children's lives today while continuing to work on clean water, improved sanitation, and nutrition.

But how much do we really know about the consequences of mass treatment with antibiotics? Of concern are the bacteria being targeted, but also other resident bacteria that can potentially cause serious infections. Some studies have tried to answer this question (Doan 2018; Keenan CID 2018; Skalet 2010). After a total of 130 children with trachoma and their household contacts who were children received a single dose of azithromycin, some of the children had nasopharyngeal (nose and throat) cultures to look for resistant *Streptococcus pneumoniae* up to 6 months after the antibiotic treatment. Before treatment less than 2% carried resistant strains of *S. pneumoniae*. This increased to more than half 2 to 3 weeks after treatment. At 6 months after the single dose it was almost 6% and still higher than baseline (Leach 1997). Another study in Ethiopia involving 12 communities of children who received treatment of azithromycin for trachoma control also found that resistant nasopharyngeal (nose and throat) *S. pneumoniae* increased (Skalet 2010). In children who received azithromycin, resistance increased from 3.6% at baseline to almost half of children at month 12. In a control community that did not receive azithromycin, azithromycin resistance was 9.2% at month 12.

Other recently published studies assessed the effect on resistance of different frequencies of mass treatment for trachoma control. One study that looked at this systematically compared communities that had received mass treatment with azithromycin, a macrolide. Twelve communities received mass treatment once a year, and another 12 communities were treated twice a year. Before the communities received mass treatment the level of macrolide resistance was 20%, and it was similar in those who received mass treatment once and twice annually. At 24 months the level of macrolide resistance was 60% in the communities that received treatment twice yearly versus 40% in the communities that received it once annually. This clearly showed a relationship between the frequency and amount of antibiotic consumption and the presence of resistance.

How are antibiotics used in the human population? Who receives them?

In most higher-income countries at least 80% of antibiotic use is in outpatients and about 20% is in hospitals and other health care facilities. Dentists prescribe 3% to 10% of antibiotics used. In the United States, outside of hospitals, prescriptions for antibiotics are given by physicians, physician assistants, dentists, and nurse practitioners. An expanding type of medical consultation in the United States today is the use of direct-to-consumer telemedicine. These consultations frequently result in antibiotic prescriptions. No current data are available to show what portion of antibiotic use comes from these interactions. Many countries do not require a prescription for antibiotics, which can be obtained at local pharmacies or elsewhere (Auta 2018).

Today only about 60% of outpatient antibiotic prescriptions are written in medical offices and emergency departments because of the growing use of urgent care centers, retail clinics, and other alternative sites. A study of antibiotic use in outpatient adults younger than 65 years in 2014 found that antibiotics were prescribed for almost 40% of 2.7 million urgent care visits and 36% of retail clinic visits. These percentages were substantially higher than the percentage of patients receiving antibiotics during emergency department visits (about 14% of 4.8 million visits) and medical office visits (7% of almost 150 million visits). This study found that inappropriate prescribing for respiratory infections was highest in urgent care centers (almost 46%) (Palms 2018).

In the United States 50% to 60% of hospitalized patients receive an antibiotic at some point during a hospital stay. In the United States during the years 2006 to 2012 about 55% of all patients received at least one dose of antibiotic during a hospital stay (Baggs 2016). The overall days of antibiotic treatment were estimated to be 755 per 1,000 patient-days. From 2006 to 2012, there was a significant increase in use of broader-spectrum antibiotics and a decrease in the use of fluoroquinolones, like ciprofloxacin. The United States uses more broad-spectrum antibiotics in hospitalized patients than the United Kingdom does. About 50% of inpatient antibiotic use is for lower respiratory tract infections, like pneumonia. In the United States there has been a trend toward use of more broad-spectrum antibiotics and fewer narrow-spectrum antibiotics, like penicillin.

What are the main reasons that antibiotics are prescribed?

Many studies give snapshots of antibiotic use during different years and in different settings.

About half of antibiotics used in humans in the United States are for respiratory infections. Acute respiratory conditions include ear infections, sinusitis, pharyngitis (sore throat), viral upper respiratory infection, asthma and allergy, bronchitis, influenza, and viral and nonviral pneumonia. In one large study the most common specific reason for an antibiotic being prescribed in the United States was sinus infection. About half of prescriptions given for respiratory tract infections are considered to be inappropriate (Fleming-Dutra 2016). Most of these are caused by viral infections, for which antibiotics do not work.

In the ambulatory setting children under the age of 2 years are the most likely to receive antibiotics (>1,000 prescriptions per 1,000 population per year), and those aged 20 to 39 years old are the least likely to be given prescriptions. It has been estimated that a third or more of antibiotic use overall is inappropriate.

The second most common reason for antibiotic use is for diarrhea or gastrointestinal infections. These include infections caused by bacteria such as *Shigella, Salmonella,* and

Campylobacter but also many infections caused by viruses, such as rotavirus and norovirus. A smaller percentage in the United States are caused by parasites, such as *Giardia, Cryptosporidium,* and *Cyclospora.* Some of the bacterial infections will benefit from antibiotic treatment; the viral infections will not. A general estimate is that only about 25% of diarrhea episodes are caused by bacteria, but this varies greatly by geographic area, age, and level of sanitation.

Besides diarrhea, other common reasons for outpatient antibiotics are urinary tract infections and skin and soft tissue infections.

A study of outpatient antibiotic prescriptions over a 3-year period (2013–2015) in the United States found that the most commonly prescribed antibiotics were azithromycin, amoxicillin, amoxicillin/clavulanate, ciprofloxacin, and cephalexin (Durkin 2018). During the 3-year period studied, the researchers found no change in the overall prescribing level despite many recent efforts to reduce inappropriate antibiotic prescribing through educational and other programs. The number of prescriptions per 1,000 persons per year was 826. This means that on average, more than 8 of every 10 people received an antibiotic prescription during a 1-year period, but antibiotic use is not evenly distributed in a population and a small proportion may receive the majority of the repeat courses. It is notable that antibiotic use has clear seasonal peaks that correspond with peak influenza season. In one study, for example, antibiotics were 42% more likely to be prescribed during February than September. Most of the increase likely reflected antibiotics given for viral respiratory infections.

Why is antibiotic use so common for respiratory infections?

There are many reasons. People are sick and know they have an infection and hope that an antibiotic will help them feel better faster. Many people do not distinguish between viruses and bacteria. Rapid, accurate, inexpensive tests to distinguish between a viral infection and a bacterial infection are generally not available, especially for individuals who do not have severe illness, so treatment is given without a specific diagnosis. Tests are widely available to diagnose influenza, one of the viruses that causes respiratory infections, but are not routinely available for most of the other viruses (except in research and academic institutions).

Another reason antibiotics are prescribed is that patients request them. It is faster for a health care provider to write a prescription for an antibiotic than to explain the reasons that it is probably unnecessary and potentially harmful to take an antibiotic. A recent study of more than 13,000 telemedicine consultations for respiratory infections found that visits were shorter when patients were given an antibiotic prescription. Antibiotics were prescribed in two-thirds of the visits. Another study found that physicians were more likely to prescribe an antibiotic for an inappropriate reason during the end of a clinic session than during the first hour, reflecting decision fatigue. Patients are generally more satisfied with the health provider (i.e., rate the provider higher) if they receive a prescription for an antibiotic instead of being advised how to manage without one (Martinez 2018). Taking an antibiotic gives the patient the impression that something active is being done.

There may be financial incentives to prescribing antibiotics in some settings. In China, at least in the past, health providers have gotten a large portion of their income from selling antibiotics to patients, so there was an economic incentive for doctors to prescribe antibiotics.

In countries where prescriptions are not required for antibiotics, community use of antibiotics for fevers and other illnesses is common. A study in Manilla (the Philippines) in a low-income population found that among patients visiting an emergency room for fever, about 40% had already taken an antibiotic before the visit. In this patient population the most frequent cause of fever was dengue fever (a viral infection) followed by other viral infections including measles, mumps, and rubella, for which antibiotics are unnecessary and inappropriate.

Does antibiotic use vary by region or by country?

Globally vast differences exist in amounts of antibiotics used by a country, a region, or a specific population. In some countries more than 40% of the population on average receives an antibiotic prescription each year. In other countries it is less than 20%. There are also regional differences, including within the United States (Hicks 2015). The Centers for Disease Control and Prevention (CDC) website shows a map that displays community antibiotic prescriptions per 1,000 population by state for 2015. These range from more than 1,000 prescriptions per 1,000 population for some states in the Southeast to less than half that in some states in the western United States. Differences in antibiotic use can reflect differences in the number and types of infections from one population to another—the burden from infectious diseases. Some populations need more antibiotics because they have more infections. Differences in use can also reflect differences in access to antibiotics. Some populations use antibiotics less often because they cannot afford antibiotics or gain access to them. There are also marked differences in prescribing habits and guidelines.

Globally with antibiotics we are simultaneously dealing with the issues of excess (inappropriate) use in some areas and lack of access in other populations. Ramanan Laxminarayan, who heads the Center for Disease Dynamics, Economics and Policy, and others have highlighted the need to find a better balance between access to antibiotics and excess use (Laxminarayan 2016; Mendelson 2016).

Residents of low- and middle-income countries have a much higher burden from infectious diseases and much less access to antibiotics than residents of high-income countries. Globally the infectious diseases on the list of the top 10 killers include lower respiratory tract infections (fourth), diarrhea (eighth), and tuberculosis (ninth). In the WHO African region, however, infections are responsible for 5 of the top 10 causes of death, including the top 3 (lower respiratory tract infections, HIV/AIDS, and diarrhea). In Europe and the Americas, lower respiratory infections are the only infectious disease category in the top 10 causes of death.

While excess antibiotic use is a major problem, especially in high-income countries, lack of access to antibiotics is a major problem in many low-income countries—or in poor populations in many countries. Although antibiotics are relatively cheap as far as pharmaceuticals go, the price of the drugs or the visit to a clinic may exceed what some can afford. It is estimated that many die because of lack of access to antibiotics to treat infections that could be cured with antibiotics. In some areas, the only antibiotics available—the older, cheaper ones—may no longer work because the bacteria have become resistant to them. According to the WHO, fewer than half of children in low-income countries with symptoms of pneumonia are taken to an appropriate health care provider. Children in sub-Saharan Africa are over 15 times more likely to die before age 5 than children in high-income countries, and at least half of these deaths are due to preventable or treatable infections.

An analysis of community-acquired pneumonia across 101 countries in children younger than 5 years of age found that an estimated 445,000 deaths could be averted if antibiotics were available to all (Laxminarayan 2016). This would be a 75% reduction in deaths from pneumonia. Another approach, scaling up the use of currently available vaccines to prevent pneumonia and respiratory infections (pneumococcal and Hib vaccines, for example), could decrease by almost 50% the number of days on antibiotics.

In the United States chronic diseases like heart disease, lung disease, stroke, Alzheimer's disease, and diabetes mellitus are now the biggest killers. Injury, suicide, and, increasingly, drug overdoses are also major killers (US burden of disease collaborators 2018). The leading infectious disease cause of death in the United States in 2014 was lower respiratory tract infections (like pneumonia). These infections accounted for more than three-quarters of the deaths from infectious diseases in the United States (Bcheraoui 2018). Between 2000 and 2014 in the United States, the only infectious disease that increased in mortality was diarrhea, which accounted for about 7% of overall deaths. The increase was probably related to increases in deaths from *Clostridioides difficile* infections (see discussion of *C. difficile* in Chapter 3). Deaths from *C. difficile* in the United States increased almost fivefold between 2000 and 2014. *C. difficile* is now the leading cause of deaths from gastroenteritis in the United States, responsible for almost half (48%) of these deaths and 83% of gastroenteritis deaths in those 65 years and older. *C. difficile* infections are largely a consequence of antibiotic use.

In a study that analyzed deaths from infectious diseases within the United States by individual county, striking geographic differences were clear (Bcheraoui 2018). Some reasons for differences include poverty, air pollution, access to medical care, and use of opioids. Use of potent, long-acting, high-dose opioids increases the risk of serious pneumococcal pneumonia (Wiese 2018) and several other bacterial infections, including bacterial endocarditis. These may be contributing to an increase in deaths from infectious diseases in some regions in the United States.

As noted previously, there are also regional differences in antibiotic use within the United States. Rates of antibiotic use are much higher in the United States than in many other countries. For comparison, Sweden dispensed 328 courses of antibiotics per 1,000 population in 2014 (vs. >1,000 per 1,000 population in some regions of the United States in 2015).

Is antibiotic use increasing or decreasing?

Global use of antibiotics is increasing. High-income countries generally have the highest levels of antibiotic usage, but rates of use are increasing most rapidly in some low- and middle-income countries. Between 2000 and 2015, global consumption of antibiotics in humans increased 39% despite all of the publicity about excess use.

Researchers analyzed consumption of antibiotics with pharmaceutical sales data for 76 countries between 2000 and 2015 and found a 65% increase in a measure called defined daily doses (DDDs) and a 39% increase in the rate of consumption—the number of doses per 1,000 people per day (Klein 2018). Most of the increase in antibiotic consumption between 2000 and 2015 was in low- and middle-income countries. Increasing use in these countries was correlated with economic status (gross domestic product per capita growth): more money, more antibiotics. The countries with the highest increase in consumption (as measured by DDDs) between 2000 and 2015 were India, where consumption almost doubled, and China, where consumption increased more than 50%. Because of the size of these countries, their contribution to overall global antibiotic use is large.

The level of consumption in high-income countries increased only 4% (and decreased in a few), but the level of use in high-income countries was already substantially higher than in most low- and middle-income countries, where the burden from infectious diseases is much higher than in high-income countries. There was also an increase in use of the so-called last-resort antibiotics—those used when all other drugs fail, presumably reflecting the increasing rates of antibiotic-resistant bacteria. These are drugs such as glycylcyclines (like tigecycline), oxazolidinones (like linezolid), carbapenems (like meropenem), and polymyxins (like colistin). Most of these are on the WHO "reserve" list of antibiotics and are unavailable or unaffordable in many areas. Globally there are an estimated 214,000 deaths from infections in young infants each year caused by bacteria resistant to first-line antibiotics where alternatives are unavailable.

In 2015 the leading consumers of antibiotics among high-income countries were the United States, France, and Italy; the leading consumers among low- and middle-income countries (LMICs) were India, China, and Pakistan. Between 2000 and 2015 the antibiotic consumption rate (DDDs) of antibiotics per 1,000 population increased from 8.2 to 13.6 in India, from 5.1 to 8.4 in China, and from 16.2 to 19.6 in Pakistan. These are still substantially lower than rates in high-income countries, where the antibiotic consumption rate decreased slightly between 2000 and 2015 (27.0 to 25.7 DDDs per 1,000 inhabitants per day), versus an increase of 8.6 to 13.9 per 1,000 inhabitants in lower- and middle-income countries.

Given the burden from infections in LMICs and increased access to antibiotics, these data suggest that global antibiotic use will continue to increase in the absence of changes in policy. A 15% increase in global consumption of antibiotics has been projected for the period 2015 to 2030 (Klein 2018). LMICs account for about 85% of the global population. Even modest increases in antibiotic use by these populations will have a major impact on global consumption.

The summary of the analysis masks important details. Some high-income countries, such as the Netherlands, Japan, Sweden, and Norway, have low rates of antibiotic consumption, low rates of infections, and low mortality from infectious diseases. They can serve as models to show that good health care and good health can be achieved with substantially lower use of antibiotics than in many high-income countries (Klein 2018). The United Kingdom with its active program around antibiotic use was able to show a 13% drop in antibiotic prescribing in primary care settings between 2013 and 2017.

How much is spent on antibiotics?

Antibiotics are big business. In 2009 expenditures for antibiotics for humans totaled $10.7 billion. A review of expenditures in the United States by class of antibiotic and health care setting from 2010 to 2015 found that expenditures had actually decreased from $10.6 billion in 2010 to $8.8 billion in 2015, but this was not necessarily related to reduced use of antibiotics (Suda 2018). Shifts had occurred with increasing use of intravenous antibiotics in the community. Over the 6-year period, antibiotic expenditures for human use totaled $56 billion, almost 60% of which was related to use of antibiotics in the outpatient setting. The top expenditures for antibiotics overall during 2010 to 2015 were for doxycycline, daptomycin, and linezolid—the latter two are expensive, newer antibiotics. An analysis in 2009 found that quinolones were the top antibiotic class by expenditure but they had decreased by 91% during the study period, probably because levofloxacin and moxifloxacin had come off patent and generic versions became available at low cost. A major increase in expenditures for the tetracycline class was probably not related to a major change in usage but rather issues related to manufacturing doxycycline. Problems arose with manufacturing in January 2013, leading to limited availability and an increase in the wholesale cost of doxycycline. The production issues were resolved, but the high purchase costs persisted.

In 2015 the proportions of expenditures for each antibiotic class were as follows: tetracyclines (19.2%), penicillins (16%), cephalosporins (12.2%), macrolides (10.7%), oxazolidinones (6.9%), quinolones (2.3%) and miscellaneous, including daptomycin and vancomycin (21%). Expenditures for quinolones dropped from 21% of total expenditures in 2010 to just 2.3% in 2015. This probably reflects primarily a decreased price. These figures do not deal with the cost of development of new antibiotics. Drug development and clinical trials are extremely costly. This is discussed in chapter 8.

3

CONSEQUENCES OF USE

ADVERSE EVENTS ASSOCIATED WITH USE OF ANTIBIOTICS IN HUMANS

What is the difference between an allergic reaction and an adverse reaction? What are the signs and symptoms of an allergic reaction?

All allergic reactions to a drug are adverse drug reactions, but adverse drug reactions also include many other kinds of reactions. Every antibiotic can potentially have adverse consequences. Every decision to take an antibiotic should include weighing the risks and benefits. Because antibiotics are so familiar and common in our lives, we sometimes forget to consider the harmful side of the balance. Frequently comments are made such as: "We are not certain what is causing the problem, but antibiotics might help, and what harm could there be from them?" The answer is that there is always potential harm.

It is true that most antibiotics are pretty safe, but all can cause adverse reactions, though at varying rates. The antibiotics available today are much safer than the early crude products that were often contaminated with impurities. We also have the benefit of decades of experience with many of the antibiotics and so have learned more about the range of side effects, how to monitor for them, and how to identify the individuals who might be more likely to suffer serious reactions to specific drugs. Although drugs are tested extensively before they are approved by the US Food and Drug Administration (FDA) for general use, adverse events that occur only a few times in every million courses of the drug may not be linked to a drug until it has been taken by hundreds of thousands or millions of individuals. Adverse events that are distinctive and serious are more likely to be picked up than ones that resemble common symptoms, such as achiness, nausea, and headache.

Patients often do not take just a single antibiotic but may be taking multiple drugs simultaneously. If they develop a rash, is it caused by the antibiotic or another drug they are taking? Specific tests are usually not done or available to determine if a specific drug caused a specific reaction. More often conclusions are reached about the likely cause of an adverse event based on when the patient started taking the drug, the potential risk factors for an adverse event, and the drug's profile. Every drug (and antibiotic) has a profile that is based on the clinical trials that were done before the drug was approved for general use; this is expanded and refined as experience with the antibiotic accumulates. This drug information is communicated from pharmacists and in drug prescribing information, in educational sessions in hospitals and clinics, informally among clinicians, at professional meetings, in scientific publications, and occasionally via drug warnings or alerts or changes in the drug label or the full prescribing information available for each drug. Table 2.1 in the previous chapter shows the kinds of data available.

Drugs also develop reputations. A high-visibility adverse event—communicated through medical journals, the public media, or social media networks—can influence subsequent use of an antibiotic. These events can also drive decisions to do additional studies or to change recommendations about how the drug should be used.

Factors that influence the likelihood of an adverse drug reaction are many. These include genetics, age, sex, coexisting medical problems, other drugs taken simultaneously, dose, and duration. For example, a high percentage of patients who have infectious mononucleosis (a viral infection; antibiotics provide no benefit) who take ampicillin (or amoxicillin) will develop a rash. Patients who are taking allopurinol (a drug for gout) who take ampicillin are much more likely to develop a skin rash than if they were just taking ampicillin alone.

What is an adverse drug reaction? It is defined as a harmful reaction, an injury, or an unwanted or undesirable effect of taking the drug. Many people will have mild nausea, a queasy stomach, or stomach upset as a side effect from an antibiotic. The term *adverse drug event* or *reaction* typically refers to something that makes a person unwell and, in many instances, unable to continue taking the antibiotic or leads to a need to change the dose. Sometimes there is damage to tissues or organs. Adverse events range from trivial, self-limited events to irreversible and fatal effects. See Table 3.1 for examples of types of adverse drug reactions.

Table 3.1 Examples of Common and Serious Antibiotic Adverse Drug Reactions

Type of Reaction	Examples	Frequency and Outcome
Allergic, idiosyncratic	Anaphylaxis	Rare; can be fatal
	Severe cutaneous adverse reactions (includes Stevens-Johnson syndrome and toxic epidermal necrolysis [TEN]); can involve internal organs	Rare; can be fatal
	Skin rash	Common; usually self-limited
	Fever	Will disappear when drug is stopped
	Hematologic (low white blood cell counts, low platelets, anemia)	Usually reversible when antibiotic discontinued; could be irreversible with chloramphenicol, drug used in past

(continued)

Table 3.1 Continued

Type of Reaction	Examples	Frequency and Outcome
Toxic/ metabolic	Liver damage; liver failure	Rare; can be fatal
	Kidney damage	Often dose related; can be irreversible
	Ototoxicity; decreased hearing; vestibular injury	Can be irreversible
	Cardiac rhythm disturbances	Fatal arrhythmias; rare
	Tendinitis and tendon rupture	Achilles tendon rupture
	Peripheral neuropathy	May be irreversible
	Central nervous system effects, like depression, hallucinations, agitation	Usually reversible
	Exacerbation of muscle weakness in patients with myasthenia gravis	During antibiotic administration
	Alternations in blood glucose (high and low blood sugar)	During antibiotic administration; rarely lead to coma or death
	Damage to developing fetus	Range of abnormalities
	Staining of teeth (young children)	Children younger than 9 years taking tetracyclines
Microbiological	Selection of drug-resistant bacteria	Common; changes may persist after antibiotic stopped
	Clostridioides difficile colitis	Relatively common; can be severe, fatal
	Yeast infection	Common; usually superficial infection of mouth, vagina

It is useful to think of adverse reactions related to antibiotics in three big categories. Not all adverse events fit neatly into one box, and some reactions have elements of more than one. An individual drug can often cause more than one kind of adverse event.

The first category is allergic or hypersensitivity reactions. These can be unpredictable (with what we know today), are often unrelated to the dose or amount of drug taken, and can range from trivial to fatal (see Table 3.1 and discussion). The second category is toxic and metabolic reactions. Antibiotics can damage a person's tissues and vital organs and their function. This includes damage to the kidneys, liver, lungs, tendons, and other organs and tissues. Some antibiotics affect hearing and balance. Sometimes the damage is irreversible, for example, some of the damage to the kidneys and hearing. Damage to the liver can be fatal—or require liver transplantation for survival. Some of these toxic and metabolic adverse reactions may be related to the level of the drug in the body. Some antibiotics affect the heart conduction system, causing irregular heart rhythm. Others can affect the level of blood sugar. Still others can cross the placenta and cause tissue damage or mutations that affect the developing fetus or can stain the developing bones and teeth of the fetus. Some can target the bone marrow and affect production or release of white blood cells, platelets, or red blood cells. The third category relates to the impact antibiotics have because they kill or slow the growth of bacteria. This can cause immediate or long-term consequences. Each of these will be discussed in more detail.

Allergies are one type of adverse reaction to an antibiotic. Allergic reactions can manifest in many different ways, including a skin rash, blisters, hives, itchiness, and wheezing. Its most severe form, anaphylaxis, can be fatal if immediate treatment is not provided. Anaphylaxis is a manifestation of severe hypersensitivity to a drug or other agent (like a vaccine, a bee sting, or food, such as peanuts). It is not related to the dose or number of doses of a drug. A single (even a first) dose can provoke an anaphylactic reaction. It is treated with epinephrine and medical support and can be completely reversible with prompt treatment—but can be fatal if treatment is delayed.

Other severe hypersensitivity reactions can take longer to develop but can affect the skin, mucous membranes (like the eyes and mouth), and internal organs. These are rare but can also sometimes be fatal. These include severe reactions called Stevens-Johnson syndrome and toxic epidermal necrolysis. If a patient survives one of these reactions, he or she should never again be given the antibiotic that caused it.

Many of the antibiotics that can damage the kidneys and affect hearing and balance can be used safely if the blood and tissue levels of the antibiotics are not too high. However, there is often a fine line between the amount of the antibiotic required to kill the bacteria causing the infection and the amount that will damage the patient's tissues and organs. This is true of the commonly used antibiotic vancomycin and the class of antibiotics called aminoglycosides (which includes streptomycin, gentamicin, tobramycin, and others). Often doctors will measure the levels of these drugs in the patient's blood to give enough antibiotic to kill the bacteria but not enough to damage the patient's tissues.

Reactions can be related to the antibiotic's bacterial killing properties or to other properties of the drug. There can also be adverse events related to the administration of the drug, with the development of inflammation of the vein (phlebitis) or clotting (thrombosis) related to intravenous administration. Some drugs are irritating to tissues as they are being infused.

One unusual type of adverse event has been named Jarisch-Herxheimer after the European dermatologist who first described it more than a century ago. He observed that patients with syphilis, which can cause a skin rash, developed worsening of skin rashes after treatment with mercury, one of the ways of treating syphilis before antibiotics were available. A similar kind of reaction was observed in the 1940s when penicillin became the drug of choice for treating syphilis. The reaction occurs in the first 24 hours after receiving treatment for infections such as syphilis, Lyme disease, leptospirosis, or relapsing fever. This reaction is precipitated by the rapid killing of spirochetes (a type of bacteria) and the release of toxic substances, like lipoproteins, from the bacteria that cause fever, chills, muscle aches, sometimes low blood pressure, skin rash, and other findings. It is mediated through substances, like tumor necrosis factor (called cytokines), that provoke inflammatory responses. Patients are not reacting to the antibiotic per se but to substances released because of the action of the antibiotic on the bacteria. It is typically self-limited, though fatalities have been reported, especially in young infants.

Other unusual effects of antibiotics are also related to their role in killing the targeted bacteria. Infections of the gut with toxin-producing bacteria (like Shiga toxin–producing *Escherichia coli* O157) can cause bloody diarrhea. It is sometimes complicated by development of a severe illness called hemolytic-uremic syndrome (HUS), which can be fatal. People pick up the infection by eating contaminated food (e.g., contaminated hamburgers, fresh produce). As a general rule, treating infections with antibiotics is a good idea. In infections caused by *E. coli* O157, however, use of certain antibiotics may lead to a worse outcome—with more patients developing the complication of HUS. Some antibiotics may actually increase the production and release of toxins from the bacteria.

How common are adverse reactions?

Adverse events related to antibiotics are common. Researchers at Johns Hopkins retrospectively analyzed records from hospitalized patients to find out how many had adverse events related to antibiotics (Tamma 2017). They examined records for 30 days after hospitalization for most adverse events but also checked up to 90 days after hospitalization for the development of *Clostridiodes difficile* colitis or infection with multidrug-resistant bacteria. They included only patients who had received systemic antibiotics for at least 24 hours and excluded patients who only received preventive antibiotics, tuberculosis drugs, and topical agents. They found that 20% of those receiving an antibiotic had an adverse event. The most common adverse events were gastrointestinal (42%), kidney (24%), and hematologic (or affecting the bone marrow; 15%). Every additional 10 days of antibiotic therapy led to a 3% increased risk of an adverse event.

The most frequently prescribed antibiotics in these hospitalized patients were third-generation cephalosporins (41%), intravenous vancomycin (28%), and cefepime (28%). In this study 78% of patients received at least one antibiotic during hospitalization (other studies have found that at least half of hospitalized patients receive at least one antibiotic). More than a quarter (27%) of the adverse events occurred after patients were discharged from the hospital. Among patients with *C. difficile* infections, 20% occurred after discharge. The highest rates of damage to the kidneys resulted from intravenous vancomycin and trimethoprim-sulfamethoxazole. Patients who experienced an antibiotic-associated adverse event also ended up with longer hospital stays.

Some of the studies that have assessed adverse reactions have also asked the question: Were there good reasons for giving the antibiotic in the first place? One study found that 40% of days when hospitalized patients were receiving fluoroquinolones were days when the antibiotic was unnecessary. This agrees with many other studies that have documented high rates of unnecessary and inappropriate use of antibiotics in hospitalized patients. An analysis of emergency room visits for adverse drug reactions found that 19% were related to use of antibiotics.

About 10% to 25% of hospitalized patients report an allergy to the group of drugs called beta-lactam antibiotics (Blumenthal 2018). This class includes the commonly used penicillin, amoxicillin, and the cephalosporins. Closer scrutiny or testing frequently shows that many who are labeled allergic are not truly allergic and can still receive a beta-lactam antibiotic. More attention is being paid to a careful review of patients who report a history of an allergy as part of antibiotic stewardship programs. Antibiotic alternatives to the beta-lactam antibiotics may be less effective, more toxic, more expensive, less accessible, and excessively broad spectrum. See chapter 8.

The consequences of being allergic to an antibiotic can be serious if one has a severe infection and few treatment choices are available. For some infections one or two classes of antibiotics are far superior to others. If one cannot use them because of a severe allergy, it may be difficult to provide effective treatment. It is always important to distinguish between a real and severe allergy that would preclude use of a particular drug in the future and some side effect that was annoying—or that was completely unrelated to the antibiotic.

How much antibiotic does it take to cause an adverse reaction?

Some toxic and metabolic reactions are dose related; many are not. Even one dose, including a first dose, can cause an allergic reaction. The range of potential reactions is broad and can include virtually any organ system or tissue, including the heart, brain, nervous system, lungs, muscles, tendons, eyes, blood vessels, and pancreas—as well as the more commonly observed reactions involving the kidneys, liver, blood cells/bone marrow, and skin. See Table 3.1.

Do genetic factors influence drug reactions?

Genetic factors clearly affect the likelihood of developing adverse reactions to some drugs. One mechanism is through breakdown and elimination of the drug. Some people have a genetic makeup and molecular machinery that only slowly breaks down and eliminates a drug, allowing the buildup of levels that may be more likely to cause adverse effects. Other people may have enzymes that break down a drug more rapidly, leading to low levels that may be ineffective.

One of the best-known genetic factors that affects interactions with some drugs relates to the enzyme glucose-6-phosphate dehydrogenase, or G6PD. G6PD is an enzyme in red blood cells that protects them from certain types of injury and breakdown. People who have low levels of G6PD, which is inherited, are prone to having their red blood cells break down (hemolysis), which can cause anemia. This is genetically determined and much more common in some populations than others. It is estimated to affect 400 million people worldwide and is more common in populations living in tropical and subtropical areas. Some sulfa drugs can cause problems in patients who have a deficiency of the enzyme. Some drugs used to treat and prevent malaria can also be unsafe to use in people who have inherited a low level of this enzyme. Before patients are given malaria drugs (like primaquine and a recently released drug tafenoquine), they must have a blood test to check levels of this enzyme. Individuals with severe deficiency are at risk for massive breakdown of red blood cells (a severe reaction that can be fatal) if they are exposed to these drugs.

It has been observed that patients with certain human leukocyte antigen (HLA) types are more likely to have serious adverse reactions to some drugs. This is also determined genetically. This has been most clear cut with abacavir, a drug used to treat HIV-infected individuals. The drug is safe in most individuals, but people who carry the HLA-B*5701 allele, which is genetically determined, are at increased risk for developing severe and sometimes fatal hypersensitivity reactions to abacavir. The FDA-approved drug prescribing information recommends screening people who might be prescribed abacavir for HLA-B*5701 and using the drug only in those who are negative for this genetic marker. This marker does not identify everyone who might have an adverse reaction, but it does find most of them.

A whole area of study called pharmacogenomics has developed in an attempt to better understand the genetic basis for different responses to drugs. This includes identifying individual differences in the metabolism of drugs (which may influence how well they work) but also the likelihood of severe adverse reactions. So far tools are not available to test patients before the administration of most antibiotics to identify that small subset of people who might be at risk for severe adverse reactions. This is a worthy goal for the future.

What are drug-drug interactions?

Antibiotics can potentially interact with other drugs a patient is taking, so it is always important to review all drugs that a person is taking before prescribing a course of antibiotics. Interactions with another drug can affect absorption from the stomach or upper bowel, can speed up or slow down the breakdown of the drug (leading to levels that are too high or too low), and can affect how rapidly the drug is eliminated by the kidneys. Presence of other drugs can make a patient more susceptible to some types of adverse side effects. Even nonprescription drugs or something as simple as antacids can affect absorption and drug levels. Fortunately there are now web-based programs that can allow pharmacists and others to quickly identify potential drug-drug interactions.

Does exposure to the sun make one more likely to have a reaction to an antibiotic?

Some antibiotics make a person more sensitive to the sun. Even with limited exposure to sunlight, a person on some antibiotics may develop redness of the skin. It is not an allergic reaction. The antibiotics most likely to cause sun sensitivity are the tetracyclines, quinolones (like ciprofloxacin), and sulfonamides. People taking these antibiotics should be advised to avoid sun exposure and to wear protective clothing when in the sun.

Why have side effects from ciprofloxacin (and other fluoroquinolones) gotten so much attention?

One group of antibiotics, the fluoroquinolones (like ciprofloxacin), have been used extensively because they are active against a relatively wide spectrum of bacteria, can be taken orally, and are well absorbed into the blood. This means blood and tissue levels are high enough to treat many serious infections. Because of their ease of use and apparently good tolerability, they have gained wide acceptance in the treatment of infections ranging from typhoid fever and osteomyelitis (bone infection) to pneumonia and urinary tract infections. In 2001 ciprofloxacin was the drug recommended in the United States for people potentially exposed to anthrax letters (a 60-day course was recommended). In 2015 in the United States, 32 million prescriptions for these drugs were written.

The fluoroquinolones kill bacteria by inhibiting part of the DNA cell machinery (DNA gyrase) and may have broad effects on other cells. With wide use has come growing recognition of adverse events—with Facebook and other groups discussing them on websites. Some call reactions to them being "floxed." Websites such as the Quinolone Antibiotics Adverse Reaction Forum, which has hosted thousands of posts, have played a role. Apparently by the end of 2015 the FDA had received reports from more than 60,000 patients describing adverse events associated with ciprofloxacin. This is much higher than reports of adverse events associated with most antibiotics.

One unusual adverse event associated with taking a fluoroquinolone is tendinitis (inflammation of a tendon), which can weaken the tendon (like the Achilles tendon) and predispose it to rupture. The FDA has announced a series of strong alerts about side effects of fluoroquinolones, including tendon rupture in 2008 and irreversible nerve damage in 2013. In 2016 the FDA recommended that the drugs be used only for serious infections because of concern about a potentially permanent syndrome called fluoroquinolone-associated disability. Some scientists are concerned that fluoroquinolones might be damaging mitochondria, the energy packs inside cells that evolved from bacteria-like cells billions of years ago. They have support for this from a laboratory assay that detects mitochondrial damage in cells. Other scientists have looked for a genetic reason for this toxic effect, which seems to occur in just a small percentage of recipients. A genetic mutation might be associated with poor metabolism of quinolones, allowing the drug to accumulate in cells.

Most doctors who are familiar with the fluoroquinolones (FQs) now agree that FQs should not be prescribed for minor infections, but this message has not effectively reached the broader community in the United States. However, prescriptions did drop about 10% in the United States in 2016 and may have dropped again in 2017. (See section about restrictions on use and black-box warnings in chapter 1.)

Recent studies have linked another adverse event to FQs: a type of kidney disease called acute interstitial nephritis. In one series the kidney disease was severe enough to require dialysis in about a quarter of the patients. Kidney function did not return to baseline in a quarter of patients. The patients with the kidney complications associated with FQ use had other findings that suggested a possible allergic reaction, like rash, fever, and eosinophils (a type of cell associated with allergic reactions) in the blood and the urine.

Large databases, for example, through health care and insurance organizations, are now available that have made it possible to assess data for rare events that may be linked to certain antibiotics and other drugs. A nationwide study in France that included almost 28,000 patients who had recent surgery for retinal detachment (where the retina of the eye separates from the layer behind it—without treatment patients can lose vision) found that taking a fluoroquinolone in the 10 days before surgery was a risk factor for retinal detachment. Taking a recent course of levofloxacin increased the risk of retinal detachment about two times; however, the absolute risk of someone who takes FQs developing retinal detachment is still extremely low (Raguideau 2016).

Using a nationwide registry in Sweden, researchers identified what may be an increase in rates of aortic aneurysm (ballooning of the aorta) and dissection (separation of the layers of the wall of the aorta by blood) and use of FQs (Pasternak 2018). This is plausible because FQs are known to induce degradation of collagen and components of the extracellular matrix, a process that is thought to be involved in the increased risk for tendinitis and Achilles tendon rupture. Aortic dissection is a medical emergency and can be fatal. In this instance also, however, the absolute risk is still very low.

It can take a long time to determine whether a particular event is related to a specific drug—and whether there is cause and effect. Findings can sometimes be completely unexpected.

Clarithromycin is a macrolide antibiotic (like azithromycin). Many years ago researchers in Denmark who thought that a bacterial infection (*Chlamydophila pneumoniae*) might play a role in heart disease decided to test whether giving an antibiotic would reduce cardiovascular disease. They undertook a large (4,373 participants) long-term (10 years) study in patients with stable coronary heart disease. They gave half the patients 2 weeks of clarithromycin 500 mg daily and the other half a placebo (dummy pills). The trial started in 1999/2000 and continued for 10 years. To the researchers' surprise, participants who received clarithromycin (and who were not taking statins) had increased rates of death due to cardiovascular disease and of illness due to stroke relative to those who did not receive clarithromycin (Winkel 2015). Because of these results, the FDA issued a statement advising caution before prescribing clarithromycin to patients with heart disease. They added this new warning many years after the drug was first approved. It will take additional studies to determine whether this is a consistent finding and, if so, the cause for it.

What is Clostridioides difficile *colitis and where did it come from?*

One of the most severe effects related to antibiotic use in the United States today is *C. difficile* colitis. *C. difficile* colitis, often known by its nickname, *C. diff*, has become a huge, pervasive, and costly problem in the United States and elsewhere. It is now the most common health care–associated infection in the United States. The existence of *C. diff* illness is largely due to antibiotics—and its continued spread is fueled by the use of antibiotics. Its name comes from the Greek *kloster*, meaning "spindle" (the appearance of the bacteria), and the Latin *difficile,* meaning difficult or obstinate. The bacteria were present long before commercial antibiotics were available and widely used.

    C. difficile is a bacterium found widely in soil and in the environment. *C. difficile* bacteria can also be found in the human colon in less than 2% of healthy adults without recent health care (but may be found in about 8% of patients on admission to the hospital). The bacterium is a drumstick- or spindle-shaped cell, an anaerobe that grows best at body temperatures in an environment without oxygen. It can live in the intestinal tract and cause no symptoms, especially if all of the other trillions of bacteria that make up the gut microbiota are abundant and varied. The masses of other bacteria compete for nutrients and territory and can keep it in check. If, however, the normal balance of other bacteria is disrupted, as can happen when a person receives an antibiotic, the *C. difficile* bacteria can thrive—and multiply. The term that describes this is "colonization resistance," which means that a healthy, diverse gut microbiota repels or resists the establishment of other bacteria that find their way into the intestinal tract—with food, drink, or other ingestions. Antibiotics disrupt the protection of colonization resistance. Disruption of the microbiota occurs during antibiotic treatment and can also persist after the treatment has stopped.

These bacteria have other features that are notable. C. difficile bacteria produce toxins that can cause inflammation and damage the lining of the intestine, leading to the development of what look like membranes inside the colon, the lower part of the intestines. These are called pseudomembranes because they are not true membranes. If one examines this layer under the microscope, one sees that it is made up of a collection of inflammatory cells, fibrin, and dying cells.

The toxins from the bacteria cause other problems in humans. They can cause high fevers. Inflammation of the colon (colitis) leads to diarrhea (sometimes bloody), abdominal pain, bloating, and paralysis of the inflamed part of the colon, causing it to become distended (toxic megacolon) like a balloon. The wall of the intestine can rupture allowing leakage of material from the colon and leading to peritonitis and sepsis, which can be fatal.

C. difficile bacteria are also equipped to survive harsh conditions. They can live as spores, invisible to the naked eye, and survive for months under extreme conditions. Spores can persist in hospitals on beds, bed rails, bedside stands, toilet seats, stethoscopes, blood pressure cuffs, walls, floors, the hands of health care workers who have contact with a person with C. *diff*, or materials that have become contaminated with spores. They can survive commercial laundering. The uncontrolled diarrhea that many patients with C. *diff* experience leads to widespread contamination of the local environment.

It is now known that the spores of C. *diff* are not killed by the alcohol hand cleaners that have become widely used in health care facilities. Eliminating the bacteria from hands requires handwashing—vigorous use of soap and water. Bleach is also effective in killing the spores and may be used as part of the cleaning process in hospitals—but cleaning must reach all surfaces that have been contaminated by these resilient spores. Use of disinfecting ultraviolet light has also been tried for terminal disinfection (final cleaning after the patient has left) in rooms that have been occupied by patients with C. diff. In general, it is much more difficult to successfully clean a room that has been inhabited by a patient with C. diff diarrhea than those occupied by patients with other kinds of infections. In guidelines recently published in the United States by the Infectious Diseases Society of America (IDSA), it is strongly recommended that all patients with C. diff infections be put in private rooms with their own toilet facilities (not shared with other patients). Furthermore, it is recommended that health care workers always wear gloves and gowns when entering the room of a patient with C. diff and for any contact with these patients.

How common is it? C. diff was estimated to cause almost half a million cases in 2011 in the United States and was associated with 29,000 deaths. Cost of treating these cases is more than $5 billion each year in the United States (Lessa 2015; Zhang 2018). Between 2000 and 2010, cases in the United States doubled.

From the earliest days of antibiotic use it was known that antibiotics could cause diarrhea, sometimes severe and persistent—then known as "antibiotic-associated colitis"—but in the 1970s severe diarrhea related to antibiotics was observed to become more common. Often it was related to a specific antibiotic (clindamycin) and was called clindamycin colitis—but it could also occur with other antibiotics, including ampicillin. Studies in the 1970s by John Bartlett and colleagues identified C. difficile and showed that two toxins were involved in causing pseudomembranous colitis (Bartlett 1978). Since then other toxins have been identified that are also involved in causing the disease.

C. diff cases have increased in parallel with the development and wide use of broader-spectrum antibiotics over recent decades. More disease-causing bacteria can be targeted, but these newer drugs have an even more profound effect on the resident gut bacteria. The antibiotics that are most often linked to C. *diff* colitis are the fluoroquinolones (like ciprofloxacin), the cephalosporins, and clindamycin.

What is driving the increase in cases?

Some strains of C. *diff* bacteria seem to be especially virulent (able to cause disease) and have been linked to severe outbreaks with many deaths. In the laboratory, some strains, including one called ribotype (RT) 027, can be shown to outcompete other strains of the bacteria. This particular strain was common in health care facility outbreaks between 2000 and 2003, causing at least half the cases in five of eight outbreaks. Resistance to fluoroquinolones was common. Fluoroquinolone use remains high in the United States. The severity of C. *diff* colitis seems to be increasing, which may be attributed to the emergence of specific strains. Patients infected with RT 027 are more likely to be dead at 3 months than those infected with other strains. In one unit in France, 64% of those infected with RT 027 died. One should keep in mind that hospitalized patients who develop C. *diff* infections often have multiple other medical problems and it is typically not C. *diff* colitis alone that leads to their deaths, but it can contribute to and hasten their demise.

The global epidemic of RT 027, the increase in antibiotic-resistant C. *diff* bacteria (especially those resistant to fluoroquinolones), and the continued wide use of FQs in many regions seem to be major drivers of the increase in C. *diff* infections.

In an attempt to understand other possible factors that are driving the increase in C. *diff* infections, researchers have studied many food additives (Collins 2018; Zeidler 2017). One group of investigators found that two ribotypes of C. *diff* (RT 027 and RT 078) that have caused epidemics and have increased in recent years can grow in the presence of low concentrations of trehalose, a sugar about 45% as sweet as sucrose. Trehalose has been used as a food additive (enhances stabilization and cryopreservation and improves taste and texture) in the United States since 2000. Exposure of the RT 027 strain to trehalose also increases *C. diff* virulence in mouse models. It remains to be seen whether this is an important driver in the increase in *C. diff* cases, but it is a reminder of the multiple factors that may influence the gut bacteria and potentially the development of illness. Trehalose has been used as a food additive in Japan since 1995 and was approved as a food ingredient in Canada in 2005. In Canada multiple severe outbreaks of *C. diff* colitis occurred in the early 2000s before the use of trehalose. Trehalose also can endow other bacteria with survival abilities, for example, desiccation resistance, osmo-protection, and heat and cold tolerance. Another nosocomial pathogen, *Acinetobacter baumannii*, which can be both drug resistant and a cause of hospital-acquired infections, also seems to accumulate trehalose.

In England cases of *C. diff* increased through 2006, when it was found that many of the cases were caused by bacteria resistant to the fluoroquinolones. In 2006 a nationwide policy was put in place to restrict the use of fluoroquinolones, and the incidence of *C. diff* in England subsequently declined by about 80%. *C. diff* infections did not disappear, but those related to *C. diff* strains resistant to fluoroquinolones markedly decreased when use of these antibiotics had been reduced.

In the United States a recently published study of health care–associated infections in 25 hospitals found no significant reduction in *C. diff* infections between 2011 and 2015. About 15% of all health care–associated infections identified on a single-day survey were caused by *C. diff* (Magill 2018).

What predisposes someone to Clostridioides difficile *infection* and how does it spread?

Many studies provide insights into the risk factors for development of *C. diff* colitis (Ma 2017; Eyre 2017). First and foremost is the receipt of antibiotics—especially ones in the three classes already noted: fluoroquinolones, cephalosporins, and clindamycin. C. *diff* infection can follow antibiotic use, whether the drugs are taken by mouth or by injection or intravenous route. Being older and being in a long-term care facility or hospital (or having had a recent hospitalization) also heighten the risk. Other risk factors include abdominal surgery and feeding tube use. Taking drugs that reduce stomach acid (e.g., proton pump inhibitors, antacids) can increase risk. C. *diff* spores are picked up by the oral route and can survive stomach acid, but more spores may survive if stomach acid is reduced or absent. Women are at slightly higher risk than men.

Cancer chemotherapy can increase the risk of C. *diff*. The cancer chemotherapeutic drugs may also have antibiotic activity, and the patient's immune system may be suppressed.

Other risk factors are not so obvious. Hospitalized patients who share a room with someone with C. *diff* colitis are at increased risk for developing a C. *diff* infection. If one stays in a room previously occupied by someone with C. *diff* infection, the risk is also increased. Furthermore, if a person is hospitalized, being in a bed whose prior occupant simply received antibiotics increases the risk for C. *diff* infection. Multiple studies now document how important the environment is in determining risk. Shedding of C. *diff* spores is especially high in those with acute infection but continues in those who were recently treated, even after diarrhea has ceased. Patients who are asymptomatic or are unrecognized carriers of C. *diff* can also be a source of contamination of the environment. An approach that is being tried in at least one health system is using robots with pulsed xenon and ultraviolet (UV) light to clean rooms after discharges or transfers of patients in an attempt to more effectively remove C. *diff* spores. One system reported a 49% decrease in C. *diff* infection rates at 90 days after using this protocol.

A study of long-term care facilities in 86 Veterans Health Administration health care regions found that regional rates of C. *diff* infections varied an astounding 40-fold (Brown 2016). They also found that regional use of antibiotics varied more than sixfold. Those long-term care residents who had been in an acute care hospital during the previous 28 days had a four-fold increased risk of C. *diff*. If they had received antibiotics, there was a sevenfold increased risk. Movement of a patient with C. *diff* colitis from an acute care facility into a long-term care facility also increased risk to those in the latter facility. What was most remarkable was that simply living in a region with high antibiotic use increased the risk of C. *diff*—the herd effect. Even patients who did not take antibiotics were at increased risk if they lived in a region with high antibiotic use. Antibiotics are truly societal drugs.

Although a large percentage of C. *diff* infections are acquired in hospitals or long-term care facilities, infections can also be acquired in the community because antibiotics are widely used outside of the hospital setting and patients move between hospitals and home. To assess the spread of C. *diff* spores in settings outside of the hospital, Canadian researchers collected stool or rectal samples from household contacts. They included people and pets in households of patients with C. *diff* infection. They found that 6% of adult household contacts and 35% of pediatric contacts of the patients with C. *diff*—plus about a quarter of the 15 dogs and cats—carried C. *diff*. In most instances genetic testing showed that it was identical to the strain carried by the patients.

Up to 30% of people with C. *diff* colitis will have a recurrence—and some unfortunate individuals will have multiple relapses. C. *diff* infections have increased in all regions of the United States, but multiply recurrent C. *diff* infections have increased even more rapidly from 2001 to 2012. Risk factors for multiple recurrences are similar to those for the development of the disease in the first place: older age, female, and use of antibiotics, proton pump inhibitors that reduce stomach acid, or corticosteroids within the last 90 days, as well as chronic kidney disease and diagnosis in a nursing home.

How is it treated?

Treatment of C. *diff* colitis has typically involved taking oral medications, with vancomycin and fidaxomicin being the drugs most often recommended. Metronidazole was used commonly in the past but is no longer recommended as first-line therapy. Occasionally the acute colitis is so severe that surgery is used as a last resort to remove the affected portion of the colon and save the life of the patient.

Management of a patient with C. *diff* colitis should always include stopping any unnecessary antibiotics (as it should for all patients); however, some patients with C. *diff* infections also have severe life-threatening infections for which antibiotics are essential to cure the infection. These include bacterial endocarditis (infection of one or more heart valves, which was always fatal before the availability of antibiotics), meningitis, brain abscess, infection of bone (osteomyelitis), and others. In some instances, the course of antibiotic treatment may be shortened by use of an adjunctive surgical procedure, such as draining an abscess or clearing dead tissue from a wound.

The use of probiotics has been advocated as a way to prevent C. *diff* colitis (Goldenberg 2017). Authors of recent guidelines concluded that evidence is currently insufficient to recommend the use of probiotics for prevention unless as part of a clinical trial, but a Cochrane review (a respected group that does systematic reviews of topics) concluded that there is evidence of moderate quality that finds a protective effect from probiotics against C. *diff* colitis and suggested its use for some groups of patients who receive antibiotics during hospitalization.

What is a fecal microbiota transplant?

A different approach has become more widely accepted in recent years (Andremont 2018; Hocquart 2018). Because the primary reason for the development of C. *diff* colitis is the disruption of the populations of bacteria that normally inhabit the colon, one logical approach is to repopulate the colon with a normal population of bacteria that can outcompete the *C. diff* bacteria—to restore a population of healthy bacteria in the gut. Despite initial skepticism, logistical challenges, and a certain yuck factor—in part because initial approaches involved making a slurry of feces from a healthy friend or relative and delivering it to the colon—the approach has now been effective in many patients with multiple recurrences, individuals who had run out of options for treatment. Many had been sick for months and some more than a year before considering this alternative. This approach is still considered an investigational new treatment by the FDA and long-term consequences are unknown; it is now considered an acceptable alternative treatment but typically used only for individuals who have had multiple episodes of *C. diff* colitis.

The term now used for this approach is "fecal microbiota transplantation" (FMT). If we knew the right recipe for a healthy colon microbiota, it might be possible to create the right mix of bacteria—the ideal microbial community composition—in the laboratory. The gut microbiota is complex, dynamic, and metabolically active (see section below: What is the microbiome?), and researchers have made remarkable progress in identifying the range and mix of bacteria that inhabit different parts of the gastrointestinal tract—but we are far from a point where we know enough to "compose" a healthy microbiota. Many bacteria present as part of the fecal microbiota have never been grown/isolated in a laboratory. To date, the approach that has been used is to identify healthy donors. There are even descriptions of patients self-administering fecal microbiota transplants using stool from friends or family members. Stool banks have also emerged that will ship specimens to physicians, but these are not regulated.

Feces are mostly bacteria but include cells shed from the intestinal walls, bile acids, bacteriophages, yeast, and potentially viruses from the donor. This means that potential donors must be screened for a number of infections, such as HIV, hepatitis B, hepatitis C, and syphilis, as well as other microbes that can cause chronic infections. Screening guidelines have been published that are based in part on the American Association of Blood Banks Donor History Questionnaire. This includes screening for high-risk activities as well, such as use of illicit drugs, tattoo or body piercing within the previous 6 months, history of gastrointestinal diseases, history of antibiotic use within the preceding 3 months, and use of other medications, including steroids. The potential donor's feces are tested for any evidence of parasitic infection.

The FDA has considered how to regulate FMT to ensure it is safe and accessible to those who can benefit from it. In May 2013 the FDA announced that it considered fecal microbiota a biological product and would require an investigational new drug (IND) application for its use. This would come with the requirement for extensive protocols and would make it complicated to use. Because of the immediate negative response from clinicians and patients, a few months later the FDA announced it would not enforce IND requirements and would allow physicians and stool banks to use FMT for C. *diff* infections without an IND application. Another draft guidance was published by the FDA in March 2016 saying it would require stool banks to submit an IND application before they could obtain stool samples and distribute them to physicians. Physicians and hospital laboratories could continue to collect and prepare FMT for use by licensed health care providers.

Others have proposed an alternative framework that would view microbiota from stool as a tissue. A working group has proposed a three-track regulatory approach (Hoffmann 2017). The first track would allow physicians to perform FMT using stool from someone known to the physician or patient and based on their scope of practice and relevant standard of care. If they wanted to use it for an indication other than C. *diff*, they would be required to obtain an IND application. The second track would be for stool for FMT obtained from stool banks that would be regulated in a way similar to human cell-tissue establishments. They would have to follow established rules for donor screening and good manufacturing practices. There would also be a requirement that physicians using their products report adverse events and outcomes. The stool bank would be required to report safety data to the FDA. They would also be required to report outcomes and safety data to a national registry. A third track would apply to "modified stool-based products." These products may include communities of bacteria from stool samples. They would be regulated as biological products or drugs and would have IND requirements.

These issues and regulatory dilemmas are unlikely to vanish in the near future. At present fecal transplantations are being used, but with greater appreciation for the fundamental importance of healthy microbiota, it is likely that other microbiota transplantations will be studied. Already there are reports of "vaginal seeding" of newborns delivered by cesarean section—the smearing of the newborn's skin, eyes, nose, and mouth with material on a gauze that had been placed in a mother's vagina as a way to try to expose and potentially colonize the newborn with the microbial bathing it would have experienced had it passed through the birth canal.

For FMT, donor feces are infused into the intestinal tract via a nasojejunal/nasoduodenal tube or via a colonoscope or retention enema. A recent study assessed delivery via fecal capsule in 57 patients and found it produced acceptable results. Apparently 30% of the participants described the treatment as "unpleasant, gross, or disgusting," but virtually all (97%) said they would undergo the treatment again, if necessary (Kao 2017). The donor's microbiota becomes established in the recipient.

So far the use of FMT has been effective in a large percentage of patients and has been generally well tolerated. There have been a couple of instances of transmission of norovirus (a virus that causes diarrhea) from donors with unrecognized (asymptomatic) infection. Long-term outcomes are unknown at this point, but many patients have had dramatic improvement in the short term.

One study from a group in France published in 2018 found that early use of FMT in patients with severe *C. diff* colitis reduced 3-month mortality from 42% in the group treated with usual antibiotics to 12% in those treated with early FMT. This was a retrospective study done in one institution (Hocquart 2018). The published observations are valuable, but most clinicians believe that research should continue to define the elements of FMT that make it so effective and to refine treatment approaches.

A small study from Oslo, Norway, was published in 2018. Instead of reserving FMT for patients who had failed other treatments, they used fecal microbiota transplantation as initial treatment with good results. A phase 3 clinical trial evaluating this approach is currently under way (Juul 2018).

A new agent, bezlotoxumab, a humanized monoclonal antibody that provides passive immunity against toxin B, one of the toxins produced by the *C. difficile* bacteria, has recently been approved by the FDA. It can be added to standard therapy (Bartlett 2017). Its main benefit is that it is effective in reducing the rate of first-time relapses of *C. diff* infections. It is expensive, so it is not yet clear how it will be used. However, the cost of a recurrence of *C. diff* colitis is also expensive—estimated to be more than $11,000 (Prabhu 2018). Another agent, actoxuab, provides passive protection to toxin A, but when combined with bezlotoxumab it was associated with more side effects.

Other approaches that are being tried include development of new drugs, administration of *C. diff* strains of bacteria that do not produce toxin to compete with those that do, and vaccines to protect against the action of the toxins.

Can fecal microbiota transplantation be used to treat other conditions?

The success with FMT for the treatment of *C. diff* infections has led to consideration of its use in other conditions that are thought to be caused by disruption of the fecal microbiota, sometimes characterized as dysbiosis (a term used to indicate microbial imbalance). Use of FMT has been tried in some cases of inflammatory bowel disease. It has also been studied in Poland in patients with blood disorders whose gastrointestinal tracts have become colonized with antibiotic-resistant bacteria (Bilinski 2017). These patients whose general immunity is suppressed are at high risk for bacterial infections. The bacteria that cause their infections often come from the bacteria in their own guts. If they carry extensively resistant bacteria in their guts, these bacteria may cause infections that are difficult or impossible to treat. The researchers in Poland found that 15 of 20 patients treated with FMT had complete decolonization (loss) of antibiotic-resistant bacteria. After the FMT, they had a higher abundance of bacteria found in the healthy individuals and greater bacterial richness—considered a good outcome.

A side benefit noted in another study of patients who underwent FMT for recurrent *C. diff* was a reduction in recurrent urinary tract infections (UTIs) (Tariq 2017). UTIs are one of the most common reasons for use of antibiotics. Patients with recurrent UTIs often suffer from infections that become progressively more resistant to antibiotics, requiring broader-spectrum antibiotics that put them at higher risk for *C. diff*. Patients with profuse diarrhea from *C. diff* are also at increased risk for UTIs. Bacteria that cause UTIs often come from bacteria, such as *E. coli* and *Klebsiella*, that are carried in the gut. A study that looked specifically at patients treated for *C. diff* with FMT who also had a history of recurrent UTIs found that UTIs decreased after FMT and the replacement of multiply resistant *E. coli* in the gut with more antibiotic sensitive bacteria.

FMT has also been shown to eliminate vancomycin-resistant enterococci (VRE) from the gut in almost three-quarters of VRE-positive patients in another study (Dubberke 2016). Risk factors for colonization and infection with VRE and *C. diff* are similar, and many patients are coinfected/colonized (>50% in some studies).

Why do yeast infections occur during and after treatment with antibiotics?

Another adverse event that can be associated with taking antibiotics is the development of an infection commonly known as a yeast infection or *Candida* vaginitis. This fungal infection, most often caused by the yeast *Candida albicans*, can cause itching and burning of the vagina and produce a white coating or white patches on the vaginal mucosa (lining of the vagina). The same yeast can also cause what is known as thrush, an infection of the mouth or tongue that produces a white coating or white patches. *Candida* may also be associated with diaper rash in babies. Normally small numbers of the yeast live in the mouth, throat, vagina, and gastrointestinal tract, but they are kept in check by the abundant normal bacteria that live in those areas. Yeasts and fungi are resistant to antibiotics, though there are specific antifungal drugs that can be used to treat them. Antibiotics disturb the balance of microbes and can kill or weaken normal bacteria, allowing overgrowth of the yeast, usually on mucosal surfaces like the mouth and vagina. The immune system is also important in keeping the *Candida* in check. Babies, with their immature immune systems, and individuals who are immunosuppressed because of drugs, other treatments, or infections such as HIV are especially susceptible to *Candida* and other yeast infections. In these circumstances, *Candida* can infect the throat, esophagus (*Candida* esophagitis), and gastrointestinal tract or even invade tissues and enter the bloodstream and infect other organs. In healthy individuals *Candida* normally does not get past the surface tissues unless a person has had surgery or other procedures that break the skin barrier. *Candida* and other yeasts are important causes of hospital-acquired infections because of the ubiquity of tubes, catheters, and other foreign bodies that *Candida* can cling to and the high frequency of antibiotic use.

What is the microbiome and why is it so important?

The term "microbiota" describes all the microbes that inhabit a particular ecosystem. The term is often used in reference to an area of the human body, but other animals, plants, insects, fish, soil, and water all have their own microbiota. The term "microbiome" is used to define the collection of all of the genomes of microbes in a particular environment or in an ecosystem. Although much of the focus has been on bacteria, other species are part of this functioning ecosystem—viruses, archaea, and microeukaryotes (like fungi and protozoa).

It is impossible to discuss the effects of antibiotics without acknowledging the key functions of the microbiota. Many have been taught to think of bacteria as bad, as germs, and as something to be targeted and destroyed. Prominent disease-causing bacteria, like *Streptococcus* and *Staphylococcus*, have distorted our thinking. A few bacteria are harmful, many are neutral or good, and some are essential for life. Bacteria do not need humans to survive. They existed long before humans inhabited the earth. They have survived floods, droughts, hurricanes, earthquakes, tsunamis, meteor strikes, and volcanoes. They may be locally altered by major events—at least in the short term—but bacteria and other microbes have the variety, abundance, and resilience to be able to survive most imaginable threats. Humans evolved in a sea of microbes. Trillions live in and on us. We rely on microbes for our development and function. We cannot live life as we know it today without them.

We exist in a microbial world with abundant, varied, creative, and resilient bacteria. Bacteria are much older evolutionarily than humans are and able to respond much more quickly to changes in the environment than humans can. They have strength in numbers, speed in replication, and almost infinite variety. They have shaped the earth and they shape our lives in ways we are only beginning to understand. We have coevolved with these microbes.

We should see them as partners, not foes, and should celebrate, preserve, and keep most of them. They are a valuable part of our lives. Instead of trying to disrupt and alter their communities and killing off loads of them, we should see them for the treasures they are.

Each of us carries perhaps two to three pounds of microbes. We have more bacteria in our bodies than human cells. Our bodies are a partnership of the human genome and microbial genetic material. The mouth may have more than 600 species of bacteria. By far the largest concentration of microbes is in the gut, which has a huge surface area, perhaps the size of a tennis court. Bacteria and other microbes make up a large part of the contents of the gut, especially the colon, the last part of the intestine. We call the contents waste, but important interactions and extraction processes occur before the remnants are eliminated.

A short detour is needed to describe what is included in this microbial soup. The term "microbe" typically has been used to describe organisms too small to be seen without the aid of a microscope—and traditionally has included bacteria, viruses, protozoa, and fungi as the main components. These make up the microbiota that is essential for life. A few decades ago scientists realized that some organisms that had been called bacteria were sufficiently different to warrant being designated as belonging to a different domain, the archaea. The archaea (the name comes from a Greek word meaning ancient things) are unicellular organisms that differ from bacteria in genetics and biochemistry. Their membranes are made of ether lipids. They are found in all kinds of habitats—water, soil, air, and rocks—including extreme environments (like hot springs) and are also part of the human microbiome. Bacteria and archaea are grouped together as prokaryotes. All are unicellular, lack a cell nucleus, and are microbes.

Every part of the body has its own microbial palate—a composition that is matched to that part of the body. Each person has a unique combination or network of microbes, though there is a lot of overlap from one person to another for a particular body site. The microbiota of the skin in the armpit is not the same as that in the groin. The microbiota of the right and left hands of an individual are not identical.

The gut microbiomes in hunter-gatherers are more varied than those in people living in industrialized areas, and they change seasonally in response to changes in the diet. A study of the Hadza hunter-gatherers of Tanzania that examined the microbiome profiles of fecal samples collected over more than a year found cyclical changes that reflected changes in the diet. In the wet season picking berries and eating honey were common, whereas hunting and consuming meat were more common in the dry season. These hunter-gatherers consume fiber-rich tubers year round. A higher diversity in the microbiome was observed during the dry season. Some taxa dropped to undetectable levels during the dry season but returned during the wet season. The functional capacity of the microbiome also changed with the season. Researchers found that the repertoires of antibiotic resistance genes in the Hadza were distinct from and less diverse than those found in people living in the United States. Other studies have shown that microbial diversity in South American Amerindians is about twice as great as in healthy people in the United States (Clemente 2015).

Researchers also compared the data on Hadza microbiomes with microbiome data collected from 18 populations in 16 countries around the world whose populations have different lifestyles. Overall they found that the microbiome in the hunter-gatherer population is more diverse than that in populations living in industrialized settings. The Hadza had more diverse pathways for breaking down carbohydrates and greater functional capacity for utilizing plant carbohydrates than the microbiomes of Americans. Some of the taxa that decrease seasonally in the Hadza population are now rare or absent from gut microbiomes in industrialized populations. These correspond to the microbiota that are abundant when the diet is rich in plant-derived complex carbohydrates. Other factors associated with industrialization may also affect the gut microbiome (Smits 2017).

Researchers have also studied what happens to the microbiome when people from non-Western countries migrate to the United States (Vangay 2018). They studied Hmong and Karen individuals living in Thailand and first- and second-generation immigrants in the United States. They found that after moving to the United States, the microbiome became less diverse. The migrants lost some of the bacteria that produce enzymes that break down plant fibers. They also found microbiome changes that have been associated with obesity.

Microbial lineages in humans appear to be passed vertically from mother to newborns. Among animals and other organisms, diverse mechanisms are used to provide essential microbiota to the next generation. Each human infant must assemble a gut microbiome—and mom provides the start. It is part of the legacy passed to the infant along with the genetic information in the human cells of the body. If women in industrialized countries have less diverse microbiomes than in past generations, this could influence the health and function of the next generation. In his book about the missing microbes, Martin Blaser postulates that repeated courses of antibiotics characteristic of many modern societies are resulting in a less diverse microbiota passed to newborns today than in past generations (Blaser 2009; Blaser 2014). This has many potential adverse consequences. Some lineages of bacteria that have traditionally been found in human guts may be becoming extinct. This has prompted researchers to start collecting and preserving high-diversity microbiotas from traditional peoples and creating biobanks of these before they disappear (Dominguez-Bello 2018).

The microbes that begin to form the microbiota for a newborn infant come from the mother. Babies born by vaginal delivery are covered with bacteria from the birth canal, and they can also swallow them during the birth process. Babies born by cesarean section start life with a different, less diverse set of bacteria. This has led to attempts by some to recreate the benefits of vaginal delivery by smearing babies born by C-section with vaginal contents from their mother.

If the mother receives antibiotics around the time of delivery, this can affect the bacteria that are transferred to the infant. Women who are found to carry Group B *Streptococcus* in the genital area before giving birth are typically given an antibiotic when they are in labor to prevent these harmful bacteria from infecting the vulnerable newborn.

The developing microbiota of the infant is influenced by diet (different for breastfed and formula-fed infants), the genetics of the infant, environmental exposures, and many other factors. Once the microbiome becomes established at a few years of age, it can be remarkably stable in that individual. Many factors affect it, including diet, the environment, illness, activity, genetics, medications, and, most important, antibiotics. Many pharmacologic agents, in addition to antibiotics, can affect the bacteria in the bowel. The diversity of the microbiota declines in the elderly, who also have less robust immune responses to a number of pathogens (Lynch 2016).

Studies of adults in the United States have found that an individual's microbiota is remarkably stable over time. One study sampled 37 adults multiple times over a period of up to about 5 years and showed that about 60% of the bacterial strains remained stable. Their findings suggest that bacteria that take up residence in the gut early in life—like those acquired from the mother, father, and siblings—have the potential to remain gut residents and exert their metabolic and immunologic effects for decades and perhaps for life (Faith 2013). This also occurs in animals. Researchers monitored the gut microbiota in laboratory mice for 11 generations and found that microbiota were maintained within mouse lines, transmitted from mother to offspring for the entire period (Moeller 2018).

Host genetics play a role, however, and many other factors are also important. A study of more than 1,000 healthy individuals found significant similarities in compositions of microbiomes of genetically unrelated individuals who shared the same household (Rothschild 2018). We regularly share bacteria with our close contacts and the environment. A glass of clean drinking water may have 10 million bacteria. Houses, different rooms in a house, hospitals, and other built environments also have distinct and different microbiomes.

The multiple functions of the microbiota in health and disease are just beginning to be understood. Some types of perturbations of the gut microbiota or imbalances in composition and function—called dysbiosis—are associated with bowel disease. One simplistic approach has been the attempt to replace the disordered microbiota with a healthy microbiota—a transplant of fecal microbiota, as discussed earlier in the section on *C. diff*. So far scientists do not fully understand what constitutes the best or ideal microbiota. It may vary depending on the individual, host genetics, and other factors. Treatment using specific bacteria for their specific attributes is being actively studied and could become an important treatment modality in the future.

What is the Human Microbiome Project?

An explosion of new information about the human microbiome resulted from the National Institutes of Health–directed Human Microbiome Project that started in 2008. This ambitious program, which included many collaborative laboratories and institutions, set out to characterize the ecology of human-associated microbial communities. Investigators carried out DNA sequencing of bacteria, archaea, microbial eukaryotes, and viruses. Four sequencing centers carried out the sequencing using standardized protocols and methods. This consortium was able to generate 5,177 unique taxonomic profiles (based on 16S rRNA gene sequences). For the first part of the study almost 5,000 samples from 242 healthy adults (129 males and 113 females) were collected and analyzed. Investigators collected samples from 18 different body habitats for women and 15 for men. The areas sampled included nine sites from the oral cavity and oropharynx (saliva, inside of the cheek, gums, palate, tonsils, throat, and tongue, and tooth biofilm [plaque] above and below the gum) and four skin samples from behind each ear, the inner elbows, and the nostrils. They also had samples from the lower gastrointestinal tract (self-collected stool). For women they also sampled three areas of the vagina. After taking the initial samples from each participant, they collected repeat samples several months later (mean of about 7 months). They also collected blood samples from the participants.

Rather than trying to grow the bacteria from each of these sites in the laboratory, to determine the composition of the community of bacteria, they used biomarker sequencing, in this instance 16S ribosomal RNA gene analysis. This approach provided semiquantitative results and allowed resolution at the genus level and sometimes at the species level. They also used metagenomics to gather information about functional capacity and pathways.

The results? They found astounding diversity in the composition of microbiota among the participants and by body site that was sampled. This important study provided a wealth of information about the structure and function of microbiota in healthy individuals and a basis for many additional studies. The results from the first part of the National Institutes of Health Human Microbiome Project were published in 2012. A second phase of the project will look at integrated longitudinal datasets from the microbiome and the human hosts. Three longitudinal studies will look at pregnancy and preterm birth, onset of inflammatory bowel disease as a model, and onset of type 2 diabetes.

A catalog of the human fecal microbial metagenome has now been developed based on data from 1,200 people from the United States, Europe, and China. These studies identified an aggregate of 9.9 million microbial genes across these fecal microbiomes.

The microbiome also includes fungi and protozoans. Analysis of 317 fecal samples from the Human Microbiome Project found that 98% contained detectable fungal taxa. *Candida* was one of the common fungi found in North America. Limited analysis from other geographic areas suggested that fungal composition may vary by sociogeographical settings.

As an indication of the importance and wide scope of microbiome research, the Microbiome Interagency Working Group of the National Science Technology Council (NSTC) released in 2018 the Interagency Strategic Plan for Microbiome Research FY 2018-2022 to provide overall guidance and direction for microbiome research across federal government agencies. This acknowledges the fundamental importance of microbiomes in animals, agriculture, marine environments, food production, coral reefs, wastewater management, and the environment.

Humans are not alone in requiring bacteria to perform essential services. One interesting example has come from the study of microbes in the Gulf of Mexico following the Deepwater Horizon oil spill. Ongoing study of that area shows that microbes capable of breaking down and degrading oil have flourished in that environment. How can microbes be harnessed to detoxify hazardous chemicals in other areas? Microbes play key roles in the global cycling of many elements and can also affect some climate processes. Although microbes are abundant in soil and water, they are also present in the air and can be carried by air currents. Many research projects are underway that should improve understanding of the microbiome in multiple spheres and disciplines.

What are the functions of the human microbiome?

The gut microbiome is the best studied of the human microbiomes. Scientists are trying to understand how an assemblage of microbial parts numbering in the trillions is influencing every aspect of human immunity, physiology, biochemistry, and function. This gut microbiota can be likened to another organ of the body, like the liver or kidneys. It persists throughout life but is influenced by multiple internal (genetic) and external forces and events. The gut is open to the outside world. Foods, fluids, chemicals, and microbes of all types enter through the nose and mouth daily and join the assemblage that flows through the body. It is in close communication with other parts of the body. It lies within and twists through the center of the body—and chemicals and cells leak from it. It is massive. The epithelial barrier (the intestinal wall) is constantly challenged by the gut microbiota. The surface area of the inside (lumen) of the intestine is more than 30 square meters. This is the largest and most diverse microbiome in the body, but every other skin and mucosal surface has its own microbiota. Even clean skin is not sterile.

Most of the bacteria that make up this organ cannot be grown in the laboratory by conventional isolation techniques. Their abundance and variety has been described by using approaches called next-generation sequencing and other molecular techniques. These culture-independent assays allow detection and classification of microbiota. They no longer have to grow the bacteria before they can study them. It is also possible to assess encoded genes and gene products.

The stomach and upper gastrointestinal tract region have relatively few bacteria because of the presence of gastric acid (acid can kill or slow the growth of some bacteria) and the relatively rapid movement (peristalsis) of this area. In the lower part of the small intestine (ileum), the bacterial composition becomes larger and more diverse. The colon contains the largest and most diverse bacterial population of the body.

The gut microbiota serve as both a barrier against invasion of disease-causing microbes (pathogens) and a repository of potential bacterial pathogens and of resistance genes. Resident microbiota interact with other bacteria. They may outcompete pathogens for nutrients, space, and metabolites. Resident microbiota may also inhibit or kill other bacteria via other byproducts or substances they produce, such as bacteriocins, peptides, and acids. They may even have specific functions. For example, a bile acid–producing bacterium might promote resistance to the colonization of C. *diff*. Loss of bacterial diversity of the resident bacteria (often anaerobic microbiota) can lead to overgrowth and domination of a particular strain, which can predispose to translocation (movement from inside to outside of the gut) of bacteria that enter bloodstream.

What are some of the specific functions? Some provocative results come from studies in mice and other animal models and will need to be confirmed with more complicated studies in humans. In animal studies changes in the microbiome in early life have been associated with a range of diseases, including diabetes, obesity, and asthma.

In humans key functions of the gut microbiota range from influencing the immune system to biosynthesis of vitamins. In their effect on immunity, they participate in the development, maturation, and maintenance of the immune system. They can modulate the immune response. Microbes can be a source of molecules that promote inflammation or others that can dampen it. Inflammation can increase gut permeability, allowing leakage from the gut of endotoxin and other substances produced by microbes. Microbes secrete metabolically active products that are used by and influence the composition of the local microbial community. They play a key role in nutrition and digestion. They extract nutrients from food. They produce enzymes involved in hydrolysis (breaking down) and fermentation of polysaccharides; microbial enzymes convert polysaccharides into digestible sources of energy. They are involved in bile transformation. Bacterial enzymes (bile salt hydrolases) de-conjugate (break apart) primary conjugated bile salts. They can degrade or break down toxins. They have a role in biosynthesis vitamins, including K and B vitamins, and are a source of hormones and other biologically active substances. They produce acetate, butyrate, and other chemicals that can influence the production of ghrelin, a peptide hormone produced in the gastrointestinal tract that acts in the central nervous system and can regulate appetite. They have a role in the regulation of insulin levels.

Gut microbiota may influence the development of obesity and type 2 diabetes. In one study gut microbes from obese mice and lean mice were given to germ-free mice. All mice were fed and housed under the same conditions. Mice that received lean-mice microbiota stayed thin; those given microbiota from obese mice became obese. Differences have also been observed in the microbiotas of lean and obese people. Some microbiota may be able to more efficiently extract energy from food inputs.

There is some evidence that the microbiome may play a role in the initiation and progression of atherosclerosis. Some of this evidence comes from animal models. More work needs to be done to determine if the microbiome has a causal role in humans—and much more work before understanding the implications for treatment and prevention. Can one change a person's microbiome to lessen the risk of cardiovascular disease?

Some studies suggest that reduced diversity of microbiota in infants and young children may be associated with an increase in asthma and other allergic diseases. Exposure to environmental microbes may also modulate mucosal immunity.

A disordered gut microbiota (dysbiosis) has been associated with a wide spectrum of common chronic disorders, including asthma, chronic inflammatory bowel diseases, and C. diff colitis.

Many studies are intriguing and offer potential new pathways for interventions in the future. We are now in the early stages of thinking about using specific microbial cocktails for treatment, but active research in these areas suggests that this may be an option for treatment in the future.

The composition of the gut microbiota may shape response to cancer chemotherapy. In patients treated with a kind of immunotherapy known as PD-1 inhibitors, which block a checkpoint molecule on T cells, patients who received antibiotics (which could disrupt the gut microbiome) relapsed sooner and did not live as long. Better efficacy of chemotherapy was observed in the presence of specific gut microbes. In experimental animals, investigators have been able to show that some specific bacteria may able to prime T cells, leading to a better response to chemotherapy (Zitvogel 2018).

Some bacteria may interfere with cancer treatment by metabolizing chemotherapy drugs. For example, some *E. coli* strains can metabolize (break down) and deactivate the active form of a chemotherapeutic agent (gemcitabine), and thus decrease its efficacy.

Microbiota at other body sites may also influence health and disease. A study published in 2018 that studied women from six sub-Saharan countries found that the composition of the vaginal microbiota affected their susceptibility to HIV infection. Women with a lower relative abundance of *Lactobacillus iners* (bacteria commonly found as part of normal bacteria residing in the vagina) were significantly more likely to become infected with HIV. They were also able to identify the bacterial species present in higher concentrations that were associated with becoming infected with HIV.

The skin microbiota of people with eczema, a skin problem, also differs from those with healthy unaffected skin. In people with eczema certain bacteria that are usually found on healthy skin may be missing and others present in unusually high numbers. This has led researchers to try applying "good" bacteria to the skin of individuals with eczema in an attempt to restore a healthy balance. Several of these studies are in progress.

How do antibiotics affect the human microbiome?

Antibiotics are a common cause for disturbance to the microbiome. Antibiotics lead to a decrease in numbers and diversity of bacteria and a change in composition and function. The effect can persist after a person has stopped taking an antibiotic. As background it is useful to keep in mind that in the United States today, on average children receive three courses of antibiotics by age 2 years and 10 courses of antibiotics before 10 years of age.

One study assessed the impact of a week-long course of antibiotics on the mouth microbiome and gut microbiome in volunteers in the United Kingdom and Sweden. Investigators used four different antibiotics. Repeat samples of saliva and feces were studied 12 months after antibiotic administration. In all subjects the microbiome was affected by the antibiotics, but the mouth microbiome was much more stable in contrast to the fecal microbiome. In volunteers who had received clindamycin or ciprofloxacin, changes were still apparent after 12 months. The beneficial butyrate-producing species of bacteria became underrepresented. Microbiome functions recovered faster than the microbial community composition returned to baseline, suggesting that multiple pathways may be available to provide some functions. Butyrate has been shown to have positive effects, including providing an energy source for colonocytes (cells of the colon) and inhibiting inflammation, carcinogenesis, and oxidative stress in the gut.

Researchers in Finland studied children aged 2 to 7 years attending daycare. Through a national database on prescription drug purchases, they could identify specific antibiotics prescribed and dates of use. They studied fecal specimens and had access to data about the health of the children. Most of the antibiotics used in the children were for respiratory infections. They found that early-life use of macrolide antibiotics (like azithromycin and erythromycin) was associated with reduction in bacterial diversity and composition. The bacterial populations did not fully recover even after 2 years. Early-life macrolide use was also associated with a decrease in bacteria that hydrolyze (break down) bile salts. They also found a positive correlation between overall antibiotic use with macrolides and body mass index (BMI) and asthma. More antibiotic use was associated with a higher BMI and an increase in asthma.

Use of penicillin had less effect on the composition and function of microbiota than the macrolide antibiotics.

Other studies have suggested that asthma and other allergies are increased in children who have taken antibiotics. Early-life use of antibiotics has been linked in some studies to increased risk for inflammatory bowel disease and increased body weight.

A detailed investigation of stool specimens using genetic (16S rRNA) sequencing was carried out on three individuals who took ciprofloxacin by mouth for 5 days. The antibiotic influenced the abundance of about a third of the bacterial taxa in the gut. Taking ciprofloxacin led to a decrease in the numbers of bacteria and diversity. The effect of the antibiotic varied from one individual to another. Follow-up analysis of specimens was also carried out. It was reassuring to see that the composition of the bacterial communities largely returned to pretreatment states by 4 weeks after the antibiotic treatment. At the same time it was sobering to find that even after 6 months, some types of bacteria did not recover. This study, done before the Human Microbiome Project was completed, confirmed the existence of more than 5,000 bacterial taxa in the human gut (Dethlefen 2008).

In Niger, children aged 1 to 60 months who had not been exposed to mass treatment with antibiotics for the past 6 years were included in a study. Half (40) were given a single dose of azithromycin and half were given placebo. Fecal samples were collected just before the antibiotic was administered and 5 days later. These were analyzed using genetic (16S rRNA) sequencing. The investigators identified 760 genera of bacteria in the samples. At baseline there was no difference between the two groups. After treatment, children given azithromycin had decreased intestinal microbiome diversity. Azithromycin has a long half-life (11 to 14 hours), so its activity against bacteria after a single dose can persist for days (Doan 2017).

Antibiotic use can also increase the availability of primary bile salts by eliminating or decreasing the bacteria that conjugate bile salts. *C. diff* colonization of the gut and germination (growth) can be affected by the availability of primary bile salts, so this may be another way that antibiotics can predispose patients receiving them to the development of *C. diff*.

Microbiomes have composition (specific genetic and microbial makeup) and function. Microbiomes that differ in composition can be similar in function. Many different compositions and arrangements of microbial communities may be able to achieve some of the same functions; that is, there are many ways to assemble a microbiome with specific functions. The microbial community also has functional redundancy or duplication, at least for some functions. This is especially apparent in the mechanisms that bacteria use to resist the action of bacteria (see chapter 5).

Does human use of antibiotics and other agents affect animal microbiota?

All animals, including mosquitoes, bees, and worms, have microbiota. Knowledge of this has been used to improve human health.

A fascinating story has emerged from observations with filarial worms that cause infections in humans. These parasitic worms that are transmitted to humans by mosquitoes and biting flies can cause elephantiasis (massive swelling of legs, arms, and scrotum, for example) and other severe and disfiguring illnesses. The microbiota of the worms include the bacteria *Wolbachia*, a type of Gram-negative bacteria. The bacteria are passed to their offspring (larvae) by infected female worms. The presence of *Wolbachia* bacteria is required by some filarial worms for normal development, fertility, and survival. Death of the bacterial microbiota in the worm (the *Wolbachia*) leads to death or sterility of the worm. Knowledge of this is used in treating humans who are infected with filarial worms. Drugs that are commonly used in mass treatment campaigns can kill the microfilariae, the form of the parasite in the blood that can be picked up by biting mosquitoes (and important to kill to stop ongoing transmission). However, the drugs that kill the microfilariae do not affect the adult worms, which have a long life span. They can live for years in the human body. Treating infected humans with a tetracycline antibiotic can kill the *Wolbachia* in the worm living in the human host and thus lead to the death of the worm. Use of doxycycline or other tetracycline has now been integrated into many treatment plans for filarial infections.

Mosquitoes can carry and transmit many disease-causing microbes to humans. They also have microbiota. Again, knowledge of this has been exploited to try to thwart mosquitoes' capacity to transmit infections to humans. Many insects carry *Wolbachia* bacteria normally. In nature, *Aedes aegypti*, the mosquito that transmits dengue, chikungunya, Zika, and other viruses, are not normally infected with *Wolbachia*; however, they can survive when infected with *Wolbachia*. It turns out, however, that if infected with *Wolbachia*, they may be unable to transmit certain viruses like dengue and chikungunya and other viruses that cause disease. Researchers are now studying whether they can use this information to prevent transmission. They are rearing mosquitoes, intentionally infecting male mosquitoes with *Wolbachia*, and releasing them into the wild. Male mosquitoes do not take blood meals and do not transmit infections. The released male mosquitoes mate with local female mosquitoes and *Wolbachia* is passed to the next generation via eggs. The presence of *Wolbachia* infection in the next generation of mosquitoes inhibits viruses such as dengue. Use of this technique in one area of Australia has been extremely effective in interrupting dengue transmission. Tests are also underway in other areas.

Bees also have microbiota. They acquire their normal microbial community orally through social interactions with other workers in the hive the first few days after they emerge. If they are deprived of these normal microbiota, they do not gain weight and function normally. Recent studies show that exposure to a chemical (glyphosate, a weed killer) can affect the gut microbiota of honeybees, leading to a decrease in some of their normal bacteria (Motta 2018). Young worker bees exposed to glyphosate became more susceptible to bacteria that can infect bees with weakened immune systems and were more likely to die from infection than were unexposed bees. Even though bees are not targeted by the herbicide (weed killer), their gut bacteria have the enzyme targeted by the herbicide—and killing their gut bacteria may be sufficient to make exposed bees more susceptible to infections and death.

Do other drugs besides antibiotics affect the microbiome?

Antibiotics are not the only drugs that affect the microbiome. In a recent study researchers evaluated the effect of more than 1,000 marketed drugs on the growth of 40 different bacteria, selected to be representative of those in the human gut (Maier 2018). They tested a range of pharmaceutical products from major therapeutic classes. A third were anti-infectives (antibacterial, antifungal, antiviral, and antiparasitic drugs), but the other 835 were drugs, like drugs to treat high blood pressure, that target human cells. They found that half of the antiviral and antiparasitic drugs also had antibacterial activity. Furthermore, almost a quarter (24%) of other drugs (not marketed as anti-infective drugs) inhibited the growth of the test bacteria. The drugs active against microbiome-associated bacteria included a wide range of agents with different physiologic actions: proton pump inhibitors (reduce stomach acid), 5-fluorouracil, methotrexate, tamoxifen, and amiodarone, as well as a number of antipsychotics. Those most likely to inhibit bacteria are widely used agents: calcium channel blockers (blood pressure pills) and antipsychotics. Bacteria that were resistant to anti-infectives were more likely to be resistant to human-targeted (not anti-infective) agents. These findings suggest that use of nonantibiotic drugs may also be affecting the human microbiome and microbial diversity. Many of the agents tested are taken long term for chronic conditions like hypertension.

Many other products used in daily life in industrialized populations today may be having subtle to profound effects on the microbiome, from chlorinated drinking water to toothpastes and mouthwashes with antiseptic and antimicrobial properties. For example, triclosan, an antiseptic with activity against bacteria and fungi, was used initially in hospitals when first introduced in the 1970s. It is currently used widely in thousands of consumer products, including soaps, toothpaste, mouthwash, cosmetics, cleaning supplies, and other items.

In summary, the gut microbiome is an essential part of the human host. It carries out biochemical transformations, digests food and provides nutrients for humans and microbiota, metabolizes foreign compounds including drugs and toxins, modifies host-derived metabolites including bile acids, mediates microbe-microbe interactions, and shapes the immune system. It may also influence circadian rhythms.

Can the gut microbiota be protected from the effect of antibiotics?

The gastrointestinal tract is often used as the route of delivery of antibiotics. Because of the impact antibiotics have on the gut microbiota, researchers have looked for a way to reduce the collateral damage from antibiotics on the resident gut bacteria. One approach that has been tried involves giving another product—a specially formulated product that includes a powerful adsorbent, activated charcoal—during the days that antibiotics are taken. The special product, DAV132, delivers the charcoal to the distal ileum (last part of the small bowel, before the colon), where it acts to adsorb almost all of the antibiotic that remains in the lumen (inside) of the intestine. They tested it on volunteers who were given moxifloxacin, a quinolone antibiotic. The volunteers took one dose of moxifloxacin daily for 5 days. Some of the study participants took DAV132 with activated charcoal and others received DAV132 that looked like the active product but did not contain the activated charcoal. They took the DAV132 three times daily for 7 days, continuing it after the antibiotic course was completed. When they assessed the amount of moxifloxacin that remained in the feces, they found that 99% had been removed by the activated charcoal. They also analyzed the bacteria and found that the richness and composition of the intestinal microbiota had been preserved in the participants who had received the new product with activated charcoal. They also measured the levels of moxifloxacin in the blood to see if blood levels were affected by using the new agent. They found no difference on day 1 or day 5 between the participants in the two groups. Studies on 14 other antibiotics that are commonly given as pills have also shown that this agent removes 95% to 99% of most of them. Removal of amoxicillin was slightly lower at 92%. This was a preliminary study on a relatively small number of participants. Much more work would need to be done before this could be recommended. Many patients on antibiotics are also taking other drugs. What would be the impact on those? Would this approach decrease the absorption and effectiveness of other drugs? This is just one of the ways that is being explored to try to preserve the benefits of antibiotics but reduce their impact on the human microbiota (de Gunzgurg 2018).

4

OTHER USES OF ANTIBIOTICS (NONHUMAN USE)

What are the uses of antibiotics other than to treat infections in humans?

Antibiotics are used widely in human medicine, in many other species—food animals, work and recreational animals, pets, fish, and honeybees—and on plants. They are also used in research laboratories to prevent the growth of unwanted bacteria, in some vaccines, and in other processes. We may think of antibiotics as drugs developed to treat human infections, but antibiotics and other antibacterial substances are used in many processes, including in food processing. We live in a microbial world, and antimicrobial substances are part of the ecology of life on Earth.

Key points to keep in mind are that antibiotics are widely used, and all use matters. Bacteria in our environment respond in the same way whether an antibiotic initially was given to a person, a cow, a fish, or a bee or sprayed on an apple tree.

What proportion of antibiotics produced in recent years had a nonhuman use?

The global consumption of all antibiotics in food animals in 2013 was estimated to be 131,109 tons. This amount is projected to exceed 200,000 tons by 2030 (Van Boeckel 2015).

Although the amount of antibiotic per kilogram (or weight) in food animals and humans may be in a similar range, the biomass of food animals now greatly exceeds the biomass of humans on Earth. Some numbers from China reflect the kinds of changes that are occurring. A comparison of sizes of populations of people, pigs, and poultry in 1968 and in 2005 found that the human population had increased about twofold (from 790 million to 1.3 billion). During that same period the pig population had increased almost 100-fold (from 5.2 million to 508 million) and the poultry population had increased almost 1,000-fold (from 12.3 million to 13 billion) (Osterholm 2005). In the United States about 7 billion chickens are raised and slaughtered each year.

Today many more kilograms, pounds, or tons—however you want to measure them—of antibiotics are given to animals than to humans. It is estimated that in the United States about 70% to 80% of all antibiotics produced are given to food animals. Globally it is estimated that more than half of all antibiotics produced go into food animals, but exact figures are lacking for most countries. In the United Kingdom in 2016, about 33% of antibiotics were used in food animals and 8% in companion animals (primarily pets). Some recent studies show that China uses about half of all antibiotics produced globally. With a population of about 1.4 billion, China accounts for about 18% of the global population today.

Why are antibiotics given to healthy animals?

There are three primary reasons for giving antibiotics to animals. One is to treat infectious diseases. Animals develop infectious diseases just as humans do. They are susceptible to some of the same bacteria that infect humans, but they may also become infected with bacteria that do not affect humans. Some can develop streptococcal and staphylococcal infections, which are common to both humans and animals. They can also carry microbes that do not make them sick but can cause severe illness in humans. Overall there is a lot of overlap between bacteria that cause infections in humans and animals, but each animal species has its own distinctive set of microbes that can cause disease. Many examples exist of types of bacteria (and viruses and other microbes) that cause severe disease in humans—or in one or another animal species—but not in others.

The second major reason animals are given antibiotics is to prevent infections. Food animals are often raised in herds or in settings with high density and poor hygiene. Dozens, hundreds, or even thousands of animals may be housed in a single dwelling or area. If one animal develops an infection, many others may become exposed and sick. Giving all of the animals an antibiotic by putting it in the feed or the water may prevent the chicken or pig farmer or rancher from losing the entire flock or herd. With chickens, tens of thousands of chickens may be raised in the same building. This is big business. Antibiotics are cheap. Loss of a flock or herd is costly.

The third reason is what is called growth promotion. In recent years the greatest tonnage of antibiotics given to animals in many countries has been for growth promotion. Many decades ago, shortly after antibiotics became available, it was observed that animals being raised for food, like pigs, that were given low doses of antibiotics gained weight more rapidly than those that did not receive them (Jukes 1950). This appears to be especially true when animals are grown in crowded, unsanitary conditions. Globally there has been a shift from the backyard growing of chickens and pigs to increasing use of concentrated or industrial farming operations where animals are raised in large numbers, often tightly packed together. Economically there is a benefit to the farmer from use of antibiotics. Antibiotic use in animals for many decades in the United States was largely uncontrolled and did not require prescriptions or veterinary oversight.

Studies were carried out in animals and showed that antibiotics were more effective in young pigs and could reduce deaths in nursery (very young) pigs. Since then it has been observed that benefit from antibiotics is greater when pigs are raised in environments with high density, high disease load, and poor diet than when raised under better conditions. When pigs are grown under optimal housing and nutrition conditions, the benefits from antibiotics are lower. Recent studies in the United States continue to show a small benefit in growth from use of low-dose antibiotics in nursery pigs but no benefit when antibiotics are given to older pigs. Nursery pigs, like human infants, are more susceptible to infections than older ones. Because of concerns that animal use was promoting antibiotic resistance, Denmark banned antibiotic use for growth promotion in finishing (older) pigs in 1998 and in weaning (young) pigs in 2000. This resulted in some loss of productivity in weaners (young pigs), but over the long term productivity increased. Although the ban led to a decrease in overall use of antibiotics in Danish swine production between 1997 and 2008 (from 81.2 mg/kg of pork to 48.9 mg/kg of pork), the amount used for treatment increased after 2001. This prompted new restrictions on use of antibiotics. It appears that when animal nutrition, hygiene, and genetics are optimal, the benefits from low doses of antibiotics are limited in pigs.

The European Union banned the use of antibiotics for growth promotion in food animals in 2006 and antibiotic use in animals declined 12% between 2011 and 2014. In the United Kingdom, where there has been a highly visible government strategy around antibiotic resistance, antibiotic use in animals dropped 22% between 2011 and 2014.

In the poultry industry, the ban on antibiotics for growth promotion in Denmark caused a small decrease in feed efficiency (weight gained per amount of feed). In poultry, as well as in swine, the benefits of low doses of antibiotics are less apparent with modern facilities, good environments, and optimal production conditions. Farms that have older houses and less modern equipment may see more benefit from low-dose antibiotics. Better hygienic conditions, better ventilation, better biosecurity (preventing rats, other rodents, birds, and other wildlife from mixing with the poultry), and management and use of vaccines have helped to control infections and limit use of antibiotics.

An Interagency Group on Antimicrobial Resistance convened by the UN Secretary-General has recommended that use of antibiotics for growth promotion be phased out. As of 2019 the World Organization for Animal Health (OIE) reported that at least 45 countries continued to use antimicrobials for growth promotion.

One factor driving reductions in antibiotic use today in food animals is consumer preference. Many people are willing to pay a little bit more for meat from animals that have been raised without antibiotics—though definitions as to exactly what "without antibiotics" means can be murky. What is the meaning of "no antibiotics added" or "antibiotic free" or "raised without antibiotics"? These must be clearly defined for consumers. Some large companies, such as McDonald's, have mandated the removal of antibiotics from broiler chickens sold in their outlets. Some other companies are following that lead. Publications with wide readership, like *Consumer Reports*, have provided information about use of antibiotics in agriculture and the presence of antibiotics in meat products.

What are the direct economic costs of raising animals without antibiotics? In clean modern facilities the increased wholesale prices are estimated to range from less than 1% to 2.6% higher (Teillant 2015) for the producer to raise animals without antibiotics. This does not take into account the negative societal costs from the consequences (related to resistance) of widespread use of antibiotics in food animals (see chapter 5).

A historical episode is interesting and underscores the limited understanding of the impact of antibiotics in the early days of antibiotics (McKenna 2017). When antibiotics first became available and in an era when antibiotics were viewed as totally safe, they were used in situations that would appall us today. In addition to adding low doses of antibiotics to feed for growth promotion for food animals, some producers also started a process that they named "acronize," which meant that an antibiotic, aureomycin (a tetracycline), would be applied to the outside of the chicken after it was killed and its insides removed. The term "Acronized" was trademarked by the pharmaceutical company Lederle, which produced aureomycin. Poultry producers could apply for permission to "acronize" their chickens but had to pay a fee to Lederle to do so. Ads appeared in magazines showcasing Acronized chickens and their supposed benefits (these can still be viewed online). The practice spread widely. Half of slaughterhouses obtained licenses to acronize their poultry. What were the benefits to the poultry producers? By reducing the bacteria on the surface of chickens, the chickens did not spoil as rapidly. They could be shipped longer distances and had a much longer shelf life. Producers could ship chickens to Alaska and Hawaii by sea rather than sending them by the much more expensive air transport. Pfizer, another pharmaceutical company, marketed a process called Biostat with oxytetracycline (same class of drug as aureomycin) to be used in a similar manner. The amounts of antibiotics used in the process were not regulated and were sometimes much higher than those recommended. The process was published in the Federal Register in 1955 and was approved by the US Food and Drug Administration (FDA). A similar process was also used to treat meat and fish, allowing producers to expand markets and reduce the cost of shipping.

It took several years and multiple outbreaks of serious infections in people before it was recognized that the process led to the development of resistant bacteria. The susceptible bacteria were killed by the antibiotic "bath" and the resistant ones survived and came to predominate. These resistant bacteria caused infections in chickens and in poultry workers who were handling the carcasses—and in some instances, family members. The process was stopped. Today the earlier meaning of acronize to describe this process has been replaced, according to online dictionaries, by the meaning "make a group of words an acronym" or to "turn words into acronym."

Which animals receive antibiotics?

Pigs and chickens receive most of the antibiotics given to food animals, but many food animals (e.g., turkeys, ducks, cattle, sheep, goats), fish, pets, and work and recreational animals (e.g., horses) are given antibiotics to prevent and treat infections. Many food animals still also receive antibiotics for growth promotion where it has not been banned. The volume of antibiotic use in food animals vastly exceeds the small amount that is used to treat infections in dogs, cats, and other pets. Recent data from the United Kingdom (2016) found that about 8% of antibiotic use was for companion animals, about 33% was for food animals, and the rest—almost 60%—was used in humans. Most antibiotic use in animals for growth promotion is in chickens and pigs.

Pets typically live longer than food animals and are frequently given antibiotics for illness. A study from the United Kingdom found that about a quarter of cats and dogs seen in consultation were given antibiotics. Pets also undergo surgery and other procedures that may lead to preventive use of antibiotics.

There has been enormous growth globally in food animal populations as incomes have increased in many low- and middle-income countries. People desire and can afford more animal protein. Between 1960 and 2000, global meat production increased more than threefold, milk production nearly doubled, and egg production increased by almost four times (Speedy 2003). The increases have continued since 2000. The consumption of livestock products per year globally averaged a little over 50 pounds per person in 1964–1966, but it varied from about 135 pounds per person in the high-income countries to less than 15 pounds per person per year in South Asia (FAO 2016). Consumption of animal products has increased in all countries, including the most affluent. Chicken consumption in the United States increased from 28 pounds per person in 1960 to 92 pounds per person in 2016. In 2000 in the United States, the average consumption of meat per person was about 270 pounds plus almost 50 pounds of fish per year (FAO 2016). The growth in meat production has resulted from intensive livestock production, involving especially chickens and pigs.

An important determinant of per capita meat consumption is wealth, though cultural and religious factors influence regional diets. Some affluent countries, such as Japan, have much higher consumption of fish than meat. Fish is the predominant dietary protein in some island countries, such as Iceland, Kiribati, and the Maldives.

Which antibiotics are used? Are the same antibiotics used in people also used in animals?

The same antibiotics used to treat infections in humans also work in animals, so food animals, pets, ornamental fish, and other nonhuman creatures are given many of the same antibiotics that are used to treat humans. Some of the same antibiotics are also used in fish farming.

The most commonly used antibiotics in food animals in 2009 were macrolides, penicillins, and tetracyclines. In animals, as in humans, there has been a shift to use of more broad-spectrum antibiotics.

There have been attempts to prevent use of antibiotics that are most critically important in human medicine from being used in animals. This work is ongoing. Recognizing that antibiotic use in food animals selects for antibiotic-resistant bacteria and that these bacteria and resistance genes can spread to humans, the World Health Organization has worked with other groups to develop criteria to rank antibiotics according to their importance in human medicine. This list has been revised multiple times as available drugs change, resistant bacteria appear and spread, and knowledge about the use of the drugs and possible alternatives increases. A list was first developed in Canberra, Australia, in 2005 with an international team and revised in Copenhagen in 2007 and 2009; in Oslo, Norway, in 2011; and in Bogota, Colombia, in 2013. The most recent list was made available in 2016 (Collignon 2016). The panel grouped antibiotics for human health as critically important, highly important, or important. The criteria they use are based on whether the antibiotic class is the only or one of a limited number of available therapies to treat serious bacterial infections in humans. They also considered whether the bacteria causing the infections may be transmitted to humans from nonhuman sources or whether humans might acquire resistance genes from nonhuman sources. They prioritized the antibiotics, taking into account the number of people affected and whether the antibiotic was used to treat infections from nonhuman sources.

The panel concluded that the highest-priority classes of drugs were the quinolones, the third- and fourth-generation cephalosporins, the macrolides/ketolides (e.g., erythromycin, telithromycin), and the glycopeptides (e.g., vancomycin). They also noted concerns about carbapenems and colistin, often last-resort antibiotics used when nothing else works. Ideally all of the antibiotics that have high priority for human health should be avoided or used in limited circumstances in food animals.

In the United Kingdom, where good data are available about usage, antibiotics from the group considered to be critically important for human health were prescribed in almost 40% of the instances when antibiotics were given to cats but much less often to dogs, pigs, or cattle.

In the United States the FDA is working with the Center for Veterinary Medicine to improve stewardship of antibiotics used in food animals. In the past, antibiotics, including those important in human health, could be used without requiring a prescription from a veterinarian. The aim for the future in the United States is to eliminate use of antibiotics for growth promotion and bring therapeutic use (use for treating infections) under the oversight of licensed veterinarians (requiring prescriptions for the antibiotics—as required for human medicine). It is work in progress. According to FDA commissioner Scott Gottleib in 2018, 95% of medically important antibiotics used in food animals are now under veterinary oversight. They are also working to define acceptable durations of use (recommendations listing how many hours or days a drug should be continued), which are not currently included with many of the indications for drugs that are used in food and water for animals.

In the U.S. arsenic-based drugs, which have antimicrobial properties, were used in chickens and turkeys for decades as feed additives to improve production. These were banned by the European Union in 1999. The FDA withdrew approval for two arsenic-based poultry food additives in 2013 and for one used in turkeys in 2015 (Nigra 2017). Since December 2015 there have been no FDA-approved arsenic-based drugs for use in food animals in the United States. Use of these drugs may continue in other countries. Before these were banned in the United States, studies showed that urine levels of arsenic and metabolites of arsenic were higher in people with higher poultry intake than in low or nonconsumers of poultry.

Are antibiotics used in food animals in other countries?

Antibiotics are used widely in food animals, though there are vast differences in the amounts used by country—just as there are wide differences in human use from country to country. One study published in 2017 (Van Boeckel 2017) found consumption levels varied from 8 mg/kg of animal product in Norway to 318 mg/kg of animal product in China. Global use of antibiotics has increased rapidly, driven by human population growth and massive increases in food animals. Improved economic circumstances in countries like India and China have been followed by increased demand for animal protein, resulting in intensification of food animal production—and widespread use of antibiotics. A recent analysis put the global biomass of humans at about 60% that of livestock and less than 10% of the biomass of fish (Bar-On 2018). By whatever measure, the biomass of farmed animals is large and their impact as biological systems and as a source of resistance genes is significant. The global swine population may be in the range of a billion and the poultry population a trillion.

How are antibiotics used in aquaculture?

Fish farming or aquaculture is now estimated to supply half of the fish consumed globally (FAO 2016). The per capita consumption of fish per year is now more than 20 kg globally; fish provide 6.7% of all protein consumed. Aquaculture is a rapidly growing food-producing sector and is expected to continue to grow as wild stocks of fish in more regions decline and natural areas have been overfished. More than half of the world's fisheries are now overfished. Aquaculture is practiced in many low-income countries and by multinational companies. In 2015 aquaculture produced 76.6 million tons of aquatic animals (value $160 billion; a third of which consisted of molluscs, crustaceans, and other nonfish animals) and more than 25 million tons of aquatic plants (value almost $6 billion). Almost 80% came from the Asia-Pacific region. Commercial shrimp farming, which started in the 1970s, has grown rapidly, especially in Asia. There have been serious disease outbreaks involving aquaculture in Asia in recent years.

China now leads the world in aquaculture outputs. Norway and Vietnam are the world's second- and third-largest exporters. Growth in aquaculture has also been rapid in Chile and Indonesia. India, Bangladesh, and Egypt are also in the top eight aquaculture producers. Nigeria's output increased almost 20-fold in the past 20 years.

Aquaculture can be carried out in many settings: in freshwater or salt water, in coastal areas, in tanks on land, in ponds, in pens in the sea, in fish cages, and even in artificially created reef structures. Aquaculture is not just about fish. Aquaculture involves farming aquatic organisms and includes plants, like kelp, and animals that are low in the food chain, such as herbivores, like oysters, and omnivorous fish, such as salmon. Today more than 500 aquatic species are farmed all over the world. Commercial shrimp farming, which started in the 1970s, is big business. About 75% of farmed shrimp are produced in Asia. Molluscs are also grown commercially, including oysters, mussels, and clams. Because they are filter feeders, they do not require inputs of fish and other feed and cause less disruption to local ecosystems.

Traditionally, farmed fish have been fed low-value wild forage fish as fish meal and fish oil. Globally 70% of the fish meal produced and 90% of the fish oil is fed to farmed fish. Increasingly, however, fish farmers are turning to alternative food sources, including plants and insects.

In many types of fish and shrimp farming, the animals are grown in settings with large numbers crowded together. They are also genetically similar. This combination puts them at high risk for many infections, including some caused by bacteria (and also some caused by viruses). For this reason, antibiotics are commonly used in fish farming, often to prevent infections. It is easy to see how an infected fish in a crowded pond could easily contaminate the water and spread infection to other fish. Chemical disinfectants are also used in the water. Despite the widespread use of antibiotics in aquaculture, there are no good estimates at present on the overall consumption of antibiotics in aquaculture—but anecdotal reports suggest many tons. Use of antibiotics in fish and in aquafarming appears to be largely unregulated.

A few specific examples are notable from local studies. In Chile, a country with a large, active aquaculture industry, use of fluoroquinolones (antibiotics like ciprofloxacin) in aquaculture was more than 10 times the use in human medicine during some years (Cabello 2016). A survey of 32 fish farms in Vietnam published in 2013 found that all of them used antibiotics.

Antibiotics for fish are included in their feed or administered by bath. Uneaten food along with waste excreted by fish, including unabsorbed antibiotics and their breakdown products, can be found in pond or water sediments. The antibiotic activity can persist in the water sediments for months (Cabello 2016). In Vietnam measurable antibiotic residues of trimethoprim, sulfamethaxozole and norfloxacin were found in water from shrimp ponds (Nguyen Dang Giang 2015).

Several vaccines are used in aquafarming to help reduce the risk for some infections. They have been used in finfish like rainbow trout, salmon, sea bream and seabass industries. They have not been as effective in mollusks and crustaceans, animals that lack an adaptive immune system needed to respond to current vaccines. Some bacteria that infect fish or that live in and on healthy fish can infect humans, including some of the *Vibrio* bacteria.

Among the many concerns about aquaculture are environmental damage to coastal ecosystems, including destruction of mangrove forests that have been used for shrimp farming in Indonesia and elsewhere. Many shrimp farms have been created and then abandoned because of loss of nutrients and buildup of toxins. Farm-raised fish may escape from their pens or enclosures and invade natural populations of fish. They may also interbreed with wild fish, diluting wild genetic stocks. Salmon farms can pollute coastal ecosystems when waste from salmon is discharged untreated into the aquatic environment. Waste contains antibiotics, pesticides, and heavy metals that change local ecosystems and even cause die-offs of other species. Waste can also decrease dissolved oxygen in the water, which has a negative impact on other species.

Is it OK for humans to take antibiotics that were made for fish or other animals?

People who own ornamental fish or have fish tanks may have noticed that many of the same antibiotics used in humans are also used to treat infections in fish. There are online discussions about taking fish antibiotics as they are easily available and less expensive than human antibiotics. Antibiotics for fish listed on websites include amoxicillin, ampicillin, cephalexin, ciprofloxacin, metronidazole, erythromycin, and penicillin (as well as drugs to treat fungal and parasitic infections in fish). Medication for fish dissolves in fish tanks and is absorbed and swallowed by the fish.

The main problem with people taking an antibiotic intended for fish is that fish antibiotics are completely unregulated. The FDA regulates human and some animal (companion animals like dogs, cats, and horses and food animals like cattle, pigs, and chickens) but not fish drugs. Drugs approved for animals (companion and food animals) may contain fillers, additives, and impurities that are not allowed in human drugs. Dosages of the drugs may be different in humans and animals, and formulations may vary depending on the animal involved.

There is no government oversight to ensure the quality, safety, purity, or effectiveness of these drugs that are marketed for fish. They have not been approved or indexed by the FDA. The FDA website indicates that the agency hopes someday to provide oversight for medications for "minor species" like fish that are currently unregulated.

So the short answer is that it is not a good idea to take antibiotics intended for fish.

What are the consequences of using antibiotics in animals?

There are many potential consequences of use of antibiotics, some obvious and straightforward and immediate, and others much more subtle, indirect, and potentially long-lasting. Many studies have shown that farms using antibiotics for growth promotion have a higher level of resistant bacteria (in farm workers and farm animals) than those that do not.

Being able to treat infections in animals means they will be healthier and perhaps live longer, relevant for pets and for milk- and egg-producing animals. Availability of antibiotics has made it easier to intensify food production, to raise animals in large numbers in small spaces. Use of antibiotics may also lead to decreased production costs for animals and greater availability and lower costs for food.

Consequences can be considered in several main areas. The most important is the activity the antibiotics have on the bacteria that live in and on the animals. Just as in humans, animals have bacteria that normally reside on their skin and in their mouths, their intestines, and other parts of the animal. Some of these bacteria are similar to those carried by humans; others are completely different. Each species of animal carries its own characteristic mix of bacteria (and viruses and other types of microbes). Each species also has its unique vulnerabilities and susceptibilities. A type of bacteria that normally lives in the intestine of a chicken might cause severe illness in a human but have no consequences in another animal.

Giving animals antibiotics selects bacteria (allows the survival of bacteria) that are resistant to that antibiotic (Marshall 2011). Because bacteria promiscuously share genetic information with other bacteria, the resistance genes or cassettes carrying resistance determinants may spread to other bacteria. Sometimes genetic material carries resistance to multiple antibiotics, meaning that giving an animal one antibiotic can sometimes lead to resistance to another or several other antibiotics. Although one might think that animals are on the farm and that only farmers or workers who come into direct contact might be at risk for exposure to resistant bacteria, in fact there are many pathways that connect near and distant human populations.

The link between antibiotic use in animals and antibiotic-resistant bacteria affecting humans is especially strong for common foodborne pathogens, like quinolone-resistant *Campylobacter* spp. and *Salmonella* spp. Antibiotic-resistant bacteria can also infect and cause disease in food animals.

During slaughter, flesh can become contaminated with bacteria from the intestinal tract and other parts of the body that have high bacterial loads. Animals are also processed in plants that receive hundreds or thousands of animals. Parts from one animal may contaminate others. The processing and packaging conditions are important (cleanliness, refrigeration, manageable volume, etc.). Even in modern plants, chicken, beef, and pork products that emerge are frequently contaminated with *Escherichia coli*, *Campylobacter* spp., *Salmonella* spp, and other bacteria—some of which can cause serious infections in humans. What is sold as ground beef in the supermarket may have parts of dozens or more different cows. Wrapping, transport, and storage conditions—the entire cold chain before meat reaches the home kitchen can influence the number of bacteria found on the meat.

Many studies over the years have shown repeatedly that supermarket meat products are frequently contaminated with potentially disease-causing bacteria. That is the reason for the emphasis on proper storage (don't let juice or blood from a package of raw chicken in the refrigerator drip on lettuce, carrots, or other items eaten raw), proper handling (don't cut raw chicken and raw vegetables on the same cutting board unless it is carefully washed between the two uses), and cooking. Heat and thorough cooking will kill most bacteria that contaminate meats.

Is any antibiotic still present in the meat, fish, eggs, or milk when they are sold for human consumption?

If animals receive antibiotics shortly before slaughter (especially in treatment doses that are much larger than growth promotion doses), residues of antibiotics may be present in the flesh that is consumed by people. This could be the equivalent of taking a low dose of an antibiotic and could pose a problem, especially if someone is allergic to the drug. But in the United States standards have been set defining the interval (days) that must pass between use of an antibiotic and the slaughter of an animal for consumption. These types of regulations may be nonexistent, less stringent, or less well enforced in some low- and middle-income countries. Increasingly global standards are being set and enforced for some food products.

Antibiotic residues can also be present in milk and milk products if the milk-producing cow has been given antibiotics. Again, regulations in the United States and many other countries specify what time frame is allowable for antibiotic use. Breeches do occur as is clear from testing meat and milk.

In Kenya, milk vending machines have become popular, dispensing locally sourced, pasteurized milk (and referred to locally as milk ATMs even though they are not automated teller machines). Researchers obtained 80 samples of milk from vending machines, from street vendors, and from commercial providers in Kenya and tested them for the presence of antibiotics in 2016 and 2017 (Kosgey 2018). They tested samples for tetracyclines, sulfamethazine, gentamicin, and beta-lactam antibiotics. They found antibiotic residues in 24% of milk samples from vending machines and 24% of samples from street vendors. The commercial samples all tested negative for the antibiotics. An earlier study found that 44% of milk samples from smallholder collections in nearby countries had beta-lactam antibiotic residues. In Kenya antibiotic use became widespread in the dairy industry as a way to increase productivity. Although there are regulations in East Africa that define maximum residue limits (MRLs) for veterinary drugs (from the Codex Alimentarius), adherence by small producers may be poor. Milk samples contaminated with multidrug-resistant *Staphylococcus aureus* are found twice as often from small producers as from large farms.

The Codex Alimentarius, sometimes called the "Food Code," is a collection of guidelines, standards, and codes of practice. The Codex Alimentarius Commission was established in 1963 by the Agriculture Organization of the United Nations (FAO) and the World Health Organization (WHO). The commission adopts standards. It currently has 187 member countries and many intergovernmental organizations and 16 UN agencies. It has developed hundreds of standards, guidelines, and codes. They provide guidance about permitted levels of additives, contaminants, and chemical residues, including pesticides, in food. One area where they also provide guidance is about the residues of veterinary drugs that are allowed in foods, including antibiotics. Governments may opt to follow these standards and guidelines to ensure food safety. The standards apply to processed, semiprocessed, and raw foods. They also cover guidance for import and export inspection and certification.

There is low public awareness in many countries about the use of antibiotics in food animals and fish. A national survey about antibiotics in Thailand in 2017 found that almost two-thirds of the general public did not know that antibiotics are used in food animals.

Why are antibiotics used in bees?

Bee colonies may also be treated with antibiotics. The FDA classifies bees as food-producing animals because humans consume honey and other hive products.

Bees produce honey, beeswax, pollen, and other products, but their greatest economic importance is as crop pollinators. The agricultural work of bees is estimated to be worth 10 to 20 times the total value of honey and beeswax. The value of bee pollination is estimated at about $15 billion in added crop value.

Bees are also affected by infectious diseases, with the most important one being a bacterial infection called American foulbrood caused by spore-forming bacteria called *Paenibacillus larvae* that are found worldwide (but cause no health risks to humans). It affects the larval and pupal stages of bee development and can weaken or kill entire colonies. Traditionally control of this destructive infection involved killing all the bees in the affected colony and then burning the dead bees and hive material including the wax comb, where the spores can persist.

Three antibiotics have now been approved for the control of American foulbrood. They do not cure the infection, but they can control it. The three antibiotics are oxytetracycline, tylosin tartrate, and lincomycin hydrochloride. Because these antibiotics (or ones closely related to them) are also medically important in treating human infections, the FDA now requires veterinary supervision for the use of these drugs to treat bees. In the past, the drugs for treating bees were available without prescription.

Do plants develop infections? Why and how often are antibiotics used in plants?

Plants also develop infectious diseases—and are also sometimes treated with antibiotics or given antibiotics to prevent infections. Many of these are the same antibiotics used to treat human infections.

In the 1950s, when antibiotics were starting to be used to treat many kinds of human infections, almost 40 antibiotics were tested for possible use for treating plant infectious diseases. Only a few were identified that worked. The main two used in the United States today are old antibiotics, streptomycin and a type of tetracycline. In plants, as in humans and in food animals, resistance of the bacteria to the antibiotics has shaped their use over many decades.

In contrast to humans and animals where most antibiotics are used systemically (given by mouth or injection so they can spread throughout the body), most antibiotics used on plants are sprayed or delivered to the outside of the plant. Some of the antibiotics used on plants are the same as those used in humans, but in general, plant use accounts for a tiny fraction of antibiotic use in the United States.

Most infectious diseases in plants are caused by fungi and viruses, but a few are caused by bacteria. These infections can affect ornamental (flowers and decorative) plants and food plants and have great economic importance. Many of the infections are contagious, meaning that they can be spread from plant to plant (or to a whole field, a region, or beyond). Plants can be affected by epidemics of plant infections, sometimes killing most or all of the plants (or trees). Plants don't move around like people, but there are ways infections can spread among plants. Depending on the particular infection, it may be spread by direct contact, via soil or water or wind, via insects (pollinating like bees or wasps, or others like white flies), by birds, by humans, via equipment use to prune or harvest, and other means. Some infections can also be spread in the plant seeds. Global trade in plants (and seeds) is an important mechanism for spreading of plant disease–causing microbes from one region to another.

Many of the infections respond to weather and ecoclimatic conditions, so the impact may vary greatly from year to year, depending on weather conditions. Extreme events, like drought, wind, hurricanes, and flooding, can make plants more susceptible to infections—or can kill them—and hailstorms can bruise and damage plant tissues, making them more vulnerable to infections.

Can humans pick up infections from plants?

Most of the bacteria and viruses that infect plants are not microbes that cause disease in humans. There are a few exceptions, but in contrast to animals, which carry or can be infected with a large number of microbes that infect, sicken, and kill humans, plants carry few microbes that can sicken humans. When humans become ill after eating plant food, it is typically because plants have become contaminated with microbes that have come from humans or other animals. For example, lettuce contaminated by *E. coli* O157 that causes hemorrhagic colitis (bloody diarrhea), cantaloupe contaminated with *Salmonella*, or pomegranate arils contaminated with hepatitis A virus all are a result of material—usually fecal material—from food animals or humans contaminating the produce during the production cycle. The plants do not naturally have these disease-causing microbes in and on them. Occasionally water plants will provide a home for one stage of a parasite that can be picked up if humans consume them raw—but it is not an intrinsic property of the plant. Plant foods can be contaminated by fungus (mold) that produces a potent toxin, aflatoxin. Plants can also contain toxins or can be contaminated by pesticides or other chemicals that cause illness in humans.

How can plant infections affect human health?

Besides the economic impact to growers, plant diseases can threaten food security, especially if populations in an area rely on one or a few main plant-based foods for their survival. People can starve if food plants become unavailable. Recall that the potato famine in Ireland in the mid-1800s was due to an infectious disease of potato plants. An estimated million people died due to loss of this staple food crop and another million and a half left Ireland.

The most important bacterial infection leading to antibiotic use in the United States in plant agriculture is an infection called fire blight, caused by a bacterium, *Erwinia amylovora*, that infects fruit trees. It costs growers more than $100 million each year in the United States because of tree loss and management of outbreaks. Its name, fire blight, comes from the reddish discoloration of plants that are infected. Trees have a reddish, scorched appearance. Bacteria can infect leaves, blossoms, stems, and ultimately bark—and can kill trees. It is contagious and reaches plants via open flowers, spread by insects, wind, and rain. The bacteria then migrate from the flower into the stem and branches and other parts of the tree, ultimately reaching the trunk. The bacteria can survive the winter even in cold environments in stem cankers. When warm temperatures return, the bacteria multiply rapidly and spread within the plant—and to other nearby plants. When weather conditions are favorable for spread, tree losses can be large. In Michigan in 2000, for example, a fire blight epidemic in apple orchards caused a loss of $42 million to apple growers in tree losses.

The antibiotic streptomycin (initially discovered in the 1940s and used first to treat tuberculosis) has been the mainstay for treating and preventing loss from fire blight. It was commercialized for plant agriculture as early as 1955 (Stockwell 2012) and is still used today. However, resistance of the bacteria to streptomycin was first observed in western Michigan and has been found elsewhere in North America, as well as in Israel and New Zealand. For many years the alternative used was oxytetracycline, which is less effective than streptomycin for susceptible bacteria. Streptomycin kills susceptible bacteria, whereas oxytetracycline just slows their growth. Once an orchard is infected with *E. amylovora*, the infection persists and management involves regular spraying to prevent the uncontrolled growth, damage, and spread of the bacteria. Streptomycin does not cure infections but can improve productivity and survival of the trees. In the United States in 2009, only about 15% of the area planted with apples and 40% of that planted with pears were treated with streptomycin and/or oxytetracycline.

In the US streptomycin is registered for use on apple and pear trees, celery (Florida only), peppers, tomatoes, potatoes (seed pieces), several ornamental plants – and also on tobacco plants.

Oxytetracycline is also used for the management of infections of stone fruit, such as peaches and nectarines. They are susceptible to infection by bacteria called *Xanthomonas arboricola* pv. *Pruni*, which causes symptoms that are called bacterial spot disease. The same treatment is also used in Mexico and Central America.

As noted earlier, most antibiotic treatment of plants involves surface treatment—delivering treatment to the outside of plants. Oxytetracycline is sometimes injected into the trunks of trees, like palm and elm trees, but it is expensive and labor-intensive and is generally reserved for high-value trees.

Another antibiotic, oxolinic acid, which is a quinolone, is used in some countries to manage fire blight (especially where *E. amylovora* is resistant to streptomycin) and to manage bacterial panicle blight of rice, an infection caused by the bacterium *Burkholderia glumae*. It is used to treat seeds and flowering plants in Japan. Resistant populations of *B. glumae* were identified within 10 years of its introduction in Japan, and cross-resistance to other quinolones, such as ciprofloxacin, was also observed. Ciprofloxacin and other quinolones are important antibiotics in human medicine.

In general, good data about which antibiotics are used by each country and on which crops and in what volumes are not readily available. Another aminoglycoside, gentamicin, is also used in plant agriculture in Mexico and Central America, but it is not approved for use in the United States. Other antibiotics not approved for use in the United States are used in other parts of the world, though data on the specific antibiotics are limited.

In the United States the Environmental Protection Agency (EPA) allows use of three antibiotics in plant agriculture. Streptomycin has been used since 1958 and oxytetracycline since 1972. In 2014 another bactericide containing an antibiotic was licensed for use in the United States. Antibiotics used on plants are often called bacteriocides (meaning to kill bacteria), but they are the same molecules used in human antibiotics. This latest bactericide contains 2% to 3% (varies slightly depending on the brand) of an antibiotic, kasugamycin hydrochloride hydrate. Kasugamycin was originally isolated in 1965 from *Streptomyces kasugaensis*, a *Streptomyces* strain found near the Kasuga shrine in Japan. It is an aminoglycoside antibiotic related to streptomycin, gentamicin, and tobramycin. Kasugamycin was never used in human medicine, but the other aminoglycosides have been widely used—and still are.

Although several different antibiotics (labeled as bactericides) are used on plants, the overall pounds or tons used is a tiny fraction of those used in human medicine and in animals. In 2011 use of antibiotics on crops accounted for less than 0.3% of agricultural antibiotic use. These amounts do not include the more recent use of kasugamycin.

In the United States kasugamycin is sold as Kasumin in 2-liter containers meant to be mixed with 100 gallons of water and spayed over an acre of trees. In the United States it is licensed for use on cherries and walnuts, as well as against fire blight in apples and pears. Studies have confirmed that it is highly effective for controlling the blossom blight phase of fire blight—and is an alternative for streptomycin-resistant infections. Researchers confirmed even before kasugamycin was licensed that exposures to low doses of the agent increased the risk of spontaneous mutations in bacteria that led to resistance to it (McGhee 2011).

Is food from plants contaminated with antibiotics?

Often multiple applications are given during the growing season. Biodegradation (breakdown of the antibiotic) is more than 60% at 28 days after application. The timing and the number of applications of a bacteriocide are in part determined by the weather conditions. Some states, like California, restrict the amount that can be applied or the number of applications allowed per type of crop. The label for the bactericide also specifies what is called the preharvest interval, the number of days that must pass between the last spraying and the harvest of the crop. For example, for cherries it is 30 days, for fruits like apples and pears 90 days, and for walnuts 100 days.

The preharvest interval varies by the agent used. For example, streptomycin cannot be applied within 30 days of pear harvest or within 50 days of apple harvest. The preharvest interval for oxytetracycline is 45 days. Maximum residual residues that are allowed have also been established for each antibiotic. These range from 0.20 mg/kg to 0.35 mg/kg of fruit. Studies of residues found that even at the highest levels found on fruits, dietary exposure would be 3,000 to 21,000 times lower than the dose of streptomycin used to treat infections in humans (Stockwell 2012). Regulatory oversight of these rules may be less stringent in some countries.

Kasumin is also licensed for use in Canada, and regulations in Canada allow it to be used on an even wider range of plants (e.g., greenhouse fruits and vegetables, including tomatoes, peppers, eggplant, and others) than listed for use by the EPA in the United States.

Copper is also active against many bacteria and sometimes used on plants affected with fire blight and other infections. It has a broader spectrum of activity than many of the antibiotics (and is also active against many fungi and algae). The active ingredient is copper sulfate, and it can be purchased in many forms: liquid, powders for dusting, and crystals. Some of these have been approved for use in organic products. Copper is also used in many other settings that can take advantage of its broad antimicrobial activity.

Kasugamycin is also marketed under the brand name Kasu in India (3% kasugamycin) for a wide range of grains, fruits, and vegetables, including rice, groundnuts, chili, potatoes, tomatoes, cabbage, cauliflower, other vegetables, grapes, pomegranates, etc. Many bactericides for agricultural use are also listed on websites from China. Some are labeled as broad spectrum. The amount being applied to food crops in other countries may be substantial.

Other large commercial plant crops are being threatened by infectious disease in the United States. This includes rice being affected by bacterial panicle blight (*B. glumae*). Citrus trees are also being threatened by the spread of Citrus Huanglongbing (HLB; also called citrus greening) or "yellow dragon disease," another bacterial infection caused by *Candidatus Liberibacter* spp. that was first detected in Florida in 2005 but has reached epidemic proportions and now threatens the $9 billion Florida citrus industry. It affects all citrus plants—orange, grapefruit, lemon, and lime trees. It is spread by a tiny insect vector, the Asian citrus psyllid, a nonnative insect that has infested citrus-growing areas in the United States. Quarantine and vector control have been used to try to control the spread, but already more than 130,000 acres of citrus farms have been abandoned in Florida. Output of citrus fruits from Florida has dropped by more than half in the last decade. The older antibiotics, streptomycin and oxytetracycline, as well as copper are not very effective. Among the approaches being tried is use of a combination of streptomycin and penicillin, though penicillin is not registered for use on plants in the United States (Zhang M 2011). The US Department of Agriculture has invested more than $400 million since 2009 in studying the problem and trying to find resistant plants. The infection is first apparent in yellowing of the leaves, splotchy mottling of leaves, premature death of leaves, stunting of growth, decay of roots, and ultimately death of the tree. The bacteria enter the phloem of the plant vascular system and spread throughout the plant. Copper is too toxic to be used systemically (by injection). Use and administration by different routes, including by trunk injection, of streptomycin and several forms of tetracyclines have been studied.

The United States is not alone in fighting this infection. The disease was first described in 1929 and reported in China in 1943 and South Africa in 1947. At least 33 countries reported citrus tree greening infections as of 2009.

Currently a deadly bacterial disease (caused by *Xylella fastidiosa*) is being spread among olive trees in Italy. It was first recognized in olive trees in southern Italy in 2013 and has spread from its initial focus causing a disease called olive quick-decline syndrome. It spreads from one tree to another by insects called spittlebugs. Officials are trying to contain it using quarantine, destruction of infected trees, and insecticides. They do not have an antibiotic that can cure the infection and are concerned that it could spread to other olive-growing regions in Europe.

In the long term, researchers are seeking to develop or find plants that are naturally resistant to many of these harmful plant infections, but developing such resilient plant stocks can be a slow process. In the meantime many orchards have already been severely affected. Researchers are also exploring genetic engineering approaches to develop trees that can resist infection.

Many parallels are seen between industrial farm animal production and commercial agriculture. Many food crops that provide large amounts of our nutrition today are grown commercially and often in high-density settings and with single cultivars and monocultures. If a pathogen to which this plant is susceptible invades, it can often quickly destroy the entire field or farm. Wild plants may have much lower productivity but higher genetic variety and thus greater resilience. Within a wild population there may be some plants that are resistant to an invading pathogen. Today more opportunities exist for the movement of plants and pathogens around the world through our global food supply and extensive trade networks.

To be labeled as organic, produce must comply with stringent regulations in the United States. These may vary by state. Since 2014 any fruit labeled organic must be antibiotic free. Certain other treatments, including copper, are allowed. Copper has antibacterial activity but is not an antibiotic. Also allowed is a biologic agent called Blossom Protect, described as a biopesticide, registered for control of fire blight. It contains *Aureobasidium pullulans*, a yeast-like saprophytic fungus found in plants and isolated from soil and water environments. It can be found on healthy apple and grape plants. It apparently is nourished by nonliving or decaying organic material and can antagonize several plant pathogens by competing for space and nutrients on the blossoms. It is certified for use for organic apple and pear production by the Washington State Department of Agriculture Organic Food Program. It is also certified in several European countries. It can be applied up to four times per season. It is used to prevent fire blight but also to protect fruits during storage. Because it is not a chemical or antibiotic, there is no preharvest interval (Federal Register 2015), and it is considered harmless to bees.

Theoretical concerns exist about the impact on the environment posed by the tons of antibiotics sprayed onto fruit trees and other agricultural crops. Although many target pathogens have developed resistance to the antibiotics, broad impacts on nontarget microbes and soil and water microbial ecosystems generally have not been observed, but studies are limited. Many of the antibiotics do not remain active in soil. Still these antibiotics and their residues can end up in soil and in surface waters. Their use has led to resistance among some plant pathogens, but the overall ecological effect appears to be small relative to human and animal use of antibiotics. Although each plant has a microbiome, bacteria may be less abundant and varied than what is found in the gastrointestinal tracts of humans and animals. Also, there are few bacteria that are pathogenic for both plants and humans, so we worry less about plants being a source of antibiotic-resistant bacteria that cause infections in humans.

Does feeding animals antibiotics in large production facilities (such as industrial production of food animals like chickens, pigs, and cattle) have an impact on the local environment?

There are many pathways by which antibiotic residues, antibiotic-resistant bacteria and resistance genes from food animals and plants can reach a broader environment (Marshall 2011). In animals the largest number of bacteria are shed in feces. Waste and wastewater may be used to fertilize crops and can contaminate fruits, vegetables, and other foods. Dust with resistant bacteria can be aerosolized. Birds can pick up and carry bacteria from a contaminated environment. Rats, flies, and other wildlife are also mobile and can transport resistant bacteria. Farm workers can carry resistant bacteria on skin and on boots and other clothing. Equipment used in the care and feeding of animals can become contaminated. An important source is the runoff of waste and water contaminated with it. Most agricultural facilities do not treat animal waste. It may be collected in a lagoon or at another site, which can be vulnerable to flooding and other extreme environmental events. Local streams can become heavily contaminated with antibiotic-resistant bacteria and resistance genes.

Globally animal production of feces from food animals (cattle, chickens, sheep) is about 4 times the amount produced by humans (Berendes 2018). Antibiotic residues and antibiotic resistant bacteria can be found in manure and wastewater.

Soils are a source of remarkable biodiversity. They have some of the most diverse microbiomes on Earth and play key roles in nutrient cycling and carbon cycling. The presence of antibiotic resistance genes in top soil and in ocean habitats suggests ongoing interactions and competition among the species. Soils have been an important source of substances that have antibacterial activity and have been used to develop antibiotics.

Soil samples have been archived as part of agricultural studies. At one site in Denmark, a soil archive was started in 1894 from fields with different types of treatment—treated with manure versus treated with inorganic fertilizer. Recently using polymerase chain reaction, researchers studied soils going back to 1923. They checked the levels of four different beta-lactam antibiotic resistance genes (Graham 2016). They found that beta-lactam resistance genes were significantly higher in manure-treated fields after 1940. They also found that antibiotic resistance genes significantly increased between 1940 and 2010. Soils treated with manure had resistance gene abundance that was approximately twice as high as fields treated with inorganic fertilizer. They also found that the appearance of specific beta-lactamase genes in clinical specimens matched their appearance in soils. Their findings suggest that clinical and agricultural antibiotic and resistance development are linked.

What are other sources of antibiotics in the environment?

Another source of antibiotics in the environment is through wastewater discharged from hospitals and pharmaceutical companies. Hospitals discharge wastewater heavily contaminated with antibiotic residues and resistant bacteria. In Dhaka, Bangladesh, NDM-1-positive bacteria were found in 71% of wastewater samples taken from hospital-adjacent areas versus 12% of samples collected elsewhere in the community (Islam 2017). Even after treatment with advanced wastewater treatment facilities, antibiotic resistant bacteria can persist. Many antibiotics cannot be removed completely by current wastewater treatment systems and can enter the environment as sludge and effluent (Zhang T 2011). On-site pretreatment of wastewater from hospitals and facilities with high levels of antibiotics and resistant bacteria may be needed in addition to usual wastewater treatment.

Pharmaceutical companies have been a source of antibiotic contamination of the environment in some settings. This has been reported in India, where large pharmaceutical companies produce a large share of the world's generic (sold without a brand name) drugs. To assess the nature and magnitude of this environmental contamination, researchers collected water samples near drug manufacturing facilities in southern India. They studied the samples for the presence of antibiotics and for resistance genes. They found that all environmental samples contained antibiotics, including moxifloxacin, linezolid, levofloxacin, clarithromycin, and ciprofloxacin. In some samples levels were more than 20 times the blood level of the drug needed to treat an infection in a human. The environmental samples also contained ESBL- and carbapenemase-producing bacteria and bacteria carrying multiple other resistance genes (Lubbert 2017).

Treating discharges and waste from drug manufacturing facilities is expensive. Many of the facilities in India are able produce low-cost drugs, but they may be contributing to spread of resistance genes that can incur future costs in other populations.

The 2016 Industry Roadmap for Combating Antimicrobial Resistance established a common framework for managing antibiotic factory discharges. They also developed a mechanism to demonstrate that their supply chains (source of ingredients for making the drugs) met established standards. They have also developed targets for 2020 for antibiotic levels released in wastewaters. So far at least eight large pharmaceutical companies have set discharge limits for antibiotics, but to date, none has published its discharge levels or environmental audit results.

5

ANTIBIOTIC RESISTANCE

What is antibiotic resistance?

Antibiotic resistance describes the survival of bacteria when exposed to a concentration of an antibiotic that would normally kill them or stop their growth. Although we call it antibiotic resistance, resistance is an attribute or characteristic of the bacteria. It is the bacteria that become resistant to the effect of antibiotics; the antibiotics are unchanged. It is also a dynamic process. Bacteria are alive and reproducing and responding to their environment. Antibiotics do not change. Bacteria do. Bacteria may be naturally resistant or may become resistant to one or multiple different antibiotics. Figure 5.1 displays how antibiotic resistance happens and spreads.

Antibiotic resistance is a trait of a particular type of bacteria relative to a specific antibiotic. It can vary by the particular strain or population of a particular type of bacteria. For example, one strain of *Staphylococcus aureus* may be sensitive (meaning it can be killed by the drug) to methicillin and another may be resistant. One strain may be resistant to penicillin and methicillin but sensitive to vancomycin. One type of *Escherichia coli* may be sensitive to (be killed by) ampicillin, whereas another may be resistant to it. Resistance can also change over time. A disturbing general trend globally has

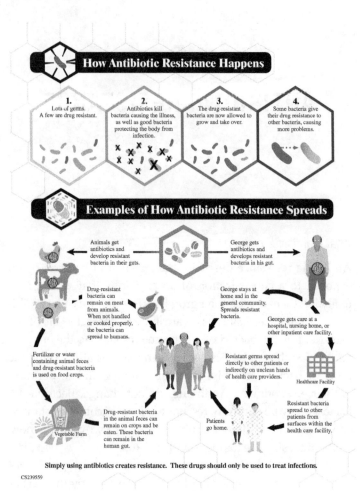

Figure 5.1 How antibiotic resistance happens and spreads.

Centers for Disease Control and Prevention (CDC). Antibiotic Resistance Threats in the United States, 2013. Atlanta, GA: CDC. CS239559, p. 14.

been the increasing appearance and spread of bacteria causing human infections that are resistant to multiple antibiotics.

Resistance is relative. There is a gray zone in which bacteria might be somewhat resistant. In some instances increasing the concentration (dose) of an antibiotic can overcome low levels of resistance. In other situations even massive amounts of antibiotic cannot overcome resistance.

Many bacteria are intrinsically or naturally resistant to many antibiotics. Because of their genetic composition, structure, or other characteristics, they can resist the effect of certain antibiotics. Even if they have never been exposed to an antibiotic, they may naturally resist the effects of many antibiotics. *Pseudomonas aeruginosa*, for example, is naturally resistant to most commonly used antibiotics. Other bacteria, such as *E. coli* and *S. aureus*, were commonly susceptible to many antibiotics in the preantibiotic era but have now become resistant to many commonly used drugs. This is one of the reasons we need to have a variety of antibiotic choices to deal with the many types of bacteria that cause human infections. Resistance to (resisting the action of) drugs and chemicals is not restricted to bacteria but is also seen other organisms, including viruses, fungi, parasites, and mosquitoes.

What is a far greater concern today is the development of acquired resistance by bacteria. In this case bacteria that were originally naturally sensitive to an antibiotic or multiple antibiotics have become resistant to one or multiple antibiotics—and in some instances to all or virtually all antibiotics currently available. Most staphylococcal bacteria were originally sensitive to penicillin at the time the drug was first discovered and used in humans. Today most staphylococcal isolates are resistant to penicillin and many also resist other related drugs, like methicillin, oxacillin, and nafcillin, that were initially developed to counteract the resistance of *Staphylococcus* to penicillin. Resistance in bacteria that infect patients can spread remarkably soon after an antibiotic is deployed for clinical use. Penicillins were first used in patients in 1943; clinical resistance was observed in patients in 1946, but the capacity to produce the enzyme beta-lactamase involved in penicillin resistance was already present in some bacteria before penicillin was ever used in humans. Methicillin was first deployed in 1960; one form of resistance was observed in 1961 and then increased and spread widely once methicillin was used. Ciprofloxacin was first deployed in 1968, and clinical resistance was observed that same year.

Resistance to a specific antibiotic may develop in one or a few types of bacteria, so appearance of resistance in certain strains of bacteria does not mean an antibiotic has immediately become useless. It may have a more limited use than initially expected. Even with the appearance of resistance among some bacteria, antibiotics may continue to be used for decades against other bacteria. For example, penicillin still works to treat some infections, even though it has been in use for more than 70 years. It no longer works against many of the bacteria it was used to treat in the 1940s and 1950s.

Many terms are used related to resistance. Some common ones are listed as follows, whereas others are defined in the Glossary:

MDR: multiple drug-resistant bacteria or multidrug resistance; describes bacteria that are resistant to multiple antibiotics commonly used to treat them

MDR-TB: refers to *Mycobacterium tuberculosis* bacteria resistant to isoniazid (INH) and rifampin, two of the first-line drugs for the treatment of tuberculosis

XDR: extensively drug-resistant bacteria; describes bacteria that are resistant to all or most of the drugs commonly used to treat them

XDR-TB: describes isolates of *M. tuberculosis* that are resistant to INH and rifampin and the fluoroquinolones (such as levofloxacin or moxifloxacin) and to at least one of the three second-line drugs given as injections (amikacin, capreomycin, or kanamycin)

PDR: describes pan-drug resistance (PDR) and typically refers to bacteria resistant to all antibiotics that have been used against those bacteria

MRSA: methicillin-resistant *S. aureus*

VRE: vancomycin-resistant enterococci

Beta-lactam antibiotics: large important class of antibiotics; includes penicillins and cephalosporins; chemical structure includes a beta-lactam ring

Beta-lactamases: enzymes produced by bacteria that break open or destroy the beta-lactam ring

Carbapenems: broad-spectrum, beta-lactam antibiotics developed to evade the action of most beta-lactamases

ESBL: extended-spectrum beta-lactamase

CTX-MESBL: cefotaxime extended-spectrum beta-lactamases

Carbapenemase: enzyme produced by bacteria that lets them survive in the presence of carbapenem antibiotic

New Delhi metallo-beta-lactamase: enzyme produced by bacteria that lets them resist almost all antibiotics

Mobile genetic elements: genetic material that can move within the genome or can be transferred from one species to another; examples include plasmids and transposons

Integrons: gene acquisition systems found in the bacteria

Plasmids: circular strands of DNA that exist in the bacterial cell, outside of the chromosome; can carry antibiotic resistance genes

Transposons: DNA sequences or segments that can change position within the genome; can replicate

Where did antibiotic resistance come from?

Antibiotic resistance is old. Bacteria have been around for billions of years, and resistance genes in bacteria are old. Resistance genes are found in bacteria that can cause disease and in those that are harmless. They are found in bacteria that live in and on our bodies and they are found in bacteria in water, air, and soil. They reside in bacteria on plants and animals. We live in a microbial world. A recent study of the biomass distribution on Earth estimated that bacteria constitute about 15% of the global biomass (Bar-On 2018). Bacteria far outnumber people on Earth—the two are not even close in number. In fact, the number of bacteria that each of us carries in and on our own bodies is more than the entire number of people living on Earth today. We each have more bacterial cells in our body than human cells. Of the estimated biomass across all taxa on Earth today—about 550 gigatons (Gt) of carbon—bacteria account for about 70 Gt of carbon (15%) and all animals (including humans) only 2 Gt of carbon. Both fish and livestock (but not wild mammals) have biomass greater than humans. We may have outsized impact, but we humans constitute a tiny fraction of the biomass on Earth. What dominates in mass? Plants are the main component, accounting for 80% of the earth's biomass.

Bacteria along with fungi and other microbes live in ecosystems in soil and in water and interact with each other in communities. Many microbes have the capacity to produce antibacterial substances. Think about the origin of many of our antibiotics. Many originated from bacteria and fungi, often from soil. Over eons bacteria also have evolved many ways to resist the action of these antibacterial substances. It is now clear that bacteria existed in nature that had the capacity to resist the action of antibiotics before antibiotics as we know them were developed and used in humans. This has been confirmed by analyzing samples from thousands of years ago—and also from studying specimens from isolated human and animal populations that had never been exposed to antibiotics. Antibiotic resistance genes are old and varied, but they were not abundant in bacteria that cause human infections until the antibiotic era—the time when humans started using antibiotics. In general, resistant bacteria have an advantage only if antibiotics are present. Resistant bacteria were not created by the development of antibiotics, but wide use of antibiotics has dramatically increased their abundance by allowing them to survive while other bacteria are killed.

The microbial world is vast, old, and diverse and has a remarkable capacity to respond to adverse environmental conditions, such as the presence of an antibiotic substance.

Bacteria can replicate rapidly (e.g., as often as every 20 to 30 minutes), so they have tremendous potential to evolve rapidly—in contrast to humans. Bacteria with a mutation that confers a survival benefit may persist. Even if a mutation occurs only once in every 10 million to 100 million replications, populations with rare attributes appear. They may not survive or thrive unless they are more fit or have a selective advantage because of the presence of an antibiotic or other special conditions. Reservoirs of resistance genes in the microbial world provide a continuing source of potential donors of resistance to bacteria that cause disease in humans.

Mechanisms that bacteria have developed to resist the effects of antibiotic substances are varied, elaborate, elegant, and well honed over eons. Bacteria employ many ways to disable, destroy, stop, or otherwise thwart the action of an antibiotic.

Antibiotics that occur naturally and synthetic ones that have been developed try to exploit any possible vulnerability of the bacteria, but the bacteria repeatedly find from their microbial network or through mutation, or through some other molecular maneuver, ways to survive in the presence of the antibiotic.

One way bacteria continue to find ways to resist antibiotics is through mutation in their genetic material. If the resistant bacteria with mutations survive, they pass the resistance to their progeny or offspring (vertical transmission of genetic material conferring resistance). This is one origin of newly resistant bacteria, but not the most common.

Widespread exposure of bacteria to antibiotics and other antibacterial substances today favors survival of progeny of rare mutants that are resistant, but most resistant bacteria today originate from horizontal or lateral transfer of resistance—side-to-side spread of resistance among bacteria rather than from one generation to the next. Horizontal transfer of resistance is common and highly efficient.

Samples of permafrost (frozen ground) from 5,000 to 30,000 years ago contain resistance genes similar to those circulating today. Resistance genes are ancient, diverse, and widely distributed. Yet another reminder that resistance genes in the environment are ancient comes from a recent study of bacteria from the deeper part of Lechuguilla Cave in New Mexico, an ecosystem that has been isolated from the surface of Earth for over 4 million years. Explorers collected samples from the cave. From these they isolated a *Paenibacillus* sp. (a bacterium) that was resistant to 26 of 40 antibiotics tested, including the newest antibiotics, like daptomycin. This bacterium also carried five new resistance mechanisms that had not been previously identified. These resistance genes were present even in the absence of any exposure to antibiotics developed by humans.

The Yanomami Amerindians in Venezuela are seminomadic hunter-gatherers, first contacted by the outside world in the mid-1960s. Recently researchers obtained samples from the skin of the lower arm, the mouth, and feces from 34 Yanomami between the ages of 4 and 50 years. They showed the highest diversity of bacterial species relative to all control groups studied. They used as controls for comparison other people who had not lived in an isolated environment. Researchers tested 131 *E. coli* strains from 11 fecal samples from the Yanomami. They found that all *E. coli* strains were susceptible to all 23 antibiotics tested. Resistance genes were present in their bacteria but were not expressed (meaning they were not actively working but could become functional if they were exposed to antibiotics).

Nonpathogenic bacteria (those that do not cause disease) in the environment carry numerous and diverse resistance genes. Nature has a large library from which disease-causing bacteria can potentially borrow resistance genes. Resistance is a natural phenomenon, but use of antibiotics has given an edge to those that are resistant. It has also become clear from studying resistance in bacteria that they often have redundant mechanisms. This means they may have many pathways to achieve the same result—to resist the antibiotic (Pawkowski 2016).

Resistance to drugs or chemicals is not a feature unique to bacteria but is a much broader phenomenon. Today, many years into the use of antiretroviral drugs, about 10% of cases of HIV being transmitted are resistant to antiretrovirals, the drugs designed to treat them. Mosquitoes in many African countries have become resistant to the killing action of pyrethroids, the chemicals that have been used to treat millions of bednets in an attempt to block the mosquito vector that transmits malaria (and many other infections). Cancer cells can become resistant to the killing effects of chemotherapeutic agents.

What are the mechanisms bacteria use to evade antibiotics?

Bacteria have evolved myriad ways to counteract, evade, destroy, neutralize, disable, and remove antibiotics and their effects on them. These fall into a few general categories, but the details and varieties of approaches are astonishing—and new ways bacteria find to evade antibiotics continue to appear and spread.

To describe the mechanisms that allow bacteria to resist antibiotics, it is useful to again consider how antibiotics work. Antibiotics have a few main approaches to killing or stopping replication of bacteria. They block the assembly of or integrity of the cell wall (cell wall synthesis inhibitors); they disrupt the integrity of the cell membrane; they block synthesis of essential proteins necessary for the bacteria (protein synthesis inhibitors); they target DNA and RNA transfer of information needed to create new bacteria (DNA synthesis inhibitors, RNA synthesis inhibitors); and they block biosynthesis of essential building blocks.

The bacteria have matched each of these mechanisms with ways to thwart the action of the antibiotic. Many bacteria do not rely on just one mechanism but may have evolved multiple approaches to avoid the action of a particular antibiotic.

In general terms, the approaches bacteria take fall into several major categories: destroy or otherwise alter the antibiotic;

prevent the antibiotic from penetrating the cell; pump the antibiotic out of the cell if it gets in; alter the target of the antibiotic (camouflage or change the target); and bypass the inhibited reaction. There are many versions and variations of each of these. The approaches bacteria have evolved to resist antibiotics are often complex, creative, and stunning in their variety.

It is worth looking at some examples in more detail to provide an idea of the range of maneuvers that are possible—and keep in mind that these are only the ones that have been identified and well defined to date.

How do bacteria destroy or disable the antibiotic?

A common approach used by bacteria is to destroy the antibiotic. Penicillin and other beta-lactam antibiotics were among the first widely used antibiotics—and remain in wide use today. The beta-lactam ring, part of the chemical structure of the antibiotic, is essential for their function. Bacteria can produce a beta-lactamase, an enzyme that destroys one of the connections in the ring, the amide bond of the beta-lactam ring, rendering the antibiotics ineffective. The enzymes split open the beta-lactam ring through a process called hydrolysis. There is now evidence that beta-lactamases are ancient. They have existed for millions of years. Penicillinase, a specific beta-lactamase that could disable penicillin, was first identified in 1940 by penicillin-researchers E.P. Abraham and E. Chain from *E. coli* before penicillin was ever put on the market.

But this specific beta-lactamase, penicillinase, that destroys the beta-lactam ring of penicillin spread quickly among bacteria once penicillins were widely used, making penicillin inactive against *S. aureus*, an important disease-causing bacterium and frequent target for treatment. The penicillinase was encoded on a plasmid (a circular strand of DNA that exists in the bacterial cell) that spread widely among *S. aureus* strains. In response to this, scientists developed new beta-lactam antibiotics, like ampicillin and methicillin, that were less susceptible to the penicillinase. This was followed by the appearance of new plasmid-encoded beta-lactamases that could break open these beta-lactam rings and resist these antibiotics as well.

Multiple generations of beta-lactam antibiotics have been developed, and more and different beta-lactamases have appeared that can hydrolyze the beta-lactam ring. The genes encoding beta-lactamases spread among bacteria through multiple mechanisms. They have been found in the chromosome of some bacteria and on mobile genetic elements, including plasmids. They can be part of integrons (or gene acquisition systems found in the bacteria). They are widespread and varied. More than 1,000 different beta-lactamases have been identified to date.

Although penicillinase production by *S. aureus* (a Gram-positive bacterium) was prominent in the early days of penicillin use, today beta-lactamases are the most important resistance mechanism in Gram-negative bacteria, like *E. coli* and other *Enterobacteriaceae*. Gram-negative bacteria can produce and secrete these enzymes when antibiotics are in the environment. It has been difficult for scientists to find or create antibiotics faster than bacteria in nature can find ways to disable them—whether from their repertoire of already existing genes or through new mutations.

The most common beta-lactamase in Gram-negative bacteria is named TEM-1, first identified in 1963. At least 140 other TEM-type enzymes have now been described. It was named after the patient from Athens, Greece, Temoniera, from which it was first identified in 1963. More recent conventions for naming beta-lactamases sometimes use the place of first identification, for example, VIM for Verona integron-encoded metallo-beta-lactamase, first reported from Verona, Italy, and NDM-1 for the New Delhi metallo-beta-lactamase first described from New Delhi in 2009.

The abundance and variety in the names of beta-lactamases reflect the extent, maturity, and duration of this antibiotic-bacteria duel. The extended-spectrum beta-lactamase (ESBL) first detected in 1979 describes the enzyme that can hydrolyze (make ineffective) third-generation cephalosporins and aztreonam. ESBLs are often encoded on plasmids; these plasmids often carry genes that encode resistance to other important classes of antibiotics, like the aminoglycosides.

The history and origin of CTX-M, a plasmid-encoded ESBL (named for activity against the beta-lactam antibiotic cefotaxime) often found in *Klebsiella pneumoniae* and *E. coli*, is especially interesting. The best evidence suggests plasmid acquisition of beta-lactamase genes from the chromosome of an obscure bacterium, *Kluyvera* sp., that is usually found in water, sewage, and soil and rarely reported in clinical infections. More than 80 CTX-M enzymes have now been described. They have spread globally and greatly complicate the treatment of infections because they confer resistance to multiple antibiotics.

A class of antibiotics called carbapenems were developed and initially reserved for treatment of serious infections caused by bacteria resistant to other antibiotics. They prevent cell wall synthesis by attaching to proteins (called penicillin-binding proteins) in the bacterial cell wall. Imipenem, a carbapenem, was approved for use in 1985 and others in the same class have become available since then. These drugs were not affected by the ESBLs, but plasmid-mediated imipenem carbapenemases were identified in Japan in the 1990s—and then spread to other countries. Other types of carbapenemases, including the Verona integron-encoded beta-lactamase, which emerged in the 1990s, have also spread. Some of the enzymes known as metallo-beta-lactamases (because they utilize a metal ion as a cofactor in the attack of the beta-lactam ring) were discovered more than 50 years ago encoded by genes in the chromosomes on bacteria that did not cause disease. This is yet another example of the capacity of bacteria to share genetic material in ways that allow them to survive in the presence of antibiotics.

The enzyme New Delhi metallo beta-lactamase (NDM-1) is notable. The gene for it has been found on several different plasmids that move readily among different species of Gram-negative bacteria. Many of these are important disease-causing bacteria, such as *Vibrio cholerae* (the cause of cholera), *P. aeruginosa, Salmonella,* and many *Enterobacteriaceae.* In some isolates the gene bla_{NDM-1} has been carried on the chromosome of the bacteria. The mobile genetic elements encoding for NDM enzymes frequently carry genes that encode resistance determinants for other antibiotics. Many of the isolates have been resistant to virtually every antibiotic. Unfortunately, it has spread rapidly.

How can bacteria change an antibiotic to resist it?

A second major mechanism of resistance bacteria use is to alter the antibiotic. Bacteria can produce enzymes that introduce changes in the antibiotic molecule. The enzymes do not destroy or break apart the antibiotic as occurs with the beta-lactamases—but these chemical changes can alter the activity of the antibiotic against the bacteria. These changes decrease the avidity (attachment, binding, or affinity) of the drug for its target in the bacteria or capacity to interact with its target. This mechanism is used by both Gram-negative and Gram-positive bacteria.

One example is the aminoglycoside-modifying enzymes that disrupt the recognition of the 30S subunit RNA binding site. This makes the antibiotic unable to inhibit protein synthesis. The genes for these enzymes are usually on mobile genetic elements but have also been found as part of the chromosomes of some bacteria. Some work to thwart the action of all aminoglycosides; others are active only against some aminoglycosides.

How can bacteria prevent antibiotics from getting through the cell wall of the bacteria?

Another major pathway bacteria use to resist an antibiotic is to prevent the antibiotic from reaching its target inside the bacterial cell. Many antibiotics must penetrate the bacterial cell to reach the target, which may lie within the cell or in the inner membrane. Many antibiotics exploit water-filled diffusion channels, called porins, to cross the cell wall barrier. Porins are specialized proteins that cross the cellular membrane and act as a pore. They are found on the outer membrane of Gram-negative bacteria and on some Gram-positive bacteria. They are involved with transport of hydrophilic (water-loving) molecules across the membrane.

Several antibiotics, such as beta-lactams, tetracyclines, and some quinolones, use porins to cross the cell membrane. Bacteria can produce proteins that can alter outer membrane porin proteins in ways that can restrict the entry of molecules from the outside or can alter the number or size of the pores within the channels. These may be associated with low-level resistance. This type of resistance may exist along with other types of resistance mechanisms.

How do bacteria manage to pump antibiotics out of the bacterial cell?

Another major mechanism of resistance is employed by bacteria that can pump antibiotics out of the cell before the antibiotic can kill them. These are called "efflux pumps." Among the earliest described in the 1980s was the system used by *E. coli* to pump tetracycline out of the inside (cytoplasm) of the cell. Since then many other efflux pumps have been described in both Gram-negative and Gram-positive bacteria. The efflux pumps are often found in bacteria that also use other mechanisms to resist antibiotics. As with genes for encoding other resistance mechanisms, genes encoding efflux pumps can be located in the chromosome or found on mobile genetic elements. Two of the most common are *tet* efflux pumps for tetracyclines and *mef* genes for macrolides. They are also clinically relevant for beta-lactam and fluoroquinolone antibiotics. More than 20 different *tet* genes have been identified, most carried on mobile genetic elements. Many of the proteins in the cytoplasmic membrane of bacteria that are involved with the efflux process are also engaged in other physiological roles. Of note, bacteria that normally produce antibacterial substances (that have sometimes been a source for antibiotics) use efflux pumps to remove antibiotics from inside the cell (in cytoplasm) to avoid buildup of toxic levels in the bacterial cell. Although in the antibiotic era these pumps found in bacteria have played a role in helping the bacteria survive in the presence of antibiotics, in evolutionary history these pumps had other important roles. In the human gut, for example, they may pump out bile salts that their human host secretes into the intestine.

These pumps are well developed, and there are five evolutionally distinct families that are found in bacterial membranes and work as pumps. They require energy because they are pumping against a concentration gradient. In Gram-positive bacteria the single-protein pumps are embedded in the cytoplasmic membrane. Gram-negative bacteria, which have two membranes to cross, have three-protein pump machineries to bridge all the barriers.

How can bacteria alter the target of antibiotic action in the bacteria?

Another mechanism of resistance is to make the target of the antibiotic action unrecognizable or unavailable. In contrast to the approach that some bacteria use to alter the antibiotic so that it will miss its target, this involves changing the antibiotic target in the bacteria—but only enough to avoid the action of the antibiotic. The bacteria still have to survive, replicate, and remain functional. Several types of target modification can be used. One is a target protection mechanism that is widely distributed among many kinds of bacteria. This involves bacteria that produce proteins that interact with the ribosome (key structure for making proteins) and dislodge the antibiotic (like tetracycline) and release it from the ribosome. The event alters the ribosome in ways that prevent rebinding of the antibiotic to the ribosome. Other proteins can displace the antibiotic molecule from the ribosome and allow protein synthesis to resume.

Mutations in genes encoding changes in the bacterial ribosome can result in decreased affinity (less able to attach) of a drug for its ribosomal target. Bacteria can produce enzymes that alter the target site. An enzyme encoded by *erm* (erythromycin ribosomal methylation) genes leads to methylation of the target ribosome and impaired binding of the antibiotic, which results in erythromycin resistance. No binding means loss of activity for the antibiotic.

How can bacteria bypass key functions to survive despite the presence of antibiotics?

Another resistance mechanism is to replace or bypass the target site. *S. aureus* can acquire the capacity to produce new penicillin-binding proteins that can perform the same function as the original penicillin-binding proteins but are not inhibited by methicillin.

The replacement-and-bypass strategy is also used by bacteria to prevent the action of vancomycin. With enterococci, vancomycin resistance involves acquiring new genes that encode biochemical machinery that remodels the synthesis of peptidoglycan, the essential cell wall material that is the target of vancomycin. By preventing vancomycin binding to cell wall precursors—materials used to build the cell wall—the enterococci can resist the action of vancomycin.

High-level vancomycin resistance of *S. aureus* was first described in 2002. This resulted from a MRSA strain acquiring a *van*A gene cluster from a VRE (*E. faecalis*) isolate. Fortunately this has been rare.

Another example of a bypass strategy is reflected in resistance of trimethoprim-sulfamethoxazole (TMP-SMX). This antibiotic, which was introduced in 1968, combines two different agents: sulfonamides and trimethoprim. Each inhibits a different key enzyme in the synthesis of folic acid, which is necessary for the bacteria to survive. When the drug was developed, it was believed that the combination of two drugs would prevent the development of resistance. This has not been the case. Multiple mechanisms of resistance have been identified, including efflux pumps and target modification. Genes encoding the overproduction of the enzymes have also been identified. These overwhelm the capacity of the antibiotic to block folate synthesis.

These examples show that bacteria have an extraordinary capacity to harness a wide range of molecular maneuvers to survive. And these just describe some of those that have been identified so far. Populations of bacteria are dynamic, interactive, and resilient. They share genetic information with each other and borrow bits of helpful machinery from neighboring bacteria, and these do not even have to be closely related bacteria.

Using an antibiotic to treat an infection begins an interaction with many populations of cells. It is not just a matter of killing off dumb bacteria. Bacterial cells are highly sophisticated biological entities and have many factors in their favor—speed of reproduction, huge numbers, and eons of experience adapting to a wide variety of environments.

What else can bacteria do to avoid being killed?

Bacteria also have other maneuvers to avoid the action of antibiotics that do not involve antibiotic resistance in the usual sense. They can form spores—creating an armor or fortress around them. Under unfavorable environmental conditions or a lack of nutrients, some bacteria have the capacity to form an endospore within the bacterium. In this state the bacteria can survive drying, heat, ultraviolet radiation, and chemicals that would kill most bacteria. Some bacteria have been shown to survive for centuries. Some well-known bacteria that are able to form endospores include *Clostridium tetani* (the cause of tetanus), *Bacillus anthracis* (the cause of anthrax), *Clostridium botulinum* (the cause of botulism), *Clostridium perfringens* (the cause of gas gangrene), and *Clostridioides difficile* (the cause of colitis, frequently following antibiotic treatment). These bacteria can exist in two states. One is a vegetative or active, reproducing growth state when nutrients are available and conditions are favorable. During times of starvation or nutrient insufficiency, they form endospores and become inactive but also difficult to kill. *C. difficile* endospores can survive 2 years (see section on *Clostridioides difficile* in chapter 3), but endospores of some bacteria have been reactivated after centuries of no active growth. For example, endospores found in Egyptian tombs were, when exposed to favorable conditions, able to activate, germinate, and grow.

Bacteria can play dead. They can enter a state of slow metabolic activity during which they are not actively growing and replicating. Many antibiotics depend on active growth and replication to do their work. A quiescent bacterium may be unaffected or only slowly affected by an antibiotic. This is true of the *M. tuberculosis* bacteria in patients with latent or inactive tuberculosis. Infection can remain latent or inactive for years or decades before reactivating. Treatment to prevent latent tuberculosis from becoming active requires a longer course of medication than treatment for most infections, which can be treated with a few doses or days of antibiotic.

Another survival mechanism is through the development of biofilms. This can occur in the human body or outside the body, on an inert surface, like a drain pipe. Bacteria can aggregate in densely packed communities—like cities of bacteria. They share nutrients and can communicate with other bacteria about the size of the population through chemicals (quorum sensing). They generate and secrete extracellular polysaccharides that protect them from host immune responses. Antibiotics cannot easily penetrate the slime-like matrix to reach them even if the bacteria are intrinsically sensitive to antibiotics. Biofilms are common in nature and are involved in dental plaque (the sticky film on teeth made up of masses of bacteria) and many chronic infections, such as lung infections in patients with cystic fibrosis. Biofilms form on plastic intravenous catheters, in artificial joints, and on other foreign material that may be implanted or inserted into the body. They are challenging to treat because antibiotics cannot easily reach the protected bacteria.

How does one test bacteria for resistance to antibiotics?

Laboratory tests can determine whether an antibiotic can kill or stop the growth of bacteria and the amount required. When an antibiotic that previously was effective in treating a particular infection, like a staphylococcal skin infection, fails to work or is slow to clear an infection, clinicians may suspect the bacteria have become resistant to the antibiotic, but this must be confirmed with laboratory testing. In general, there is extensive laboratory work that goes on before an antibiotic is ever approved for clinical use and this continues for the life of the antibiotic.

Before an antibiotic is ever marketed, scientists test it in the laboratory and then do clinical trials in people. They test a potential antibiotic against a whole range of bacteria that are known to cause infections in humans. They may first do studies in animals and test various concentrations to determine which types of infections might be effectively treated with the drug in concentrations that are safe to give to humans.

When an antibiotic is approved by the FDA, it is approved for specific clinical indications, for example, for urinary tract infections or skin and soft tissue infections and for infections caused by specific bacteria or types of bacteria. Based on laboratory testing and clinical trials, information about how well it works (its efficacy) against various infections is also made available at the time of FDA approval. This means that clinicians have reasonably good guidelines about what to expect when they use the drug.

Microbiology laboratories in hospitals test material from patients. Samples of blood, urine, sputum, cerebrospinal fluid, and other specimens from patients with suspected or documented bacterial infections can be sent to the laboratory for testing. Depending on the infection and the laboratory, the laboratory technicians may be able to grow the bacteria causing a person's infection. If they grow the bacteria ("culture" or "isolate" the bacteria), they can identify the bacteria (for example, *E. coli*, *S. aureus*, *K. pneumoniae*) and test it against whole panel of antibiotics and relay results to the clinician. This is especially important when bacteria are found in the bloodstream, usually indicating a serious infection.

Clinicians might suspect that bacteria have developed resistance to an antibiotic when treatment does not work—when the patient does not get better despite treatment that should be effective. They would also suspect resistance when specimens, like sputum or urine, continue to show growth of bacteria despite treatment with an antibiotic that should work. The laboratory can also run tests to determine if the bacteria are sensitive to an antibiotic. In the past a method called the Kirby-Bauer approach was used. Traditionally testing was done by growing the bacteria, spreading a thin layer of the bacteria on a large agar plate (shallow plastic dish containing a layer of agar that provides nutrients for bacteria), and placing multiple small discs on the plate, each impregnated with different antibiotics (see Figure 2.1 in section on How does one decide which antibiotic to use?). The antibiotic discs contain a concentration of antibiotic that would correlate with the level of antibiotic that could be achieved safely in the human body. The agar plate is placed in an incubator overnight to allow growth of the bacteria. The antibiotic from the discs diffuses into the agar surrounding each disc and the highest concentration of the antibiotic is immediately adjacent to the disc. Discs are placed far enough apart so that the agar around each disc has only one antibiotic in it. After allowing time in the incubator, the agar plate is examined for growth of the target bacteria and any clear zones—zones where bacterial growth has been prevented—around each antibiotic disc are measured. In areas with no visible growth, the bacteria have been inhibited by the presence of the antibiotic. Minor variations of this approach have been used in clinical laboratories for many decades—and this approach is still used in some areas.

In most hospitals in the United States there are now automated systems that have replaced the traditional disc diffusion approach (Kirby-Bauer) used in the past. Results must be interpreted when reports are sent to clinicians. Standards and official guidelines are available to assist in the interpretation of results. For example, at what minimum inhibitory concentration (MIC) of antibiotic is a bacterial isolate considered sensitive, intermediate, or resistant to an antibiotic? Whether an antibiotic will work for a particular infection may also depend on the location of the infection in the body. A bacterial infection in the urinary tract may be effectively treated with an antibiotic that on laboratory testing shows marginal activity if the particular antibiotic is one that is eliminated from the body by the kidneys and is present in the urine in high concentrations.

The laboratory staff must decide which antibiotics to test and which results to report to clinicians. Some hospitals restrict the use of some antibiotics because of expense, toxicity, or other factors. In choosing an antibiotic to treat an infection, clinicians typically look over the list of antibiotics tested on the bacteria and pick one that is marked as "sensitive."

Laboratories play an important role in deciding which information to report and how to display it. Laboratories also collect and analyze data about bacteria isolated and resistance patterns for that institution and can review and communicate trends over time. They can provide what are called antibiograms—a profile of resistance patterns for various bacteria and antibiotics in that particular hospital or region. Laboratories can also alert clinicians when they identify an isolate that is extensively resistant—a situation in which isolation of the patient or other special precautions may be warranted to avoid spread of the bacteria. The laboratory staff may be the first to identify a cluster of identical bacterial isolates from an intensive care unit or neonatal care unit or from the community suggesting an outbreak that may need to be investigated to determine the source and means of transmission. Microbiological laboratories can play an important role in providing essential information for the antibiotic treatment of infections.

How does antibiotic resistance spread among bacteria?

The capacity of bacteria to resist the effect of an antibiotic can spread to other bacteria via two major mechanisms. The first is relatively straightforward; the second is much more complicated and more common.

The first occurs through genetic mutation in the bacteria. If a genetic mutation occurs in the chromosome of the bacterium that allows it to survive in the presence of an antibiotic, the surviving bacterium will pass the mutation to future generations, to its offspring or progeny (vertical transmission). An example is mutation in a gene encoding the target for the antibiotic. In some instances, bacteria with mutations conferring resistance to an antibiotic are less fit (less able to reproduce), so they may not survive at all—or may be able to survive only or primarily in the presence of the antibiotic that kills other bacteria (that are competing for nutrients in the same environment). Resistance that works through many different mechanisms can occur via genetic mutation. Some types of resistance require multiple sequential mutations. In many instances progeny resulting from mutations do not survive because of the fitness cost of resistance—they cannot compete with nonmutants. If they do survive, they may become the predominant population and may displace antibiotic-susceptible populations of the same bacteria. This is vertical gene transfer.

As noted earlier, mutations may be rare events, but bacteria, because of their short generation time (can replicate in as short a time as 20 to 30 minutes) and their large numbers, have many opportunities for mutation. The frequency of spontaneous mutations leading to antibiotic resistance has been estimated to arise in 1 in every 100 million to 1 in every 1 billion replications, but this varies with the antibiotic-bacterium pair. More mutations in bacteria are required for resistance to develop to some antibiotics than others.

The second major category or way of becoming resistant involves the bacteria acquiring foreign DNA. The process is called horizontal or lateral gene transfer. This is a process whereby packets of DNA that can confer resistance are transferred from one bacterium to another—and then can continue to be spread in the progeny (offspring) of the recipient bacterium. Critically important, this type of gene transfer can occur between different species of bacteria. It can occur in nature and in humans and animals. The process often involves what are called mobile genetic elements that can move within and between cells and helps to spread resistance.

There are three main ways that horizontal gene transfer occurs: transformation from free DNA, transduction from a bacteriophage (a virus that infects a bacterium), and conjugation. Transformation from naked DNA is the least common and involves uptake of free pieces of DNA from the environment, usually from nearby dead bacterial cells. The DNA becomes part of the DNA of the host bacterium and is passed to progeny (offspring).

Another main pathway is transduction, which involves infection of the bacterium by bacterial viruses or bacteriophages (phages). The phage can inject DNA into the bacterial cell. One possible outcome (alternative to death of the bacterium) is that the phage can find a place on the host chromosome and excise some host cell DNA. Bacterial genes can accompany the phage genes and spread through populations. Phages regularly infect Gram-negative and Gram-positive bacteria.

The last process is conjugation or what is sometimes called bacterial sex, whereby DNA is transferred between live bacteria. This involves direct physical connection between one bacterium and another. It is the most common mechanism for spread of resistance among bacteria and it often involves plasmids. Plasmids are small, circular, self-replicating, extra-chromosomal pieces of DNA. They carry supplemental genetic information, often including antibiotic resistance genes. Multiple plasmids can reside in the same cell. Plasmids can carry multiple antibiotic resistance genes and are frequently transferred via conjugation. The presence of plasmids in bacteria is old, but a study of clinical specimens of intestinal bacteria from the preantibiotic era found that the plasmids at that time did not carry antibiotic resistance genes. They do now. Plasmids are found in bacteria in soil and marine samples. Many of the beta-lactamases that inactivate many antibiotics are carried on plasmids. Through conjugation, bacteria can transfer plasmids rapidly and to unrelated bacteria. This can often happen in a hospital setting and in the human gastrointestinal tract.

Other systems are used to transfer resistance genes. A resistance gene (or a few) can reside on bits of DNA called transposons. These can jump from a plasmid or chromosome on one bacterial cell to another. Integrons are another system that aids in the horizontal transfer of genetic material that can move resistance elements from one bacterium to another. Integrons are genetic platforms that allow whole cassettes of mobile genetic elements to move among bacteria, again helping the bacteria adapt rapidly to a changing environment that includes antibiotics or other substances that threaten their survival. Because of the massive amounts of antibiotics and other antibacterial substances used, these mobile genetic units are now widespread.

It has been observed that taking one antibiotic can lead to resistance to a different antibiotic. Taking amoxicillin to treat gonorrhea (in the past, when it still worked) could be shown to increase resistance in fecal *E. coli*. Use of a single antibiotic can lead to the appearance of bacteria resistant to multiple antibiotics. Resistance determinants encoded together can spread to other bacteria. Resident bacteria in the gut can harbor resistance genes that they can pass to other bacteria and can share with bacteria that can cause disease (pathogens). It is important to recognize that the antibiotic resistance genes are not limited to the bacteria that make us sick or to the bacteria that are found in and on our bodies.

Where does this transfer of resistance genes among bacteria take place?

Bacteria have multiple mechanisms to transfer resistance genes from one bacterium to another as described earlier. They can exchange resistance determinants not only with their own species of bacteria (like *E. coli* to *E. coli*) but also to unrelated bacteria. They can transfer whole cassettes at one time that lead to resistance to multiple antibiotics, as noted earlier. This can occur in humans, animals, the environment, and any place where multiple species of bacteria reside together and comingle. The presence of an antibiotic in the environment can eliminate some of the background bacteria and make it easier for bacteria resistant to it to survive and thrive. As a reminder, we talk about antibiotic resistance, but it is the bacteria that are resistant, not the antibiotic. Bacteria can rapidly evolve, mutate, and change to become resistant. The antibiotic stays the same, but it can become ineffective over time if the bacteria change.

In the human body by far the greatest number, variety, and density of bacteria reside in the gut—and this also provides a relatively protected environment in which bacteria can be transported from one geographic region to another. Humans provide mobile homes for the transport of bacteria and resistance genes from one area to another. Humans provide food (nutrients) and shelter for the bacteria. The bacteria are alive, dynamic, metabolically active, and constantly undergoing creative swaps, exchanges, and acquisitions that contribute to the enormous variation in bacteria. Bacteria with a doubling time of 20 to 30 minutes can adjust to a changing environment.

The difference between a pathogen (microbes that cause disease) and other bacteria (like the resident bacteria that live in our guts and provide essential services for our well-being and survival) is often not clear-cut. Bacteria exhibit a spectrum in their capacity to cause disease—and context matters a lot. Some bacteria, like the bacteria that cause plague, normally never colonize or reside in or on the body without causing disease. Other bacteria, including several that have the potential to cause severe disease, like *Neisseria meningitidis* (cause of severe meningitis), can sometimes be carried in the throat without invading or causing disease or any symptoms. Others, like *E. coli* and many bacteria found in the gut, normally do not cause disease but have the capacity to cause severe disease if they are found in certain locations (urinary tract or peritoneal cavity) or if human host defenses are severely compromised, as occurs in patients on chemotherapy.

So bacteria have multiple channels for spreading genetic elements that confer resistance among each other—but how do they travel the world? It is worth examining their multiple potential avenues for spread.

How do resistant bacteria and resistance genes spread globally? What is the role of travel in the movement of resistant bacteria and resistance genes globally?

Humans carry bacteria and facilitate their movement through multiple channels. We have seen many of the mechanisms that bacteria use to resist antibiotics and how resistance genes can spread vertically in bacteria (from parent to offspring/

progeny) and horizontally from bacteria to other bacteria that they come into contact with. But today we are seeing bacteria that resist multiple antibiotics in most parts of the world. How does that happen? How do resistant bacteria move globally?

Multiple processes continue in parallel. For example, bacteria continue to mutate and pass resistance to progeny as they replicate; they also continue to acquire resistance genes from other neighboring bacteria. Resistant bacteria can acquire additional resistance genes—and sometimes an entire cassette of genes encoding resistance. They are also moved around the world by some of the means described later—but all processes continue in parallel and interact to permit the wide distribution of multiply resistant bacteria. Some strains are more fit (can survive better) and are better able to spread widely and rapidly. Hospitals are often a site where resistant bacteria accumulate and spread to especially vulnerable populations.

Living creatures are extensively connected today. Humans have always migrated and explored new lands throughout history, but the volume, distance, and speed of travel by humans today is unprecedented. More than a billion people travel across international borders each year (>1.2 billion in 2015). People travel by air, land, and sea—and can now reach virtually any part of the earth within a day or two. Travel by foot, horseback, and sailing vessels has been expanded by multiple options for rapid transport, including air travel. Networks of roads, tunnels, railroads, and trails cross borders and bridge rivers, mountains, and ecosystems that were once a barrier to the movement of people, animals, and microbes.

Human travel is an important channel for the flow of resistant bacteria and resistance genes around the world. When people travel, their microbial residents accompany them. Humans provide a mobile home for bacteria and other microbes—and antibiotic resistance genes. People provide food, shelter, and transport for this microbial organ, which is how some have described the gut microbiota, allowing microbes to reach the most distant places on Earth. People may pick up and drop off new microbes en route or at their destinations. They may carry new bacteria home with them—whether or not they have any symptoms that would suggest a change in their microbial composition.

Techniques available today make it possible to determine whether two microbial isolates are identical. This is important in tracing the origin and spread of infections. Many bacteria may appear similar superficially when identified in the laboratory, but genetic sequencing and other analyses allow clinicians to find out whether isolates that are both *E. coli* or both *Salmonella*, for example, are identical or not. This information can be critically important in investigating an outbreak of infection or determining the origin and spread of an infection. Today with the volume and rapidity of travel, cases from outbreaks with the same origin may appear on two or more continents over a short time span. Without genetic testing of the bacteria—and surveillance and communication channels—it may be impossible to establish linkage and take the steps necessary to interrupt ongoing dissemination.

We live in a world in motion, and human travelers are a key part of this global movement. The world is heterogeneous in biological diversity, and risks of exposures to many bacteria vary from one place to another. Some bacteria are geographically focal and found in only limited areas; others, like *Staphylococcus* and *Streptococcus*, are found worldwide. Most of those that are found only in focal areas can be carried anywhere by travelers. Travelers can carry pathogens—bacteria that cause disease, like Group A *Streptococcus*—and they can also carry resistance genes, often silently. If resistance genes transfer to pathogens, it can make them more difficult to treat.

Travelers serve many roles. One is as victim. In the early years of exploration of new areas, especially in the tropics, they often died from infections for which they had no immunity, such as yellow fever and malaria, that did not exist in their home communities. Today with vaccines and preventive medications, travelers going to new places can be prepared for exposures to unfamiliar microbial threats like malaria, typhoid fever, and Japanese encephalitis.

Travelers can serve as sentinels (Wilson 2003). They sample the local environment they visit. They eat, drink, breath, swim, bathe, have sex, and interact with the local humans, animals, and ecosystem. They can become infected or colonized (carry bacteria without symptoms) with bacteria in this new environment. Thus, they can serve as a sentinel population, providing biological material from their bodies upon return—bacteria, viruses, parasites, resistance genes, or antibodies—that help to define the microbes that are found in the areas they have visited. This can be valuable in mapping the global distribution of various infectious diseases. A global network, the GeoSentinel Surveillance Network, has been systematically collecting and analyzing data from travelers for more than 20 years. The network now has 71 sites around the world where GeoSentinel health providers evaluate ill travelers who have returned or are in transit. The database now includes more than 300,000 records from travelers who have visited many destinations worldwide. GeoSentinel health providers see sick travelers and diagnose and treat whatever the problem is and then report the findings in a standard way to a central database. This is analyzed and summarized and shared through publications and other channels (Leder 2013). Having knowledge of which infections occur in various locations (and making this information available to health providers globally) allows providers to educate future travelers about local risks and provide vaccines or suitable preventive measures. When a provider evaluates a returned ill traveler, this knowledge of disease distribution also helps to guide diagnostic testing and initial treatment. Data from these sentinel travelers can thus guide recommendations about interventions.

Travelers often return to areas that have sophisticated laboratory testing that is unavailable in many low-income countries where an infection may have been acquired. This allows for antibiotic susceptibility testing and detailed analyses of microbes that cause disease. A clinical laboratory in Toronto may be able to define the serotype, genetic sequence, or other characteristics of a bacterium or virus causing an outbreak in Uganda because a traveler has carried it home to Toronto.

In addition to being sentinels, travelers can also be carriers of infection and a source of microbes that can spread to local populations. This is not new. The plague, a bacterial disease that devastated Europe starting in 1347 and killed 30% or more of the population, probably originated in China and traveled along the Silk Road. It was later carried throughout the Mediterranean and Europe by fleas and rats that were regular passengers on ships.

Columbus and those who followed brought infections to the New World that were new to local populations. Infections such as measles and smallpox decimated populations of local residents who lacked any previous exposure to these infections. The historian Alfred Crosby discussed the biological and cultural consequences in his book *The Columbian Exchange* published in 1972.

Travelers continue to introduce infections into new areas, but today the volume, reach, and speed of travelers is much greater than in past centuries. Although many of the infections moved by travelers in recent decades are caused by viruses— such as severe acute respiratory syndrome (SARS), Middle East respiratory syndrome (MERS), HIV, Zika, and chikungunya— these outbreaks in new populations document the ongoing microbiological exchange among populations (Wilson 1995). Travelers also move bacterial infections and resistance genes, as will be seen in some of the examples discussed later.

How do travelers pick up multiply resistant bacteria? Where are the resistant bacteria found?

A 2010 study from the United Kingdom published in the medical journal *Lancet Infectious Diseases* made headlines (Kumarasamy 2010). Gram-negative bacteria (in the general family *Enterobacteriaceae*) from India and Pakistan and from patients in the United Kingdom were found to be resistant to virtually every antibiotic ever developed. Most carried a resistance gene on a plasmid that could readily be transferred to other bacteria. The enzyme was named the New Delhi metallo-beta-lactamase-1 using the convention to name resistance mechanisms after the place where they were first found. The first published report naming the resistance gene in 2009 described infection in a Swedish man of Indian origin who had traveled to India in 2007 and was hospitalized in India with an infection. He had surgery in New Delhi in late 2007 and received multiple antibiotics. When he returned to Sweden in early January 2008, he was found to be infected with multiply resistant bacteria that carried a resistance gene and produced what was later characterized and named the New Delhi metallo-beta-lactamase-1 (NDM-1).

Other researchers worked to find out where bacteria with this resistance gene were found and the extent of its spread. By 2010 it was found in bacteria from multiple places in India, Pakistan, and Bangladesh. But it was also found in multiple different bacterial isolates in the United Kingdom. When researchers tried to determine where the resistant bacteria in those patients had originated, they found that among 29 UK patients with the resistant bacteria for whom they had information (32 isolates in total), 17 had traveled to India or Pakistan within the previous year and 14 had been hospitalized during their trips. Reasons for hospitalization were varied and included kidney or bone marrow transplantation, dialysis, cosmetic surgery, road traffic injury, and burns.

Some of the same researchers returned to India in the fall of 2010 to assess how widely dispersed these resistant bacteria were in the environment (Walsh 2011). They collected 50 samples of tap water (public water supplies used for drinking, washing, and food preparation) and 171 samples of seepage water (e.g., pools of water found in streets) in New Delhi within a 12 km radius of the city center and carried them back to the

United Kingdom. There they tested them along with samples of water from Cardiff Wastewater Treatment Works in Wales as controls. They looked for bacteria by checking for growth of bacterial colonies on agar that contained multiple antibiotics so that only extremely resistant bacteria could grow.

They then tested bacteria for the presence of NDM-1. They found that NDM-1-positive bacteria were present in 2 of 50 tap water samples and 51 of 171 seepage water samples from New Delhi and in no samples from Cardiff, Wales. The resistance gene was found in multiple different species of bacteria, including in bacteria in which it had not previously been reported. These included *Shigella boydii* (which can cause shigellosis manifested as dysentery), *Vibrio cholerae* (the cause of cholera), and *P. aeruginosa*. Most of the bacteria carried the resistance gene on plasmids, although two carried it on their chromosomes. The researchers did other laboratory tests to determine how easily the resistance genes could spread. They found that the resistance plasmids could easily be transferred to other bacteria. They tested it at different temperatures and found that the transfer of resistance genes was more efficient at 30°C (about 86°F) than at higher or lower temperatures. The average peak daily temperature in New Delhi reaches 30°C, a temperature within the daily range for 7 months of the year. These ideal temperatures for the transfer of these resistance genes are commonly found in tropical and subtropical regions.

The publication of the paper from India led microbiologists to examine their collections of bacterial isolates for the presence of this resistance mechanism in the past—at a time before it had been characterized and named. The earliest date bacteria were found that carried this resistance gene was in 2006 in Indian hospitals. In tertiary care (referral) hospitals in India and Pakistan, NDM-1-positive bacteria were found in outpatient stool samples and in higher prevalence in inpatients and patients in intensive care units. Studies of archived (saved) bacterial specimens identified isolates as early as 2009 in China from four different provinces and from a tertiary care center in Nairobi, Kenya, between 2007 and 2009.

The enzyme NDM-1 does not cause illness, but the bacteria that carry the gene that encodes the enzyme can make people sick—and this genetic element has been found in many types of bacteria that cause severe disease and can kill. The gene can be carried by bacteria that are found in healthy people and would cause no symptoms—unless those bacteria caused infection or transferred the genetic element to bacteria that can cause disease.

Although we will never know with certainty exactly when and where this novel mechanism for resistance first occurred, we know when the first patient was identified with such an infection and a report published in the medical literature. Use of the name New Delhi metallo-beta-lactamase-1 has created controversy, with some people in India claiming that the name tarnishes India's reputation for safe medical care and unfairly blames India for its emergence. It is true, however, that many of the initial reports of infections were in people who received medical care in India. The bacteria with this resistance gene have since appeared in many parts of the world. By 2010, bacteria with NDM-1 had been reported in the United States, Israel, Turkey, China, India, Australia, France, Japan, Kenya, Singapore, Taiwan, and the Nordic countries—presumably carried to those countries by travelers. Other countries have reported its presence since then.

NDM-1-positive *E. coli* were reported from municipal wastewater in Jeddah, Saudi Arabia. Wastewater was sampled five times over a period of a year from 2012 to 2013. Researchers found the NDM-1-positive bacteria in concentrations of 10,000 to 200,000 per cubic meter of water and found them throughout the sampling period. The authors reporting this finding expressed concern because Jeddah does not have a sanitary waste system with the capacity to capture all of the sewage. Only about 50% of the city of Jeddah is connected to a centralized wastewater treatment plant. The rest of the waste is managed with septic tanks that discharge partially treated wastewater (Mantilla-Calderon 2016). Saudi Arabia is a critically important location because of the Hajj. Each year Jeddah is the entry point for up to 2 million pilgrims who are arriving from more than 180 countries. See discussion of mass gatherings later in this chapter.

A study published in 2014 from China described the presence of bla_{NDM-1} genes in water that had been treated at wastewater treatment plants. The resistance genes survived several parts of the treatment, including disinfection by chlorination. The resistance genes were also found in high concentrations in dewatered waste sludge that was used to apply to soils, raising the possibility of another avenue for resistance genes and resistant bacteria to reach humans—that is, through the food supply of plants gown in these soils (Luo 2014).

A different study from China looking at estuaries also found widespread environmental pollution with antibiotic resistance genes. Researchers sampled water from 18 estuaries along 4,000 km of the east coast of China (Zhu 2017). They analyzed the specimens using high-throughput polymerase chain reaction (PCR) to look for antibiotic resistance genes. They detected 259 antibiotic resistance genes—on average 118 per estuary. These conferred resistance to most classes of antibiotics used in humans and animals. They found vancomycin resistance genes in all estuaries. They also found residues of common antibiotics in the water, including tetracyclines, sulfonamides, fluoroquinolones, and macrolides. They found a positive correlation between the presence of antibiotic residues and the presence of resistance genes. This study showed the wide distribution of resistance genes in areas with large populations of humans and animals. Water is used for irrigating food crops, for raising fish, and in other ways that can potentially provide pathways for resistance genes to reach humans.

A few studies have assessed what happens after people pick up multiply resistant bacteria. Once people pick up the resistant bacteria, they can persist, usually in the gastrointestinal tract (but sometimes also in a chronic wound infection). One woman who carried NDM-1-positive bacteria in the intestinal tract and was tested for it over time carried it until she died 13 months later.

Because of the cases of travelers carrying unusual and resistant bacteria, the Centers for Disease Control and Prevention (CDC) now recommends that clinicians in the United States should consider screening for multiply resistant bacteria (particularly carbapenem-resistant *Enterobacteriaceae* [CRE]) in patients who report recent health care exposures outside the United States or in regions of the United States with a high incidence of CRE. In the fall of 2016 a woman developed septic shock (life-threatening complication of infection) in Nevada (Chen 2017). She had previously had multiple hospitalizations in India related to a thigh bone fracture complicated by a bone infection. She was infected with an NDM-1-producing *K. pneumoniae* that was resistant to 26 antibiotics. The only drug to which it was relatively sensitive was fosfomycin, but that drug was approved in the United States at that time only as an oral treatment for uncomplicated bladder infections. An intravenous formulation is available in some other countries. The patient died from the infection. She had been placed in a private room with contact precautions. After she died the staff carried out active surveillance studies to see if the bacteria had persisted or spread, but no evidence of spread was detected.

In caring for patients with multidrug-resistant infections the goals are twofold: finding effective treatment for the infected patient, which may include surgery and antibiotics, and preventing spread to the hospital environment, health care providers, and other patients.

How often do travelers pick up resistant bacteria? Do they spread them to others?

These highly visible examples led researchers to assess how often this was happening. For example, how often do travelers to another country pick up and carry home resistant bacteria without knowing it? Do they spread to others? Can they make them sick?

Researchers have now done multiple studies to try to answer some of these questions. A study published in 1990 by researchers studying diarrhea in travelers showed that US travelers to Mexico picked up resistant bacteria even if they did not take antibiotics. A later study (published in 2010) assessed Swedish volunteers who provided rectal swabs before and after travel. These were cultured in the laboratory and checked for the presence of resistant bacteria. As an aside, Sweden, along with some of the other northern European countries, has a low background rate of antibiotic resistance.

On average, these travelers spent about 2 weeks abroad. In this study the researchers found that almost a quarter of the travelers picked up a type of multiply resistant *E. coli* (called ESBL-producing *E. coli*) during travel and carried it home. All three travelers who took the antibiotic ciprofloxacin for diarrhea acquired the resistant bacteria. The likelihood of picking up the resistant bacteria depended on the country visited. Among those who traveled to the Indian subcontinent, eight of nine (88%) acquired the resistant bacteria. Rates of picking up resistant bacteria were lower for other regions. At 6 months after return from travel, almost a quarter of those who had resistant bacteria on return from travel continued to carry the ESBL-producing *E. coli*.

Many additional studies, some much larger, have followed, including one that studied travelers from New York. Many have studied European travelers, but others have looked at residents from North America, Asia, and Australia (Kantele 2015; Kantele 2016). Some have had longer follow-up and others have assessed whether there is onward transmission of resistant bacteria to close contacts. The best single study was a prospective multicenter study that assessed more than 2,000 Dutch travelers and 215 household members and had follow-up for 1 year after return (Arcilla 2017). In this study the researchers found that about a third of all travelers acquired ESBL *Enterobacteriaceae* during travel. Among those who traveled to southern Asia, 75% acquired multiply resistant bacteria. Factors that were associated with picking up resistant bacteria were using antibiotics, developing travelers' diarrhea that persisted after return, and having pre-existing chronic bowel disease. The median duration of carrying the resistant bacteria after return was 30 days, but more than 11% continued to carry resistant bacteria at 12 months after travel. In 12% of cases the resistant bacteria spread to another household member.

Consistent findings across many studies are high rates of picking up resistant bacteria especially during travel to parts of Asia, increased risk with use of antibiotics, and increased risk with development of diarrhea. Other studies have found that taking the antimotility (antidiarrhea) drug loperamide (Imodium) along with antibiotics increased the risk of resistance carriage (higher than antibiotics alone). Some studies have found that a longer duration of travel and older age increase the risk. The increased risk of carrying antibiotic-resistant bacteria in those taking antibiotics may reflect the phenomenon known as colonization resistance. The normal healthy bacteria in the gut may make it difficult for a new strain or species of bacteria to become established. This can apply to bacteria that cause disease as well as those that live in the gut as normal resident bacteria. The normal bacteria can provide useful and healthy competition for outsiders.

Antibiotic resistance in general has increased over time, and carriage of resistant bacteria by travelers has increased over time. A map displaying the pooled prevalence of fecal carriage by ESBL organisms by World Health Organization (WHO) region of the world and the rates of carriage in travelers to those areas shows marked similarities. This means that the microbes that the travelers carry home reflect the microbiological situation in the geographic region visited. Travelers mirror the local environment. Travelers eat and drink and sample the local environment. In areas with poor sanitation, common in many low-income countries, travelers are even more likely to consume fecally contaminated food and drinks. This manifests as what has long been called traveler's diarrhea.

One can and should ask what difference it makes if one is carrying bacteria in the gut that are resistant to multiple antibiotics—especially if one is healthy and feels fine. As noted earlier, resistant bacteria in the gut can be totally silent. Most people who carry multiply resistant bacteria do not become sick from them—and most have no reason or way of knowing they are carrying them unless they are part of a medical study. However, many kinds of infections that make us sick come from and involve bacteria that are already in our bodies. When a person develops a urinary tract infection, often it is caused by bacteria that were in the gut. These antibiotic-resistant bacteria may become predominant if one has to take an antibiotic for an unrelated reason, such as for strep throat. The origin of bacteria causing other types of serious infections, such as bloodstream infections, is often those already carried in the gastrointestinal tract.

What is medical tourism? Are travelers who receive medical care abroad at risk for infections with resistant bacteria?

Those who have been hospitalized during travel or have traveled with the goal of receiving medical care (medical tourism) have a particularly high risk of becoming infected or colonized with multidrug-resistant bacteria, especially in some low- and middle-income countries where antibiotic resistance rates are high.

Medical tourism or health tourism is travel to another country to receive health care (Chen 2013). It is hard to get accurate numbers on how common this is, but it seems to be increasing, and worldwide it is a multi-billion-dollar business. Common procedures are dental work and cosmetic surgery, but major procedures, like kidney transplantation, cardiac surgery, reproductive care, and joint surgery, are also done.

Common destinations include Thailand, Mexico, Singapore, India, Malaysia, Cuba, Brazil, Argentina, and Costa Rica.

The financial rewards from medical tourism are sufficiently large that some countries have developed robust systems to facilitate the travel of medical tourists. Hospitals can now seek accreditation through the Joint Commission International (JCI), and hundreds of international hospitals have done so. As of 2013, Singapore alone had 22 JCI-certified hospitals.

Why do people travel outside of the United States for medical care? Reasons are many, but lower cost is often a key motivating factor. Other reasons include long waits for or unavailability of a procedure in the home country, higher quality, legal or cultural restrictions at home, privacy and the opportunity to recover away from home, and a desire to combine exotic vacation with a medical procedure.

But medical tourism raises many financial, legal, ethical, and health-related issues. Quality is highly variable, and regulation is lacking in many areas. Outcomes may be poor and complications frequent. Other concerns include exploitation of local donors for organ transplantation (e.g., for kidneys and other organs or tissues), diversion of skilled specialists to hospitals serving medical tourists and away from local populations, and fragmented follow-up care for travelers who undergo medical care and surgical procedure care abroad.

Medical tourism has become so common that many professional societies and organizations provide internet resources about quality and safety and accreditation of health care abroad. These include the CDC, the American Medical Association, the American College of Physicians, the American Society for Plastic Surgery, the International Society of Aesthetic Plastic Surgery, the American Dental Association, the Global Observatory on Donation and Transplantation, and the WHO. Several organizations provide health care standards and accreditation internationally, including the International Organization for Standardization, the International Society for

Quality in Health Care, and the Canadian Council on Health Services Accreditation (Chen 2013).

Many of the countries that have developed medical tourism programs lie in tropical and subtropical areas. Many are low- and middle-income countries. Many of the types of procedures done involve the use of antibiotics, and most can be complicated by the development of infections. Patients in hospitals often become infected with the bacteria that are present in a particular hospital environment and carried by the hospital staff. Studies of returned travelers who require medical care show that being hospitalized and receiving medical care in some countries is a risk factor for carrying multiply resistant bacteria.

Travelers also often undergo unplanned health care during travel because of injury or the development of an acute medical problem, like a heart attack, or an illness, such as acute pneumonia. There are limited data on how often this happens. Illness is common during and after travel, especially after travel to low-resource areas, but most illnesses are diarrhea, respiratory tract infections, or skin ailments—and most of these resolve without the need for hospitalization. One review of multiple studies found that of travelers with illness or injury, less than 1% to 3% ended up being hospitalized during travel.

Are mass gatherings an important source of infections and spread of infections or resistance?

Mass gatherings are events that bring large numbers of people together usually from many parts of the world. Individuals often spend time in close proximity—and then they typically return home, perhaps carrying some extra bacterial (and viral) baggage. The best-known examples of mass gatherings are the Hajj, the Olympic games, and Kumbh Mela. For the annual Hajj held in Saudi Arabia, 2 million to 3 million individuals gather from more than 180 countries. For the less well-known

Kumbh Mela in India, as many as 120 million Hindu pilgrims gather and bathe in holy river water. These events provide conditions that could allow the sharing and spread—and subsequent global dispersal—of disease-causing microbes or resistance genes.

Several years ago an uncommon serogroup of the bacterium *N. meningitidis* (cause of meningococcal meningitis, which can be fatal) appeared at the Hajj, spread among some of the pilgrims, and was carried back to home countries (in the throat)—again showing the capacity of bacteria to hitch rides with humans. Although it was not multidrug resistant, it was not prevented by the vaccine that was the main vaccine used at that time. A change in vaccine recommendation was subsequently made in response to those events. Another notable feature was that it could be carried silently. Not everyone who picks it up gets sick. As a consequence, there were instances when people who had not traveled to the Hajj picked it up (and got sick) from those who had traveled to the Hajj but were unaware that they were carrying it because it was not causing symptoms.

For the Hajj, certain vaccinations are required for those planning to attend—but no vaccines are available for many infections that can be a threat.

What is wastewater epidemiology?

One of the more interesting approaches to surveillance for antibiotic resistance genes (and another study that confirms that resistance patterns vary by geographic region of the world) involved the metagenomic analysis of toilet waste from airplanes—or what one can call the airplane poop study (Petersen 2015). Researchers identified 18 long-distance flights destined for Copenhagen, Denmark, where they lived and had laboratory access. The researchers worked with members of the transportation and airline industry—or whoever gives permission for such a study. They arranged to collect samples from the toilet waste storage tanks at the end of each of the 18 flights originating in major cities in Asia or North America. Apparently each long-distance flight generates about 400 liters of waste. The researchers took samples of the waste to a research facility where they used state-of-the-art equipment to extract and analyze DNA from the waste samples and look for markers of antibiotic resistance.

What they found was a significantly higher abundance of antibiotic resistance genes among samples from South Asia, North Asia, and all Asian samples compared to North America samples (flights originating from North America). Norovirus (virus that causes diarrhea) and *Salmonella enterica* (bacteria that can cause diarrhea) were detected in higher amounts from South Asia than in samples from North America, whereas *C. difficile* (the cause of *C. difficile* colitis) was most abundant in samples from North America. The researchers propose that this approach could be used as a way to monitor resistance genes as well as identify disease-causing microbes in real time. They explained that at the point of origin of the flights, the toilets were rinsed and disinfected, so the material tested came from just that one long-distance flight. This novel approach could potentially be used for surveillance and monitoring of levels and types of resistance and pathogens globally.

An approach called wastewater-based epidemiology is already used in some settings. Wastewater can be analyzed for the presence of many substances, including viruses, bacteria and other microbes, antibiotic resistance genes, and residues of antibiotics and other drugs, including illegal drugs. It has been used to look for polio viruses in many areas working to eradicate polio transmission. Apparently some cities in China are analyzing sewage for traces of drugs or their metabolites excreted in urine. This potentially can be used to track down drug users or drug manufacturers. A study in eight European cities found correlation between the amount of cocaine in wastewater and drug seizures. These investigations raise privacy and other issues that are beyond the scope of this book.

How does resistance spread in health care facilities?

People and their microbes and resistance genes move within regions and globally. Hospitals and health care settings, including long-term care facilities, are places where multiply resistant bacteria are preferentially found. Why does this happen? Several factors contribute. Hospitalized patients often receive antibiotics. Some patients are in the hospital because they have infections that are being treated with antibiotics. Others are suspected of possibly having an infection and are given antibiotics "just in case," and others are given antibiotics to prevent an infection in a high-risk situation, such as a patient who is undergoing a surgical procedure like a total hip replacement.

Hospitalized patients are especially vulnerable to infections because of tissue injury; surgical wounds; placement of catheters, central venous lines, and other artificial materials; and immunosuppression because of underlying disease or drugs, radiation, or other interventions. Contamination of a wound can occur at the time of a procedure (surgery or placement of a device), but continued presence of an intravenous catheter, Foley catheter, drain, or chest tube can provide a potential entry point for subsequent contamination and infection.

Resistant bacteria may develop from a patient's own bacteria, particularly when a patient has been given multiple courses of antibiotics that may eliminate many of the bacteria that are sensitive to the antibiotics, leaving those that can survive in the presence of antibiotics (antibiotic-resistant bacteria).

Resistant bacteria may also spread from other patients who happen to carry resistant bacteria whether or not they have an obvious infection. These resistant bacteria may be spread by contact with the hands of health care workers who may not adequately wash hands between care of different patients or who fail to use barrier protection, such as gloves. Bacteria from other patients may also contaminate a shared environment— toilets, sinks, drains, bed rails, bedside stands, and equipment such as blood pressure cuffs and stethoscopes.

Instruments used in the health care system may become contaminated with bacteria, including multiply resistant ones. Many illustrative examples exist. A detailed investigation may be needed to determine the source of infection in the event of an outbreak in a health care setting. Today the availability of genetic sequencing of bacteria makes it easier to pin down the exact source of an infection if a cluster of patients have been infected. This is especially valuable when infections are caused by bacteria, such as *S. aureus* or *C. difficile*, that are commonly found in the hospital environment.

Infections can spread within a hospital, but health care institutions are not isolated places. Increasingly hospitals are part of health care systems and networks that involve ambulatory care settings, chronic care facilities, and multiple hospitals. This allows multiply resistant bacteria to spread regionally through patient transfer. Patients may be silent carriers of resistant bacteria and can be a source of an outbreak in a new institution (Toth 2017).

Chronic care facilities, in particular, are sites where multidrug-resistant bacteria frequently infect or colonize patients. Residents often have had long hospitalizations and multiple courses of antibiotics.

In Illinois in 2013, the Department of Public Health made a particular type of resistance (CRE) reportable to a registry (XDRO registry, which stands for extensively drug-resistant organisms; http://www.xdro.org). Why was this important to track? CRE infections have become increasingly common. Up to 50% of patients who develop infections with these multiply resistant bacteria can die. Patients can also carry these bacteria silently (colonization) and they can be a source for spread to other patients in health care facilities.

When investigators analyzed CRE data for the state of Illinois, they found that CRE rates were higher in hospitals with higher connectedness to other hospitals and strong connections to long-term acute care hospitals (Ray 2016).

One type of CRE is the NDM-producing bacteria. As discussed previously, it was first identified and named in 2009 when multiple cases were reported, especially linked to exposures in India. It has been uncommon in the United States; however, in 2013 an outbreak was identified in a tertiary care hospital in northeast Illinois. Thirty-one cases were reported through the XDRO registry mentioned previously. The spread of the resistant bacteria was traced to a contaminated duodenoscope (a tube inserted via the throat into the upper part of the gastrointestinal tract beyond the stomach that allows clinicians to look at the tissues and potentially take samples of fluid and/or tissue). As an aside, these delicate instruments have multiple compartments and are difficult to clean and sterilize and have been the source of transmission of infections in other settings.

In an investigation of the outbreak, researchers found that of the 31 infected patients who were identified at the primary hospital, 19 were admitted to 13 other hospitals during the next 12 months. This shows the extent of connectedness among hospitals and the potential for the movement of resistant bacteria and resistance genes. The researchers carried out a social network analysis to better understand sharing patterns among health care facilities and identify those facilities most likely to share patients with the primary hospital. The entire patient-sharing network for Illinois includes 210 hospitals, but using network analysis, they were able to identify the nine hospitals the outbreak patients would most likely visit. This allowed them to be more efficient in focusing public health resources on these high-risk facilities.

Are there ways resistant bacteria spread that do not involve movement of humans?

Massive global travel and migration is one part of the conveyor belt that is mixing and moving microbes and their resistance genes. But there are many others.

People are not the only moving species. We move animals around the world—massive numbers of live animals and pieces and parts of them—as part of the globalized food supply. Each animal carries its microbiota. Many animals today have been raised in industrialized farm animal production systems. This is especially true for swine and chickens. Many have received antibiotics for growth promotion or to treat or prevent infections. Many of the antibiotics given to animals are the same classes of antibiotics or even exactly the same drugs as those given to humans. In animals, as in humans, treating with antibiotics leads to selection of resistant bacteria. These can be present even if the animals are not sick. Even though official regulations require that any antibiotic must be stopped for a set period of time before slaughter so that the meat does not contain antibiotics, the effect of an antibiotic in selecting resistant bacteria can persist. Even with modern slaughterhouses and rapid refrigeration, meat is frequently contaminated with bacteria that come from the gut of the animal or from the processing system.

Food animals can carry antibiotic-resistant bacteria in the absence of obvious disease. They are more likely to carry antibiotic-resistant bacteria if they have received antibiotics. Some particular strains of antibiotic-resistant bacteria have been found in food animals—for example, methicillin-resistant *Staphylococcus* on pig farms in the Netherlands and elsewhere—and have caused infections in farm workers.

Hens that appear healthy may be infected with salmonella and can lay eggs that contain salmonella inside, even though the shells are intact. Shells of eggs can also be contaminated with poultry feces containing salmonella. If they are not cleaned before breaking them, the fecal residue can contaminate the eggs.

We also move massive quantities of fruits, vegetables, nuts, spices, and other foods around the world. The food chain is very long, and produce from multiple countries may end up in the same package. These come with their own microbes—and sometimes are contaminated by wastewater with runoff from animals. Manure used on fields and that reaches produce may also contain bacteria—and resistance genes. Multiple outbreaks underscore the risks of fecal contamination of food with outbreaks of *Salmonella, Campylobacter*, and *E. coli*. This is yet another indicator of the movement of feces and bacteria from one region and one population to another.

Resistance genes in bacteria in water and soil can also reach humans and animals. Humans eat fish raised in these waters and produce grown in soils irrigated with this water.

Birds migrate and can carry microbes over long distances. Probably the most important microbes carried by birds are the influenza viruses, but birds can carry *Salmonella* and *Campylobacter* and other potential bacterial pathogens.

Wildlife (wild mammals) can also carry antibiotic resistance genes, but because they are less likely to be exposed to antibiotics than pets and food animals and usually have less intimate contact with humans, and because their biomass is small relative to that of livestock, they probably play less of a role in spreading antibiotic resistance genes than livestock and food animals.

Do pets carry antibiotic-resistant bacteria?

Pets can also carry methicillin-resistant *Staphylococcus* and other potential pathogens. There is good documentation of the spread of pathogenic bacteria from pets to people with whom they have close contact—and from people to pets.

In the United States there was a multistate (18 states) outbreak of diarrhea from 2016 to 2018 caused by *Campylobacter jejuni*, an infection often traced to contaminated food. It involved 118 people whose ages ranged from younger than 1 to 85 years. About a quarter of those infected were sick enough that they were hospitalized. The infections were unusual because the bacteria were resistant to all of the antibiotics that are typically used to treat *Campylobacter* infections. Because of the unusual nature of the outbreak, the CDC investigated it. One feature that provided an early clue was that 29 of the people infected worked in pet stores. After a careful investigation, the source of the outbreak was found to be puppies that had come from different breeders but had had contact with each other at distributors, during transport from various facilities, and at the pet stores. The puppies carried the *Campylobacter* in their feces. The investigation uncovered (for the 149 puppies whose records were available) that 95% had received antibiotics before or while at the store. In 55% of cases the puppies were not sick and were given antibiotics anyway for prophylaxis (prevention) only—apparently to make certain the puppies would appear healthy and would sell. The median duration of antibiotic treatment was 15 days. In this case the extensive use of antibiotics (that most would consider to be inappropriate) in animals was discovered only because it resulted in a severe outbreak of infections in humans, leading to many hospitalizations and an investigation. The antibiotic-resistant bacteria in the puppy feces spread to people who had direct contact with puppies or the environment where they were housed (Montgomery 2018).

Reptiles (snakes), turtles, and baby chicks kept for pets often carry *Salmonella* in their feces, and this can contaminate the outside of the animal. Some strains may be antibiotic resistant. Regardless of resistance patterns, these can be transmitted to their owners who handle them. Handwashing after handling these pets or having contact with their environment can help to prevent spread.

What are other routes of spread of bacteria from animals to humans?

Resistant bacteria can spread between humans and pets through direct contact or through shared materials as described previously.

People swimming in surface water (freshwater lakes, streams, rivers) contaminated with untreated waste and wastewater runoff from farms may become infected with bacteria from animals, such as *E. coli* O157:H7, which can cause severe bloody diarrhea. Cattle waste is a primary source of this specific strain of toxin-producing *E. coli*, but it can also be carried by deer, sheep, goats, and other animals. Several outbreaks have been reported in swimmers.

Does antibiotic resistance ever disappear?

Examples exist of reductions in the prevalence of specific types of antibiotic resistance in response to removal or marked reduction in the use of antibiotics. In situations where extremely resistant infections have been identified in hospitals, use of barriers (like gloves and gowns), isolation of patients, and enhanced cleaning and disinfection have sometimes eliminated the source and spread of a specific multiply resistant pathogen. Some multiply resistant bacteria are less fit than other bacteria and may be unable to survive in the absence of favorable conditions.

Resistance as a general phenomenon will not disappear. A reservoir of resistance genes is found in environmental bacteria. This supply will not be exhausted. Resistant bacteria will be favored in an environment with wide use of antibiotics and other antimicrobial substances, which is the current global situation.

Which bacteria have developed resistance?

All major types of bacteria that cause illness can become resistant to antibiotics, but this occurs more rapidly with some bacteria than with others. It is worth describing two key examples of bacterial infections that have different routes of spread and have different clinical consequences. Both have a global impact. Current and increasing antibiotic resistance complicates their management.

Why does tuberculosis remain such a serious global problem?

Among the most important of the bacteria globally that are drug resistant is *M. tuberculosis*, the cause of tuberculosis, also known as TB. Although TB is not a common infection in the United States, it remains a serious global problem—and antibiotic resistance is complicating its treatment.

In 1900, tuberculosis was a leading cause of death in the United States. As a single agent, it claimed more lives than any other specific infection. Other top causes of death were all causes of pneumonia and influenza. Tuberculosis was feared. It could attack and kill people at any age, including those in the prime of life. Also known as "consumption," it was visible, causing those infected to waste away, often over months or years. It carried social stigma. Many believed that it was inherited. It was untreatable with medications available at that time. Robert Koch described the bacteria that caused tuberculosis (leading it to sometimes be called "Koch's bacilli") in 1882; he was awarded a Nobel Prize in Medicine or Physiology in 1905 for his work on tuberculosis.

Tuberculosis is a bacterial infection caused by *M. tuberculosis*. In contrast to staphylococcal or streptococcal and most other familiar and rapid-onset bacterial infections, tuberculosis is usually a slow infection. The bacteria that cause staphylococcal and streptococcal infections can double every 20 to 30 minutes. If you do the calculations, you quickly realize the numbers of bacteria become enormous very quickly. *M. tuberculosis* replicates at a deliberate pace, requiring 15 to 20 hours to double. It can take weeks for visible growth of the bacteria to appear on an agar culture plate in the laboratory. TB has other characteristics that make it formidable to recognize and treat. It can mimic many other common infections. Although it typically enters the body through the respiratory tract (inhaled with air) and takes residence in the lung, it can enter the blood-stream and spread silently to other parts of the body. It can be quiet and slow. It can infect a person and cause no symptoms for a lifetime, as it does in the majority of those infected. In fact, it is estimated that a quarter to a third of all people in the world are infected with TB. Occasionally it can progress directly to an active form, usually causing fever, cough, sweats, and weight loss. Often the onset of symptoms is insidious, coming on slowly, and the person is able to continue to work or go to classes. Symptoms may continue for weeks or months and wax and wane. If tuberculosis infection is unrecognized and untreated, the infection may be spread to others in the household or at work and to anyone who shares the same air. Tuberculosis is one of the infections that can spread through the air with the greatest of ease, the bacilli floating in tiny particles called droplet nuclei that can remain suspended in the air. In fact, one does not have to have face-to-face contact with (or even see) someone with tuberculosis to pick up the infection.

The long lag between exposure to infection and the start of symptoms after infection (weeks, months, years, or never) led to the uncertainty in the past as to whether tuberculosis really was a contagious infection, one transmitted from person to person. People understood that infections like influenza or streptococcal infections could spread from person to person because they observed other cases or outbreaks that might occur a few days or a week or so after exposure. Tuberculosis was more subtle and vague because the onset of symptoms would take a minimum of weeks—and the majority of people who are infected (85% to 90%) never develop symptoms.

The scientific studies that showed without a doubt that tuberculosis was spread through the air involved guinea pigs and some Baltimore patients with active tuberculosis (Riley 1957). Guinea pigs are extremely susceptible to tuberculosis. Even one or a few inhaled bacteria (tubercle bacilli) can cause infection in them. A scientific study in the 1960s using a rotating drum to create droplets containing bacteria showed that disease-causing tubercle bacilli could float as tiny particles (droplet nuclei) in the air for 6 hours or longer. Researchers working at a Veterans Administration hospital in Baltimore planned a study. They placed guinea pigs in an area that was created to receive the air from a six-bed ward housing patients with suspected tuberculosis. The guinea pigs were never in the same room with the patients with TB and only received air from their room. Lo and behold, the guinea pigs became infected with tuberculosis, showing that infection could spread where there was only air contact.

An episode in 1965 on a navy vessel, the USS *Byrd*, also supported these research findings (Houk 1968; Houk 1980). One of the men on board the ship developed active tuberculosis with a large cavity in his lung (where the TB infection had destroyed normal tissues), a type of TB that is usually highly contagious. His infection was initially diagnosed as a viral infection and he continued working for about 6 months, despite having symptoms like a cough and sweats. Once tuberculosis was diagnosed, all of those on board the ship were evaluated to find out if they had become infected. The staff had detailed information about where the men worked and slept when on board the ship. They also reviewed the ventilation system of the vessel. Among the men who shared a bunking (sleeping) compartment with the infected man, 80% had picked up TB infection (converted tuberculin skin test from negative to positive). Another 81 men had little contact with the infected man and slept in a separate compartment; however, three-quarters of the ventilation in that compartment came through interconnecting ducts from the first compartment. Of the men in the second compartment who did not work with the infected man, 54% had skin test conversion (indicating recent infection). Although this was not designed as a formal experiment, the layout of the ship provided ideal conditions for analyzing spread by air contact only. The men were infected in roughly the same proportion as the amount of TB-contaminated air that they breathed.

With the development of the antibiotic streptomycin in the 1940s, followed by isoniazid and other antituberculosis drugs, tuberculosis became a treatable, curable infection. In fact, Selman Waksman, who discovered streptomycin and received a Nobel Prize for it in 1952, made the jubilant comment in his Nobel address that "The conquest of the 'Great White Plague' [which is what TB was called], undreamt of less than 10 years ago is now virtually within sight." By the early 1950s, tuberculosis dropped out of the top 10 causes of death in the United States. In 2017 there were only 9,093 new cases of tuberculosis reported in the entire United States, just 2.8 new cases of tuberculosis for every 100,000 people, the lowest rate ever in the United States (Stewart 2017). The majority (>80%) of the new cases of TB in the United States today are from reactivation of inactive (latent) infection, not from new transmission, and the majority are in the foreign-born who picked up infection before coming to the United States.

While the United States is working to eliminate tuberculosis, the global picture is much bleaker. Some countries have rates of TB that are more than 100 times higher than the US rate. Today tuberculosis remains one of the top 10 killers globally. In 2016 it was the sixth most common cause of death in low-income countries—and it remains one of the top 10 causes of death in children globally. In 2015 almost a quarter of a million children younger than age 15 years died from tuberculosis, most of them younger than 5 years and living in Africa and Asia. Most of the deaths were in children who were not receiving tuberculosis treatment.

Although we have a TB vaccine, BCG (bacille Calmette-Guerin), that is used widely in many parts of the world, it has not been effective in halting the spread of TB. Globally more than 10 million new cases occur each year and 1.6 million die from infection. Today TB kills more people than malaria or HIV. In Africa TB kills about 25% of patients with HIV/AIDS.

TB has always affected the most vulnerable populations. Among those infected with the tubercle bacillus, up to 90%

will never develop symptoms. A small percentage develop symptoms a few weeks after becoming infected. In the majority the bacteria will persist in a silent, latent form, often in a small focus in the lung. If infection becomes active, it most often involves the lungs (70% to 80%) but can appear at any site in the body (e.g., lymph nodes, kidneys, bone, central nervous system, gastrointestinal tract, liver). TB reactivates when a person's immune system is unable to contain the infection. HIV/AIDS is one of the most potent factors making individuals susceptible to TB and at risk for reactivation if latent TB is already present. Other conditions that predispose to active disease or reactivation include extremes of age (very young and very old); malnutrition; immunosuppression from steroids, chemotherapy, or other agents; diabetes mellitus; and other chronic illnesses. In 2015 diabetes, alcohol use, and smoking globally accounted for about a quarter of deaths and disability from tuberculosis. Globally 16% of those with active TB die from the infection.

The HIV pandemic has made TB more difficult to control, and TB has worsened the impact of HIV infection. Each infection adversely affects the other. Individuals who already have inactive TB are at high risk for reactivation if they become infected with HIV. Although HIV is a potent risk factor for tuberculosis, the vast majority of TB deaths globally are in HIV-negative individuals.

TB control is hobbled by lack of good diagnostics—as is true for many other infectious diseases. Compounding the problem of tuberculosis control is the lack of a rapid, bedside or in-the-field, accurate, inexpensive diagnostic test that could be made widely available. Pulmonary tuberculosis is usually diagnosed by examining a sputum specimen, but a sputum sample may not be available, especially in young children; women may be reluctant to cough and spit out sputum. The testing still done in many parts of the world requires the use of chemical stains, a microscope, and a trained person to examine the specimen. The staining process still used in some places (Ziehl-Neelsen stain, named after two German doctors) was developed in the 1880s. The TB bacteria do not show up on Gram's stain (used to see many bacteria under the microscope) because of a waxy cell wall. The Ziehl-Neelsen process stains the bacteria red, while the background of cells, mucous and debris, will stain blue. Even if a smear suggests the presence of bacteria that look like TB bacteria, the test will not provide details of what drugs are likely to work. Unless TB bacilli are abundant, they may be difficult to find on a smear, so 50% or more of infections can be missed by smear but picked up by a positive culture. Traditional cultures take weeks to become positive.

A newer test that requires an investment of money and space but can provide rapid (within hours) preliminary results and indicate whether the bacteria are resistant to one drug is called Xpert MTB/RIF. This is an automated, PCR-based assay that can diagnose the presence of tuberculosis and determine whether it is likely to respond to rifampin, one of the key drugs used in the treatment of tuberculosis. Another version assesses sensitivity to isoniazid. An even newer version of this device, called Xpert MTB/RIF Ultra, has been useful in diagnosing tuberculous meningitis, an infection that is difficult to diagnose (smear microscopy is positive in only about 15% of cases; cultures take weeks and find only 50% to 60% of cases). Its use has been recommended by the WHO. Development of this test is a step in the right direction, but much more investment is needed in health systems to diagnose and treat TB.

Tuberculosis is typically slow to develop. It also requires prolonged treatment. Not only can TB be difficult to diagnose but also treatment typically requires taking multiple drugs (usually at least four) for months to years. This is in contrast to many common bacterial infections that can be treated effectively with a few days of antibiotics. Some drugs are available only in injectable forms. It is hard work to complete a full course of treatment, and there are many hurdles to overcome. Many of those infected have other vulnerabilities—such as being homeless, HIV infected, living in extreme poverty, incarcerated, or living in conflict zones where drug supplies are often interrupted.

In the United States approximately 96% of persons diagnosed with active TB disease complete therapy, but that is in the context of a strong public health care system with providers who monitor treatment. Globally an estimated 83% are successfully treated. A recent review of treatment of tuberculosis in India found that only 45% of patients with any form of tuberculosis had completed treatment by 1 year. Among those with multidrug-resistant TB, the completion rate was only 14%.

Multidrug-resistant/extensively drug-resistant tuberculosis

Resistance in tuberculosis is characterized as MDR for those TB isolates that are resistant to rifampin and INH, two of the mainstays of TB treatment. Extensively drug-resistant (XDR) tuberculosis describes resistance to INH and rifampin and also a fluoroquinolone plus one or more of the three injectable second-line drugs (amikacin, kanamycin, or capreomycin). People can develop MDR or XDR tuberculosis because of inadequate or incorrect treatment that favors the selection of resistant bacteria or because they become infected from someone who has MDR or XDR TB. About 4% of new TB cases are MDR; about 19% of those that have been previously treated are MDR, though this can vary widely from one region to another.

Antibiotic resistance is a global problem. Drug-resistant tuberculosis is a disaster and is getting worse (WHO 2017). By 2014, XDR TB had spread to 105 countries. The WHO estimated that in 2016 there were almost 600,000 new cases of MDR tuberculosis, almost half of them in India, China, and Russia. In 2016 approximately 240,000 died from MDR and rifampin-resistant tuberculosis. The success rate in treating MDR TB is only 54%. It is also extremely expensive to treat, and those infected may not be able to afford the drugs unless they are available through the public sector. Effective drugs are also toxic and may cause severe side effects. Drug-resistant tuber-culosis infects an individual, but if it is not effectively treated, it can also be transmitted to others. When someone with MDR or XDR TB transmits it to another person, that other person will also be infected with MDR or XDR TB. In some settings, infection with XDR TB is virtually a death sentence.

In 2016, among those with MDR TB, infection was XDR in 6.2%. Treatment was successful in 54%, 16% died, and many others were lost to follow-up. Data are often incomplete and unreliable because drug susceptibility testing is not available in many areas. When drug susceptibility testing is available, it can take 6 to 16 weeks to obtain the results.

When people talk about antibiotic resistance, they are often talking about common infections like *Staphylococcus* and *Streptococcus*, but globally antibiotic-resistant TB remains a major killer that is often underestimated or forgotten.

Resistance of the TB bacteria almost always occurs because of a mutation in the chromosome of the bacteria (Gillespie 2002). These mutations are now known to occur at a predictable rate—and the rate that leads to resistance varies by the drug. For example, for streptomycin, the first drug that was discovered that was active against TB, mutations leading to resistance to the drug occur about once every 200 million replications of the bacteria—a rare event. However, if a person has an active lung infection that contains 100 million bacteria, there is a good chance that as these replicate, a mutation will occur. Assuming the mutated bacteria continue to grow and divide despite the presence of the drug, the patient will ultimately end up with in-fection dominated by the resistant bacteria. Although resistant bacteria may be less fit initially, they can lose any fitness def-icit associated with the resistance mutation as they continue to multiply. The rates of mutation are known for each of the drugs used to treat tuberculosis, but they typically occur once per tens to hundreds of millions to billions of replications.

People who have severe, extensive infection (may have billions of bacteria) or have infection in tissues that are protected from the action of the drug (bacteria found in cavities or areas that are walled off by the body) may be particularly at risk for developing resistant bacteria while on treatment. Once bacteria become resistant to a particular drug, it does not reverse and return to a sensitive state.

The ongoing mutations in the bacteria making them resistant to the drugs are the reason that treatment of tuberculosis typically involves starting with four different drugs. The likelihood that bacteria can survive the presence of all of these drugs at the same time is extremely small. Unfortunately, over time many TB bacteria have become resistant to two, three, four, and more drugs, and these resistant bacteria are spreading in some areas.

Useful results have come from a study just published in 2018 (Collaborative group for the meta-analysis 2018). A meta-analysis of more than 12,000 patients with MDR tuberculosis from 25 countries treated between 2009 and 2016, some of whom were given newer or repurposed drugs (drugs initially developed for a different reason but found to be active against TB), found that 61% were treated successfully, 14% died, and 8% failed treatment. The study showed which drugs were associated with better outcomes. These drugs included linezolid, levofloxacin, carbapenem, moxifloxacin, bedaquiline, and clofazimine. The first four of these drugs are not typically considered anti-TB drugs. The investigators also learned that two drugs often included in TB treatment, kanamycin and capreomycin, were associated with worse outcomes. These results will lead to changing some of the approaches and testing of new treatment combinations.

The resistance of mycobacteria to linezolid and fluoroquinolones (levofloxacin and moxifloxacin) appears to be related in part to pumps (efflux pumps) that remove the drugs from bacterial cells. Verapamil, a drug long used to treat hypertension, has been shown to inhibit these efflux pumps. Adding verapamil to anti-TB drugs might improve their activity. So far, this has been studied only in mice, but it should be tested as a possible approach to improving treatment outcomes in humans (Pieterman 2018).

Why is gonorrhea so hard to treat?

The story of the epidemiology and treatment of gonorrhea highlights the development and spread of resistance in another important widespread bacterial infection.

Gonorrhea, caused by the bacteria *N. gonorrhoeae*, is a common sexually transmitted infection that is found worldwide. The bacteria that cause gonorrhea cannot survive well outside of the human body. There are no reservoirs of the bacteria in animals or in the environment. A person cannot become infected from a toilet seat! Infected humans carry the bacteria and transmit infection to another person through direct physical contact, through touching. Like many other bacteria, those that cause gonorrhea have preferred niches or tissues within the human body and do not often stray outside of those areas. *N. gonorrhoeae* bacteria are well adapted to infect genital tissues—the urethra, the cervix in women, the vagina in girls before puberty, and the rectal tissues. It has been remarkably successful in surviving and spreading in all countries through sexual contact.

Infection in women can be complicated by the spread of infection from the cervix (cervicitis) into the lining of the uterus (endometritis) and into the fallopian tubes (salpingitis) and the peritoneum (peritonitis). Infections can cause scarring and be associated with infertility and ectopic pregnancy (fetus outside of the womb) in women. The bacteria can also infect the throat and the conjunctivae (lining of the eye) and can cause blindness if not treated. Occasionally the bacteria enter the bloodstream and can infect joints, skin, and other tissues, but most infections remain localized to the genital tract—the urethra in men and the cervix in women. Common symptoms are a discharge of pus from the urethra and burning on urination in men and an abnormal vaginal discharge in women. The pus typically contains white blood cells and large numbers of bacteria.

Clinicians are required to report to public health departments certain infections of public health relevance, such as gonorrhea, syphilis, measles, and diphtheria, among others. Gonorrhea is the most commonly reported notifiable infection in the United States. More than half a million infections were reported in the United States in 2017. Globally it is estimated that there are 80 million infections each year. Unfortunately, the rate of gonorrhea is increasing in the United States, along with other sexually transmitted infections, which have increased for 4 straight years. Gonorrhea diagnoses have increased 67% since 2013.

One reason this infection is so common is that it spreads easily. Most people who are infected do not have severe symptoms and can continue their usual activities, including working, traveling, and having sex. About 40% of infections in men and more than half of those in women cause no symptoms. Individuals who are totally unaware of the presence of infection can easily spread it through sexual contact. Untreated infection can persist for weeks or longer, so a single individual with multiple sexual partners can potentially pass the infection to multiple people. Infection does not make people immune, so people can be reinfected, sometimes multiple times. Infants born vaginally can come into contact with the bacteria in the birth canal. In the United States a topical eye ointment containing erythromycin is recommended for all newborn infants to prevent eye infection (neonatal conjunctivitis) with *N. gonorrhoeae*, which can cause perforation of the cornea and blindness.

Before antibiotics were available, infection was prevented by avoiding sex or use of barriers, like condoms. Multiple other interventions were also used in attempts to clear the infection. Compounds of arsenic, antimony, bismuth, gold, silver, and mercury were tested. During World War I, soldiers apparently were supplied with packages that contained condoms but also mercury and silver compounds. Urethral irrigations were used for men using substances like mercurochrome. Use of heat was tried utilizing a fever cabinet that a person would sit in with only the head outside of the heated chamber. This is reminiscent of deliberately causing malaria infection, which caused high fevers, to treat syphilis.

When the sulfa drugs were discovered in the 1930s, they were used to treat gonorrhea. Initially they cured 80% to 90% of cases, but the benefit did not last long and by the late 1940s more than 90% of gonococcal samples in some areas were resistant to them. Some forms of sulfonamides, especially when combined with trimethoprim (an inexpensive combination), continued to be used in low-resource areas for several decades (Unemo 2014).

Penicillin was documented to be active against gonorrhea in the early 1940s and became the favored treatment into the 1970s. Initially low doses worked; the recommended dose had to be progressively increased as the bacteria became more resistant. During the 1960s other antibiotics, tetracyclines and spectinomycin, were also available to treat gonorrhea.

Each chapter in the history of gonorrhea treatment is uncannily familiar. A drug was used, low-grade resistance in bacteria appeared, the dose was increased and the higher dose worked, bacteria became more resistant and then totally resistant to the drug, resistant forms became widespread, and a shift to a new drug was necessary to cure infection.

The initial resistance of gonorrhea to penicillin was because the bacteria produced a beta-lactamase, the enzyme that destroyed the beta-lactam ring of penicillin. It was encoded on plasmids that spread easily among the bacteria. These beta-lactamases appeared in 1976 in Southeast Asia and rapidly spread internationally. Chromosomally mediated resistance to penicillin emerged later in the United States and led to the discontinuation of penicillin as first-line treatment. Today both kinds of resistance are found globally.

Tetracyclines provided good treatment of gonorrhea for people allergic to penicillin until high-level resistance developed in the mid-1980s. These resistant bacteria also spread internationally.

Spectinomycin was an antibiotic synthesized in the early 1960s specifically for the treatment of gonorrhea. It is related to the aminoglycosides (like gentamicin) and is produced in nature by *Streptomyces spectabilis*. As early as 1967, spectinomycin resistance was first reported in the Netherlands. Spectinomycin was used in Korea in military personnel starting in 1981, but within 4 years it was failing in more than 8% of cases. Resistance was also reported in the United Kingdom. Spectinomycin was abandoned as a first-line treatment for gonorrhea and is now unavailable in most countries.

The fluoroquinolones, such as ciprofloxacin and ofloxacin, were highly effective when they were first introduced and were widely used to treat gonorrhea. Low doses of 250 mg worked initially but had to be doubled by 1990. Ciprofloxacin-resistant strains were first reported in the Asian and Western Pacific regions in the 1990s. In the United States fluoroquinolone-resistant strains were reported first in Hawaii and then spread to the West Coast and then to rest of the United States. The CDC removed ciprofloxacin from recommended treatment for gonorrhea in 2007.

Azithromycin, developed in 1980, is another agent active against gonorrhea—but it is a drug that is also widely used for many other infections. Because decreased susceptibility to it has developed in many countries (initially reported in 1990s), its use is now recommended only when combined with another drug.

The cephalosporins, in active clinical use since the 1960s, have played a prominent role in the treatment of gonorrhea. The oral agent cefixime was recommended in the United States until failure rates became unacceptable. The current US treatment recommendations, which have been updated many times in recent decades, include use of azithromycin (orally) and an intramuscular injection of ceftriaxone.

Recent reports cause concern. In Seattle 5% of men who engage in homosexual relations and contract gonorrhea had infections with reduced susceptibility to azithromycin. In 2017 a woman in Canada was reported with ceftriaxone-resistant gonorrhea after having sexual contacts during a trip to China and Thailand.

Use of whole genome sequencing (allowing comprehensive genetic analyses of multiple strains; the entire genome of a bacterium is sequenced) has allowed much more detailed mapping of the spread of infections. Investigators in England used this technique to show the sustained transmission of one clone of azithromycin-resistant *N. gonorrhoeae* across England (Fifer 2018). Failures of azithromycin-ceftriaxone combination therapy have also been reported in UK men who acquired the infection in Asia. China has reported an increase in gonococcal strains resistant to azithromycin and with decreased susceptibility to ceftriaxone reaching 3.3% in 2016. In eastern Chinese cities, azithromycin resistance in gonorrhea was reported to reach 32% in 2014.

N. gonorrhoeae cannot travel alone. It accompanies its human host and can be transmitted in a new environment. Although widespread antibiotic use can lead to the independent emergence of antibiotic resistance to a particular antibiotic in more than one geographic region, genetic markers continue to highlight the important role of travelers in the global dissemination of resistant strains/clones of gonorrhea. HIV spread globally, largely through sexual activity, although it also has alternative routes of spread. Sex with a new partner is common during travel. One review estimated that the prevalence of casual sex was about 20% among foreign travelers. Identification of resistant gonorrhea infections in returned travelers has been one way to identify locations where resistant infections are circulating.

It is important to keep in mind that resistance of gonorrhea to antibiotics is reported from countries and locations with good surveillance and the capacity to monitor treatment outcomes and do susceptibility testing. Today virtually all infections with gonorrhea are diagnosed without growing the bacteria. There are many regions of the world where there are no laboratories with the capacity to grow (isolate) bacteria and test for drug susceptibility. Data available almost certainly underestimate the global extent of resistance.

Paradoxically, the improved treatment for HIV and use of and availability of pre-exposure prophylaxis (PrEP, which means taking anti-HIV medication preventively before having sexual contact) have led to decreased use of condoms and increased risk for other sexually transmitted infections, such as gonorrhea and syphilis, which have increased in many areas. A study from Australia found that regular use of condoms by gay and bisexual men dropped rapidly with the introduction of PrEP (46% in 2015 to 31% in 2017). They did not observe any significant decrease in condom use among HIV-negative men who were not using PrEP (Holt 2018).

It is likely that gonorrhea will continue to become resistant to widely used antibiotics, leading to failed treatment and the need to find new options. Sadly, it is a recurring theme. A phase 2 trial published in late 2018 found that a new antibiotic (zoliflodacin) that inhibits DNA biosynthesis was effective in treating urogenital and rectal gonococcal infections with a single oral dose (Taylor 2018). It has received a "fast track" designation from the FDA for development only as a treatment for gonococcal infections. It may be useful in the shortterm, but past events suggest that yet one more antibiotic is unlikely to provide a longterm solution for treating gonorrhea.

Are antibiotic-resistant bacteria found in all countries?

Yes. Resistant bacteria are found in all countries, but levels of resistance vary widely. Even bacteria in isolated human populations that have not been exposed to antibiotics have bacterial resistance genes, but levels of antibiotic resistance in such unexposed populations are low.

Are levels of resistance influenced by the amount of antibiotic used in a region or country?

Marked differences can be observed in the levels of antibiotic resistance by country and also in regions within countries. In some areas these seem to correlate with the amount of antibiotic used. In Europe the lowest levels of resistance are generally found in northern European countries, which also have the lowest levels of antibiotic use. Regional differences have been observed within the United States in limited studies. Levels of resistance are also influenced by spread of resistant bacteria. Some low- and middle-income countries with relatively low antibiotic use have high rates of resistance because resistant bacteria can spread easily because of poor sanitation and waste disposal.

A recent analysis explored the role of the temperature of the local environment and levels of antibiotic resistance, which vary regionally in the United States (MacFadden 2018). It found that higher local temperatures and increased population density were associated with higher levels of antibiotic resistance. They raise the question whether warming temperatures in some regions of the world could provide another driver for increasing antibiotic resistance. More research is needed to clarify the role of eco-climatic variables in the emergence and spread of resistant bacteria.

What can be done to slow or stop antibiotic resistance?

The main driver of antibiotic resistance is use of antibiotics. All of the interventions to reduce the need for antibiotics by reducing infections and reducing use by eliminating inappropriate and unnecessary administration in humans, animals, fish, and plants will potentially be useful. Treating or containing antibiotic-containing waste (from humans, animals, and pharmaceutical production facilities) can also reduce environmental contamination with antibiotics and their impact on soil, water, and other environmental bacteria. Once bacteria develop resistance to antibiotics, dissemination of resistance genes is more rapid and widespread in low-income countries. Resistance genes spread easily in areas that lack clean water and sanitary treatment of waste.

Two complementary approaches are needed to slow the increase in resistant bacteria: control the drivers that increase the appearance of resistance in the first place, and slow or stop the spread of resistant bacteria and resistance genes once they have appeared.

6

CONSEQUENCES
OF ANTIBIOTIC RESISTANCE

*What are the most important consequences of having
infections caused by antibiotic-resistant bacteria?*

Several major consequences stand out. Infections caused by
antibiotic-resistant bacteria lead to more deaths and disability
than infections caused by antibiotic-sensitive bacteria. They
cause more suffering through longer hospitalizations and
more adverse events. They cost more to treat than infections
caused by sensitive bacteria. They also compromise the benefit
of preventive antibiotics that many medical procedures now
depend on.

The Centers for Disease Control and Prevention (CDC)
estimates that in the United States each year, at least 2 million people develop serious infections caused by antibiotic-
resistant bacteria and at least 23,000 die from them. The
number of deaths from antibiotic-resistant infections in Europe
(European Union and European Economic Area) in 2015 was
estimated to be 33,000 (Cassini 2019). A 2014 report estimated
that globally about 700,000 people die each year from resistant
infections. The burden from antibiotic-resistant infections is
much greater in low- and middle-income countries than in
high-income countries. This is because the burden from infectious diseases generally is greater in low- and middle-income
than in high-income countries. One study estimated that in

India alone, 58,000 newborns die each year from antibiotic-resistant infections. A study from Thailand published in 2016 suggested that the rate of deaths from antibiotic-resistant infections in Thailand was four times higher than that in the United States.

Antibiotic-resistant infections are more expensive to treat than antibiotic-sensitive ones. The drugs are more expensive, hospitalizations are longer, patients have more adverse reactions, and outcomes may be poor.

The situation is getting worse. A recent analysis of deaths and disability caused by antibiotic-resistant bacteria in the European Union and the European Economic Area (Cassini 2019) found that the burden from these infections has increased since 2007. The burden was highest in infants and people age 65 years and older. The burden as measured by disability-adjusted life-years (DALYs) was huge—almost as high as all of the disability from influenza, tuberculosis, and HIV combined. The burden was greatest in Italy and Greece.

After thoughtful review of the available data, economist Jim O'Neill, who has studied antibiotic-resistant infections extensively (Hall 2018; O'Neill 2016), has given his best estimate of 1.5 million deaths annually from antimicrobial-resistant infections globally. These estimates include deaths from drug-resistant tuberculosis and from the parasitic infection malaria. Both of these numbers are substantial and contribute to the high number. To put the numbers into perspective, the 1.5 million estimate puts the number of deaths in the same range as deaths globally from diabetes mellitus and higher than deaths from road injuries. Some projections put estimated annual global deaths from antibiotic resistance as high as 10 million by 2050. Better estimates may be available in the future from the Institute for Health Metrics and Evaluation. There is general agreement among multiple sources that problems related to antibiotic resistance are worsening and are likely to continue to worsen in the foreseeable future.

In the United States the estimated cost of drug resistance is $20 billion per year for direct costs. Decreased productivity related to antibiotic resistance is estimated to add another $35 billion in costs annually.

O'Neill has done economic analysis taking into account the additional health care costs incurred by drug resistance, the lost productivity of patients affected by these infections, and the social cost of illness or death. This leads to an estimated global cost to health systems of $57 billion, with an additional estimate of $174 billion for lost productivity. Modern medicine today relies on effective antibiotics. Removing that pillar—or even chipping away at it—is extremely costly.

Recognizing the potential major economic impact of antibiotic resistance, other groups, including the World Bank, have developed models for projected costs. The consequences of antimicrobial resistance could decrease world economic output (gross domestic product) by as much as 2% to 3%. Although the estimates and projections vary, they are all large and suggest a substantial economic impact of antibiotic resistance.

Are infections caused by antibiotic-resistant bacteria less severe, more severe, or the same?

Infections caused by antibiotic-resistant bacteria can be similar in severity, more severe, or less severe than infections caused by antibiotic-sensitive bacteria. It depends on the specific bacteria and even the specific strain. Antibiotic-resistant bacteria are not necessarily more able to produce toxins, invade tissues more readily, or spread more easily than antibiotic-sensitive bacteria. The capacity to resist antibiotics and the capacity to cause disease are two distinct and separate characteristics of bacteria. Transmissibility—or the capacity of bacteria to spread or transfer from one person to another or from one host to another (like from animal to human)—is yet another attribute of bacteria. Bacteria that can cause disease are described as pathogenic. They often have virulence factors, like the capacity to produce toxins, that allow them to invade, damage, or destroy cells or tissues. Bacteria that are normally considered nonpathogenic (unable or unlikely to cause disease), like some of the staphylococci that live on our skin (*Staphylococcus epidermidis*) or streptococci that live in our mouths, can cause serious infections under the right circumstances.

So-called nonpathogenic bacteria can be extremely resistant to all or most antibiotics. Extremely nasty or virulent ones, like Group A *Streptococcus*, can be sensitive to penicillin and many other antibiotics. Extreme antibiotic resistance plus virulence and easy transmissibility in the same bacterium is the worst possible combination of attributes. The bacteria that caused pneumonic plague (the form of plague that infected the lungs; the Black Death) and killed about a third of the population in Europe was highly transmissible and highly virulent. This outbreak occurred before antibiotics (or vaccines) were available. The cause of the deaths and means of spread were not understood at that time. In a contemporary outbreak in Madagascar in 2017, there were more than 2,300 confirmed and probable cases of plague and more than 200 died, even though the bacteria were not resistant to most antibiotics. Plague is highly transmissible and rapidly progressive, and early diagnosis and treatment are required to save lives.

Some bacteria that pick up resistance genes become less fit (strong) and less able to compete with other bacteria and may cause less severe infection. However, many antibiotic-resistant bacteria keep their full capacity to produce severe disease. Antibiotic-resistant bacteria can also acquire new virulence traits.

Are outcomes worse for antibiotic-resistant infections?

Being infected with resistant bacteria leads to worse outcomes in many instances. Effective treatment may be delayed. Often the bacteria are not known to be resistant when treatment is started—so people are initially treated with an antibiotic that doesn't work against the bacteria. Patients have all the potential side effects from the antibiotic and no benefit from it. So it is like having no treatment—and perhaps worse if there are side effects from the drug. There may be a delay in getting results from susceptibility testing and identifying what alternative drug might work. If the bacteria have not been cultured in the laboratory, an inactive antibiotic may be continued.

Often the alternative drugs are more toxic, less effective, less accessible (there may be a delay in getting access to them), and more expensive. Patients may be unable or unwilling to pay for them. Clinicians may be unfamiliar with the drugs, their administration, and their side effects. In some instances, no alternative antibiotic options exist. Clinicians can review whether any other interventions, such as surgery, draining infected fluid, removing artificial material, giving immune therapy, or stopping drugs like steroids that adversely affect the capacity to control infection, might be useful adjunctive treatment.

Patients with carbapenem-resistant *Enterobacteriaceae* (CRE) in their blood have poor outcomes. In one study 22% died within 14 days—and these patients overall were 4.5 times more likely to die than someone infected with antibiotic-sensitive bacteria (Tamma 2017). Hospitalization also often ends up being longer—and more expensive—and there is more time for complications to develop from being in the hospital. In India patients infected with multiply and extensively resistant bacteria like *Escherichia coli, Klebsiella*, and *Acinetobacter baumannii* were two to three times more likely to die than other patients (Gandra 2018). Many of these patients have severe underlying diseases.

The alternative drugs used to treat patients infected with resistant bacteria may have toxic side effects. Among the more serious are those that can lead to hearing loss (which can be permanent), kidney failure (which can require kidney dialysis), and liver failure (which can be fatal—or can require liver transplantation). The longer course of antibiotic treatment may increase risk for *Clostridioides difficile* infection (see section on *C. difficile* in chapter 3).

What are the consequences of being colonized or having these multiply resistant bacteria present on the skin, in the gut, or on superficial wounds? As has been noted earlier, most people who carry these multidrug-resistant bacteria in their intestines are unaware of it and do not have symptoms. However, the bacteria in the gut provide a reservoir or pool of bacteria that sometimes escape and cause infections in other parts of the body, for example, urinary tract infections (UTIs). In a study from Norway (a country with low background prevalence of multiply resistant bacteria), researchers analyzed patients with UTIs caused by multiply resistant bacteria (extended-spectrum beta-lactamase [ESBL] positive). They identified 100 patients who had community-acquired UTIs caused by ESBL-positive *E. coli* or *Klebsiella* (common bacteria causing UTIs). They then found 190 other patients (controls) with UTIs who were similar in characteristics of age, sex, underlying diseases, and severity of infection and looked at differences between the two groups. Those with infections with multiply resistant bacteria (ESBL-positive) had several independent risk factors. They were more likely to have had recent travel to Asia, the Middle East, or Africa; recent use of fluoroquinolones or beta-lactamase antibiotics; and diabetes. By far the greatest increase in risk (21 times higher risk) was travel to Asia, the Middle East, or Africa within the past 6 weeks. For travel 6 weeks to 24 months earlier the increased odds for infection with these resistant bacteria were 2.3 times.

Another study showed similar findings. In the United States, patients seen in emergency rooms with pyelonephritis (kidney infection) caused by ESBL-producing *E. coli* were more than four times more likely to have traveled outside the United States in the last 90 days than those infected with non-ESBL-producing *E. coli*.

So, although most people who acquire resistant bacteria (often related to travel or recent antibiotics) do not develop problems, when they develop an infection, the bacteria often come from their own reservoir of bacteria, often those carried in the gut. People carrying resistant bacteria are more likely to have resistant bacteria that cause their infections—and these are often harder to treat.

What would be the consequences if antibiotics stopped working? What do people mean by the "postantibiotic era"?

In the preantibiotic era, several infectious diseases were in the top 10 killers in the United States. We still rely on antibiotics today to treat many serious infections, like pneumonia, urinary tract infections, sepsis, meningitis, bacterial endocarditis, skin and soft tissue infections, wound infections, and others. The burden from infectious diseases in the United States and other high-income countries decreased dramatically even before antibiotics became available because of improved sanitation, clean water, vaccination, and other factors. However, we still rely on antibiotics to treat many severe infections for which no effective vaccines or other interventions currently exist. These include everything from the common streptococcal and staphylococcal infections to rare and lethal infections like plague and tularemia. We need effective antibiotics to save lives. Health systems in low- and middle-income countries have even greater need for effective antibiotics because the burden of infectious diseases is much greater.

What medical procedures today rely on the availability of highly effective preventive antibiotics?

Modern medicine relies on antibiotics to provide support for many kinds of surgery, for chemotherapy, and for other medical interventions. Antibiotics have been called the "bedrock of modern medicine" because they also allow interventions that would be extremely risky without antibiotic support.

Antibiotics are routinely used today in surgery and medical procedures to reduce the likelihood of infections. Preventive antibiotics are used for hip fracture surgery, transrectal prostate biopsy, pacemaker implantation, spinal surgery, knee and hip replacements, cesarean section, abdominal hysterectomy, colorectal surgery, and other procedures. Antibiotics are used to support cancer chemotherapy because they treat and prevent infections that occur as a consequence of chemotherapy. An estimated 650,000 cancer patients in the United States receive chemotherapy each year. Of those, about 10% develop an infection that requires treatment.

The benefits of antibiotics can be substantial. In a recent study of 200 children with acute leukemia receiving intensive chemotherapy, the likelihood of bacteremia (bacteria in the bloodstream) was significantly lower in those receiving preventive antibiotics (with levofloxacin) than in a control group (about 22% vs. 43%) (Alexander 2018). In the same study, however, children undergoing hematopoietic stem cell transplantation had no significant benefit from levofloxacin.

Antibiotics are used in the United States for common procedures involving millions of patients annually. For example, the estimated numbers for some common procedures per year in the United States for recent years are cesarean section, 1.3 million; transrectal prostate biopsy, 1 million; spinal surgery, 796,000; hysterectomy, 498,000; and total hip replacement, 332,000.

Surgical procedures could be done without using antibiotics, but the rates of infection would be substantially higher. Infections, especially if they involve artificial material, like a prosthetic joint or a pacemaker, can be extremely difficult and expensive to treat and sometimes can require removal of the material.

A recent study analyzed the potential consequences of antibiotic resistance on surgery and cancer chemotherapy in the

United States (Teillant 2015). Based on published literature, the investigators estimated that about 40% to 50% of bacteria causing surgical site infections and more than a quarter of those causing infections after chemotherapy are already resistant to standard preventive antibiotics being used today in the United States. They then estimated what the consequences would be with increasing antibiotic resistance. If the efficacy of antibiotic chemoprophylaxis decreased even by 30%, they estimated there would be about 120,000 additional infections and 6,300 additional deaths per year in the United States.

A recent prospective study done in hospitals in Israel, Switzerland, and Serbia between 2012 and 2017 aimed to answer the question of whether patients who carried ESBL-producing *Enterobacteriaceae* in their feces before colorectal surgery were more likely than those who did not carry it to develop surgical site–related infection after surgery. None of the patients had an infection at the time of surgery, and all received prophylaxis (preventive antibiotic) with a cephalosporin antibiotic plus metronidazole. The researchers found that a surgical site infection developed significantly more often in ESBL-positive carriers than in noncarriers (almost 25% vs. 11%). Carrying these antibiotic-resistant bacteria more than doubled the risk of infection (Dubinsky-Pertzov 2018). In this study almost 14% of all patients screened had fecal cultures that were positive for ESBL-producing *Enterobacteriaceae*, predominantly *E. coli*. These bacteria are not susceptible to the antibiotics routinely used for prophylaxis for colorectal surgery. As these resistance genes become more widely disseminated, one can expect to see more failures following usual antibiotic prophylaxis.

Do we have antibiotics to use when bacteria become resistant to first-line drugs?

The list of alternative antibiotics is long, but many are slightly different versions of current drugs. A review of drugs in the antibacterial pipeline in 2018 found that it was dominated by derivatives of established antibiotics—for example, another version of a tetracycline or a macrolide or a fluoroquinolone (Theuretzbacher 2019). Some involve adding a new chemical to an old antibiotic to extend its activity and make it active against a broader array of bacteria. The number is growing, but many of the new antibiotics have fairly narrow indications and are aimed specifically at antibiotic-resistant infections. Very few target the important group of resistant infections caused by Gram-negative bacteria, the *Enterobacteriaceae* that can be multiply resistant, like *E. coli* and *Klebsiella*.

Are these other antibiotics as safe and effective as first-line drugs? Are they available and affordable?

A number of alternative antibiotics have been developed for use in situations where first- and second-line drugs do not work because of resistance or cannot be used because of allergies or other issues. Often they are approved by the US Food and Drug Administration (FDA) for specific and narrow indications, for example, complicated skin and soft tissue infections or community-acquired pneumonia.

Some have side effects or contraindications that would prevent them from being used in wide populations. In general, there is much less experience with them than with first-line drugs. Unusual and serious side effects may not have been identified. With the fluoroquinolones, like ciprofloxacin, which have been used extensively throughout the world, new adverse reactions are being identified decades after their introduction—and after tens of millions of doses have been given.

Many of the alternative drugs are extremely expensive. They may not be available in many countries or regions. A review of the new antibiotics (those considered new chemical entities and not just slightly modified drugs) approved between 1999 and 2014 identified 25 that were for systemic use. Of these, only 12 had registered sales in more than 10 countries globally. Of these antibiotics, half were approved for infections caused by antibiotic-resistant bacteria (Kaliberg 2018) and so had narrow indications for use.

Can antibiotics still be used for prevention when bacteria become resistant?

Antibiotic resistance makes it harder to prevent and treat infections. Antibiotics were initially tested for their effectiveness in preventing infections during surgery and in other settings at a time when the bacteria on the skin and in the bodies of most people were sensitive to them. As a higher percentage of people in the community carry bacteria resistant to the drugs used for prevention, like the cephalosporins, the preventive antibiotics are less likely to work—or will be less effective than in the past. One option is to escalate the choice of antibiotic to a generation or class of antibiotic (or a combination) that broader spectrum and is more likely to work. This is already done in some situations, but choices are limited. Antibiotics used for prevention also need to be extremely safe.

Are people dying today because of antibiotic-resistant infections?

The short answer is yes, but we do not know how many. The number is projected to increase. The study mentioned earlier estimated that 33,000 people in Europe died from antibiotic-resistant infections in 2015 (Cassini 2019). Many of them also had other underlying diseases, so the resistant bacteria may have been only one factor in their deaths.

Globally today more people are probably dying from lack of access to antibiotics than from antibiotic-resistant infections; however, we are also seeing deaths in people with infections resistant to all available antibiotics.

One major problem today that is likely to only worsen over time is that antibiotic choices are extremely limited for many people globally. When bacteria become resistant to the first-line, inexpensive, available antibiotics, as is happening in many areas, and when alternatives that are effective are not available, an infection can be functionally/operationally untreatable in that setting and for that patient.

The majority of deaths from infectious diseases globally today are in low- and middle-income countries. Infectious diseases account for a small proportion of all deaths today in high-income countries. Chronic diseases like heart disease, cancer, and diabetes are overwhelmingly the most common cause of deaths in the United States and other high-income countries. Deaths in all areas are expected to increase with increasing antibiotic resistance but are likely to disproportionately affect people living in low- and middle-income countries where infections are more common (poor sanitation and lack of clean water contribute to spread; poor nutrition and micronutrient deficiencies increase burden; access to medical care may be limited).

Rates of antibiotic resistance are higher today in many low- and middle-income countries than in high-income countries. Antibiotic use drives the emergence of antibiotic-resistant bacteria everywhere, but in countries that lack clean water and good sanitary facilities, antibiotic-resistant bacteria can spread easily.

Observations in travelers who pick up antibiotic-resistant bacteria simply by traveling to countries with poor sanitation confirm the ongoing fecal contamination of food, drink, and the environment with resistant bacteria in these areas.

A current, active outbreak may be a harbinger of events to come. An outbreak of extensively drug-resistant (XDR) *Salmonella enterica* subsp. *enterica* serovar Typhi (cause of typhoid fever) in Pakistan was first reported in February 2018 (Klemm 2018) after 339 cases had occurred mainly in Hyderabad, east of Karachi. During 2016–2018 5,372 cases of XDR typhoid fever were reported in Pakistan (Chatham-Stephens 2019). Five cases of XDR typhoid fever were identified in the United States in patients who had traveled to or from Pakistan. Cases have also been identified in the United Kingdom after visits to Pakistan. The current outbreak strain is susceptible only to azithromycin and carbapenems. Only one oral antibiotic (azithromycin) is effective against it—and it is expected that it will be only a matter of time until the bacteria will become resistant to that drug as well. That will make the infection untreatable with oral antibiotics. The only options for treatment would be expensive intravenous drugs that are not available or affordable for many patients in low-income countries.

The bacteria that cause typhoid fever spread through contaminated food and water; they can spread easily in areas with poor sanitation. Each year about 22 million cases are estimated to occur. Infection can lead to intestinal hemorrhage and perforation, killing up to 15% of those infected. Even though antibiotics can be effective, about 200,000 people currently are estimated die from typhoid fever each year. The number of deaths is highest in South Asia and Africa. Before antibiotics were available, typhoid fever was fatal in about a third of patients in low-income countries and about 10% of patients in high-income countries. Use of effective antibiotics reduces the typhoid fever case fatality rate to less than 2%. A recent meta-analysis suggested that the overall case fatality rate was almost 2.5%—and higher (4.45%) in hospitalized patients. If antibiotic-resistant bacteria continue to spread in the absence of other interventions, the number of deaths could rise sharply.

Fortunately, a vaccine exists that may be able to help control spread. A recently approved vaccine is effective in young children (Andrews 2018). Pakistan began a vaccination campaign in February 2018 that aims to deliver 200,000 doses of vaccine. GAVI (the Global Vaccine Alliance, which brings together public and private sectors to provide new and underused vaccines for children in the poorest countries) agreed to purchase an additional 10 million doses for Pakistan.

Over recent decades the bacteria that cause typhoid fever (and those that cause a related infection, paratyphoid fever) have become progressively more resistant to commonly used antibiotics. It appears that the current strain emerged from one that had become resistant to multiple antibiotics and then acquired an additional resistance gene on a plasmid (a circular piece of DNA) most likely transferred from *E. coli*.

Some of what we know about typhoid fever in the United States comes from travelers. Travelers pick it up by eating contaminated food. The CDC collects information about typhoid and paratyphoid fever cases seen in the United States and periodically publishes descriptions about where infections were acquired and the resistance patterns. This helps clinicians make decisions about treatment early in the course of the infection. Over the years typhoid fever became resistant to the older antibiotics that could be taken by mouth, chloramphenicol, ampicillin, and trimethoprim-sulfamethoxazole, and then to the fluoroquinolones. Recently a single event in the bacteria, the acquisition of a plasmid, was able to transform this disease-causing bacterium into a virtually untreatable one (Klemm 2018).

Why are antibiotics considered community drugs? How does my taking an antibiotic affect my neighbors and the community?

Bacteria are communal property in a sense. We share bacteria from others and from the environment, and we contribute our own to the community through activities of regular daily life. We may share more with household members, close friends, and colleagues than with more distant relations.

When some of our resident bacteria become resistant to antibiotics, the genes conferring this resistance may be shared with bacteria in other communities in the neighborhood. We do not live in isolated bubbles. Our bacteria spill into the spaces around us and we constantly sample and exchange bacteria with our surroundings.

People who have not taken antibiotics can end up carrying multiply resistant bacteria that they have picked up from other people, animals, food and drink, or from the environment.

One study in nursing homes followed residents to see how often they picked up multiply drug resistant bacteria (D'Agata 2018). It found that almost a third of 137 nursing home residents who had not been given antibiotics picked up multiply resistant bacteria over a 12-month period. Factors that were associated with picking up resistant bacteria included frequent visits from health care providers, the presence of pressure ulcers (like bed sores), and taking certain medications that could affect the gastrointestinal tract (such as laxatives and drugs that affect the stomach acid). It is worth noting that well over half of the residents of the nursing homes received antibiotics during the 12-month period.

7

INTERVENTIONS TO REDUCE NEED FOR ANTIBIOTICS AND ALTERNATIVES TO ANTIBIOTICS

Are there ways to reduce the risks of infections so that we do not need antibiotics?

We have many tools available to reduce the need for antibiotics by reducing infections. It is worth examining several of these—keeping in mind that using antibiotics drives the appearance of antibiotic resistance. Given that probably at least half of antibiotics produced globally are used in animals, this section will also comment on the agricultural and food sectors.

The big three approaches—the major categories—include providing clean water and sanitation everywhere, wider use of vaccines, and better infection control in health care. Several other approaches will also be discussed. With these interventions the need for antibiotics could be dramatically reduced.

Throughout most of history, humans lived and populations multiplied without the use of drugs that today we call antibiotics—but that does not mean that they were ignorant of some of the principles that can reduce risk of infection or spread of infection from one person or animal to another. Today, even with abundant and varied antibiotics available, many interventions are extremely useful in reducing the need to use antibiotics. Unfortunately, humans sometimes forget or find it difficult to apply these principles, knowing that antibiotics are available if they develop a bacterial infection.

How do clean water and improved sanitation reduce use of antibiotics?

At the top of the list is clean water and sanitary waste disposal. Regrettably, about a quarter of people alive today do not have regular access to clean water. They collect water from surface water, streams, or springs, sometimes after walking long distances. Often it is contaminated with bacteria, viruses, or parasites. Soap for simple acts like handwashing and bathing may be unavailable. Many infections, including most of those that cause diarrhea, are picked up by drinking unsafe water or eating contaminated food. In 2015, the World Health Organization (WHO) estimated that 71% of the global population had safely managed drinking water service on the premises (at the house or living quarters), available when needed and free from contamination. At the same time 844 million people lacked basic drinking water service. Almost 2 billion people use drinking water that is contaminated with feces. In 2015, 2.3 billion people lacked basic sanitation services (like toilets or latrines) and 892 million still practiced open defecation. These people are usually unable to wash their hands afterward or before preparing or eating food. This contributes to contaminated food and diarrhea and other infections. When these infections are severe, they are typically treated with antibiotics, even though many of them are caused by viruses or parasites that will not respond to antibiotics.

Diarrhea still remains a leading cause of death and illness in children younger than 5 years of age in low- and middle-income countries, but there has been progress. Deaths from diarrhea have dropped from 1.2 million in 2000 to 446,000 in 2016—still a very large number. The highest rates of death from diarrhea are in sub-Saharan Africa, south Asia, and Southeast Asia. It is not just the acute diarrhea episodes that take a toll on these children, but also the other consequences of these episodes of illness. Diarrhea, especially during the first 2 years of life, can affect the absorption of essential nutrients and lead to poor physical growth and impaired cognitive (brain) development. Undernutrition leads to a reduced response to vaccines and increased risk for other infections. Effects can be lifelong and can affect learning and productivity (Troeger 2018; Wierzba 2018).

One of the UN Sustainable Development Goals for 2030 (Goal 6) is to ensure the availability and sustainable management of water and sanitation for all. The WHO/UNICEF program called WASH monitors progress in the areas of water supply, sanitation, and hygiene. The WHO and UNICEF are tracking progress toward 2030 goals, which are aspirational global targets, and are working in several related areas: drinking water, sanitation and hygiene, wastewater management, water use efficiency, integrated resource management, and protection of aquatic ecosystems.

When travelers visit countries where access to clean water and sanitation is limited, they may develop so-called travelers' diarrhea, which results from consuming contaminated food or drink. This is a small problem relative to the burden of disease in low-income countries caused by lack of clean water and sanitation—but it is one of the most common problems experienced by travelers and can end up disrupting a trip (and requiring medical care in some instances). It is a marker for the frequent fecal contamination of food and water. Lack of clean water and sanitation contributes to deaths in infants and young children locally. Collateral damage from it includes the frequent use of antibiotics and its contribution to the global development of resistance. This also consumes family resources for medical care and lost productivity.

In the United States when safe drinking water through chlorination and other approaches was provided, there were major decreases in typhoid fever and other infections spread by contaminated water. This occurred in the early 1900s in most major cities—long before antibiotics and vaccines were available to treat or prevent many of these infections. Availability of clean water had a major impact on disease and deaths in the United States.

Because diagnostic tests to identify the specific cause of illness are usually not available, sick children are often given antibiotics in the hopes that they might help even when infections are caused by viruses and parasites that will not respond to antibiotics. In many countries antibiotics are readily available in local stores without a prescription or from roadside stands. Unfortunately, many of these are poor quality and may have none of the active antibiotic or a limited amount of it—or worse, adulterants or other substances that are toxic.

Lack of clean water and sanitation (or inadequate use) can also contribute to respiratory infections. A large study done in England compared adults in primary care practices. Half were assigned to a web-based internet intervention designed to increase handwashing. The other half had no intervention. The findings? The participants in the handwashing arm of the study had fewer influenza-like illnesses and fewer gastrointestinal illnesses than those who did not have the intervention. Even more impressive is that the benefits extended to the family members of those assigned to the intervention designed to increase handwashing. This showed that even in a high-income country benefits from handwashing can be shown in decreasing respiratory and diarrheal illnesses (Little 2015; van Weel 2015).

In Bangladesh and other countries, WASH programs (with focus on safe water, sanitation, and hygiene), which were developed to provide the means for handwashing, can lead to a decrease in both diarrhea and respiratory infections.

Clean water and sanitation are a basic foundation for preventing the spread of infections. Globally the most frequent illnesses leading to use of antibiotics are diarrhea and respiratory infections, so interventions to reduce their frequency could have a global impact on overall antibiotic use. Benefits are likely to be greatest in populations that lack basic access to clean water and sanitation, but studies, such as the one in England mentioned earlier, suggest that even high-income countries could benefit from attention to basics, like handwashing (Grayson 2018).

Another behavioral change that could potentially reduce the need for antibiotic treatment is for women with recurrent bladder infections to increase their daily water intake (Hooton 2018). A study in the United States found that older women with at least three urinary tract infections a year who normally had low water intake could reduce infections by 50% by simply drinking an extra 1.5 liters of water daily. The women who drank more water also ended up taking fewer courses of antibiotics (1.9 instead of 3.6 courses of antibiotics per year). This is an inexpensive intervention to reduce antibiotic use.

Poor nutrition and micronutrient deficiencies—most common in low-income countries—can also contribute to the burden from respiratory and diarrheal infection. Making populations more resilient and less susceptible to these infections can also help to reduce the need for antibiotics.

Similar benefits can be seen in the agricultural sector. Food animals that are raised in modern facilities with good hygiene, good ventilation, good nutrition, good biosecurity (preventing rats, other rodents, and other wildlife from mixing with them), appropriate vaccination for the animal and location, and optimized genetic stocks and without excessive crowding are less likely to need antibiotic treatment or to benefit from antibiotics given for growth promotion.

How can processing and handling of food affect antibiotic use?

The process known as pasteurization that is used for milk and some other products followed from work originally done by Louis Pasteur, who showed, among other things, that bacteria were responsible for the spoilage (and fermentation) of milk and other products. This knowledge was harnessed to make milk much safer. By killing bacteria that might contaminate raw milk and combining this with refrigeration to markedly slow the growth of any residual, surviving bacteria, infections associated with drinking raw milk virtually disappeared. These included infections caused by *Brucella* spp., *Campylobacter* spp., *Salmonella* spp., *Listeria monocytogenes, Escherichia coli,* and other bacteria. Making certain cows were free of certain infections also helped to make the milk supply safer. In many countries milk is not routinely pasteurized, so travelers must check the source and processing of milk and be aware that products made with milk (e.g., ice cream, yogurt, cottage cheese, butter, fresh cheeses) may have been made with unpasteurized milk and may be unsafe.

Avoiding infections related to raw milk is another way to reduce the need for antibiotics. The Food and Drug Administration (FDA) does not regulate raw milk in the United States, but it advises states not to permit the sale of raw milk. Although pasteurized milk is available everywhere in the United States, some individuals choose to drink raw milk, putting them at risk for infections. In some states raw milk can be sold on the farm or at farmers' markets, and in 12 states it can be sold in retail stores. "Cow-share" programs are allowed in some states, through which consumers combine resources to buy a cow (and consume its milk). Unfortunately, outbreaks of infections related to raw milk are still common in the United States. For example, between 2010 and 2012, there were 51 outbreaks of infections related to consumption of raw milk in the United States. In 2016 an outbreak of *Campylobacter jejuni* infections (a cause of diarrhea and other infections) was traced to drinking unpasteurized milk in Colorado. No one died, but one person had to be hospitalized. What was notable in this outbreak was that the infections were resistant to the antibiotics often used to treat *Campylobacter* infections (resistant to ciprofloxacin, tetracycline, and nalidixic acid).

Foodborne infections are common in the United States and globally. Contamination can occur at many points in the growing, production, and processing cycle. There are also many measures that can be taken that are under a consumer's control to reduce the burden from foodborne infections through safe storage and safe preparation. Although some foodborne infections are caused by viruses (e.g., norovirus, hepatitis A, other) or parasites (*Cyclospora, Cryptosporidia*), bacteria are the most common causes of foodborne infections. These include *Campylobacter, Salmonella,* Shiga toxin–producing *E. coli* (STEC), *Listeria, Vibrio,* and *Yersinia.* Many are self-limited but some are severe, leading to hospitalization and death. The CDC's Foodborne Diseases Active Surveillance Network (FoodNet) monitors cases of foodborne infections that are diagnosed in laboratories at 10 sites in the United States (covering about 15% of the US population or about 49 million people in 2015). This enables the CDC to have a general idea of the infections and trends in the United States. In 2016 FoodNet identified almost 25,000 cases, about 5,500 hospitalizations, and 98 deaths that were from foodborne infections. The most common bacteria identified in the United States were *Campylobacter, Salmonella, Shigella,* Shiga toxin–producing *E. coli, Yersinia, Vibrio,* and *Listeria.*

Globally the picture of foodborne infections is very different. The burden from foodborne infections is much greater in low- and middle-income countries and is highest in Africa and parts of Asia. Lack of refrigeration contributes to bacterial growth when food is contaminated. Overall an estimated 230,000 people died from foodborne diarrheal agents globally in 2010. A large share (40%) of the burden of foodborne infections is borne by children under 5 years of age. Food- and waterborne infections also include cholera and typhoid fever. Reducing foodborne infections, including through improved sanitation and food handling, could reduce global antibiotic use. Food can also be a source of antibiotic-resistant bacteria.

How can using vaccines reduce the need for antibiotics?

Another major intervention we can use to reduce the need for antibiotics is wider use of vaccines. We have multiple excellent vaccines, many given routinely to infants and young children and others used in older age and high-risk groups. Some prevent viral infections, such as influenza, polio, and measles, and others can prevent bacterial infections, such as *Haemophilus influenzae* meningitis and other infections (Hib vaccine), cholera, typhoid fever, and pneumococcal infections. They have saved millions of lives, prevented billions of episodes of illness, and averted serious disabilities, such as the paralysis that can follow poliovirus infections. We have not gained the maximum benefit possible from existing vaccines because many people have not received the full range of vaccines that could protect them.

Introduction of the pneumococcal vaccine has led to dramatic decreases in hospitalizations and deaths from pneumococcal pneumonia and other pneumococcal invasive infections (like meningitis and middle ear infections) in young children who have received the vaccine. Many types of pneumococci, called serotypes, cause serious infections. The 7-valent pneumococcal vaccine (PCV7) protects against 7 of these; the 13-valent pneumococcal vaccine (PCV13) protects against 13. In the United States the PCV7 was introduced in 2000 and the PCV13 in 2010. This has resulted in decreased numbers of cases of acute otitis media (middle ear infection) due to the pneumococcal serotypes included in the vaccine and an overall decrease in antibiotic use. One study published in 2008 showed a 42% reduction in antibiotic prescriptions for treating acute otitis media after the PCV7 was introduced in 2000. Even more remarkable is that use of the vaccine has been associated with decreases in pneumococcal infections in persons who have not been vaccinated, such as older populations who are at increased risk for pneumococcal pneumonia. This is attributed to the capacity of the vaccine to affect carriage of the *Streptococcus pneumoniae* bacteria in the throat. Normally many people carry strains of bacteria (the presence of bacteria in the absence of symptoms is called colonization) in the throat without knowing it. These bacteria also have the capacity to invade and cause disease.

A recent study estimated that universal coverage with the 13-valent pneumococcal vaccine in young children could avoid 11.4 million days of antibiotic use globally in children under the age of 5 (Boston Consulting Group). Globally at present coverage with this vaccine is only about 40%—so there is a major opportunity to increase coverage and reduce the need for antibiotics. Coverage with the Hib vaccine is better (about 70% globally) but should still be improved. In Iceland, use of a combination pneumococcal–*H. influenzae* conjugate vaccine reduced ear infections by 40% in children younger than 4 months (Sigurdsson 2018).

Despite use of vaccines, acute otitis media is still the most common reason for an antibiotic prescription in a young child. Although vaccine coverage of young children is generally high in the United States (despite the presence of populations that have been skeptical about their benefits and have been hesitant to receive them) and most other high-income countries, many vaccines given routinely in the United States, such as the Hib vaccine, pneumococcal conjugate vaccine, rotavirus vaccine, and meningococcal vaccine, are unavailable or unaffordable in some low- and middle-income countries. Children in many regions of the world are also at risk for infections that are rare or nonexistent in high-income countries—infections for which good vaccines exist but are not given because of the cost and lack of access. For example, cholera outbreaks continue to occur in many low-income countries, with recent examples being outbreaks in Haiti and a massive outbreak in the past 2 years in Yemen. A cholera outbreak started in Yemen in October 2016. By March 2018 there were more than 1.1 million cases with more than 2,000 deaths countrywide. A safe and effective cholera vaccine exists and should be deployed much more broadly. Cholera is easy to treat and patients can be cured with early fluid replacement and antibiotics; however, systems to provide safe treatment and clean water and sanitary facilities are often unavailable in areas with outbreaks—and many still die from these infections.

Another vaccine that could prevent disease and save lives, especially in young children in parts of Asia, is the vaccine to prevent typhoid fever. Because the bacteria that cause typhoid fever are increasingly becoming resistant to all common antibiotics, it is becoming more difficult and expensive to treat—among even those who have access to treatment. The WHO recommended in March 2018 that infants and children over 6 months old in countries where typhoid fever is endemic or epidemic receive a single dose of the typhoid conjugate vaccine. This recommendation was made after reviewing the safety, efficacy, and affordability of the vaccine and the growing rates of antibiotic-resistant typhoid fever. The highest-priority countries are those that have the highest burden of typhoid fever (countries in the Indian subcontinent) and those with a growing burden of drug-resistant infections. In countries where it is feasible, they recommended that vaccines should also be given to children up to age 15 years in catch-up campaigns. One of the advantages of the recommended typhoid vaccine is that it is a conjugate vaccine and can produce an immune response in infants as young as 6 months of age. The appearance and spread of an extensively drug-resistant strain of typhoid fever since 2018 in Pakistan makes the argument for expanding use of the vaccine even more compelling.

How can vaccines against viral infections reduce the need for antibiotics? Why does influenza, a virus, get so much attention?

It is easy to understand how using a vaccine that prevents a bacterial infection could reduce the use of antibiotics, for example, preventing pneumococcal pneumonia, meningococcal meningitis, or typhoid fever—infections that require treatment with antibiotics. But vaccines that protect against viral infections can also have a major impact on the use of antibiotics for two main reasons. The first is that many infections, bacterial and viral, cause similar symptoms. Quick and accurate diagnostic tests typically are not available to make an immediate specific diagnosis, so many people with viral infections end up getting antibiotics, even though antibiotics are totally ineffective in this setting. So children with diarrhea from rotavirus infection or fever from influenza might be given an antibiotic because they are sick. Viral respiratory infections are a common reason for unnecessary and inappropriate use of antibiotics.

The second way a vaccine against a viral infection can help to reduce antibiotic use is to help to prevent a bacterial complication of a viral infection. The influenza virus by itself can cause severe infection that can be fatal in a small percentage of cases, usually by causing severe damage to the lungs. The influenza virus infection targets tissues of the respiratory tract and disrupts normal protective barriers and also predisposes those who are influenza infected to secondary bacterial infections of the bronchi and lungs (bronchitis and pneumonia) and to bacterial infection of the sinuses (sinusitis) and middle ear (otitis media). The respiratory tract, damaged and vulnerable because of infection with the influenza virus, is especially susceptible to infection by bacteria, such as *Streptococcus pneumoniae* and *Staphylococcus aureus*, that may be found in the respiratory tract. Damage of tissues by the viral infection can allow bacteria to gain a foothold and invade. The presence of a viral infection (influenza but also other viral infections, whether symptomatic or asymptomatic) also increases the bacterial colonization and the density of the bacteria in the respiratory tract—perhaps by disrupting protective barriers or providing better nutritional conditions for bacteria with the presence of mucus and dead cells or host cell debris (DeMuri 2018). Staphylococcal, streptococcal, and pneumococcal infections can be severe and occasionally lethal infections even in young healthy individuals. Hence, preventing influenza with the vaccine will also prevent some secondary bacterial infections that follow. Influenza vaccine cannot prevent all bacterial pneumonias, but it can reduce the frequency of those that occur as a complication of acute influenza virus infection. Many of the millions of deaths from the 1918–1919 influenza pandemic were probably from these secondary bacterial pneumonia infections. The good news is that we now have antibiotics for treating bacterial infections (not available 100 years ago); the bad news is that many of these bacteria are now resistant to many of the commonly used antibiotics.

Influenza is one of the viral infections for which we also have specific antiviral drugs, though most people who are infected with influenza are not treated with anti-influenza drugs because they do not seek medical care or because the specific diagnosis of influenza is not made. Some influenza viruses have now become resistant to the anti-influenza drugs.

Influenza outbreaks occur every year in the United States during the cooler months. Although the severity of illness and number of cases vary from year to year, outbreaks occur every year. In the temperate Southern Hemisphere, outbreaks occur during their cooler months. In the tropics, outbreaks can be seen throughout the year, though patterns may also be affected by seasonal rainfall. In the United States, an estimated 12,000 to 56,000 people die every year from influenza and 140,000 to 710,000 people are hospitalized because of influenza. The 2017–2018 season was particularly severe and an estimated 80,000 people died from influenza. The numbers vary widely from year to year because some influenza strains cause more severe disease than others—and susceptibility to the viruses in the population may vary. When a new strain begins to circulate, as has happened every couple of decades or so, the death toll may be much higher.

Influenza is one of the infections that is found in every country. Global interconnectedness means that new strains travel even faster than in the past, though even a century ago the virus that caused perhaps 50 million to 100 million deaths globally spread to all continents even before the advent of rapid air travel. Influenza kills everywhere, and a recent study estimated that globally there could be almost 650,000 deaths each year from influenza (Iuliano 2017). The World Health Organization estimates that seasonal influenza epidemics cause 3 million to 5 million severe cases globally each year. The highest rates of death from influenza are estimated to be in low-income countries in sub-Saharan Africa and Southeast Asia and among older individuals.

In the United States, the Advisory Committee on Immunization Practices (ACIP), the group that makes vaccine recommendations for the country, recommends annual seasonal influenza vaccination for everyone over the age of 6 months who does not have a specific reason not to receive the vaccine. Despite publicity and campaigns reminding people about the vaccine (and now availability of the vaccine in local pharmacies), less than half the population receives it. Increased efforts are being made to try to reach certain groups, those who are most likely to have complications if they become infected— people over the age of 65 years, those with diabetes or chronic lung or cardiovascular disease, and pregnant women.

Influenza vaccination is also recommended for health care personnel because they can transmit influenza to vulnerable patients. Overall, in recent years about 47% of the entire population received the vaccine (children older than 6 months: almost 60%; all adults: 43%). Coverage is higher in those older than 65 years and in health care personnel. In 2016–2017 a survey found that 53.6% of pregnant women reported receiving influenza vaccine before (16.2%) or during (37.4%) pregnancy. Vaccination during pregnancy has the added benefit of protecting infants from influenza during their first 6 months of life when they are too young to receive the vaccine. In recent years more than 80% of pharmacists, physicians, and nurses received influenza vaccine, which is now mandated by some hospitals. Studies have shown that vaccinating health care workers not only reduces absenteeism among them but also reduces influenza illnesses and deaths in nursing home residents under their care. In a study in Veterans Administration health care systems, vaccination coverage among health care workers was 92% to 97% in those hospitals that mandated influenza vaccination and 60% to 68% in those that did not. During all three influenza seasons studied, vaccinated health workers had lower absenteeism from illness than unvaccinated workers.

An interesting study in the United States (Taksler 2015) found that in counties where younger adults (18 to 65 years old) had higher levels of coverage with influenza vaccine, the frequency of influenza in the older population (age 65 years and older) was lower. Previous studies in Japan have also shown that vaccinating children reduced rates of influenza in the older population. So vaccinating one segment of the population may help protect another by reducing the circulation of influenza virus in the community, and there may be community benefit from influenza vaccination that extends beyond the individual. Another study in Taiwan found that older patients who underwent major surgery had a lower risk of postoperative pneumonia and death in the hospital if they had received a preoperative influenza vaccination (Liu 2018). It is easy to make strong arguments in favor of influenza vaccination.

In the United States the percentage of people receiving the vaccine has increased in recent decades as recommendations for use of the vaccine have expanded. Globally, however, influenza vaccine is given to a small percentage of the population. The WHO recommends that seasonal vaccine be given to high-risk groups, but most countries globally do not have national influenza vaccine plans. At present the global capacity to produce influenza vaccine is insufficient to vaccinate everyone. The WHO estimates that 10 billion doses of flu vaccine would be needed if there were a pandemic (a global epidemic). The global potential annual production of influenza vaccine has increased from 1.5 billion doses in 2006 to 6.4 billion in 2016, but this number refers only to potential production capacity.

Currently only a few countries vaccinate 30% or more of their population (e.g., the United States, Canada, Israel, Japan, South Korea, Chile, Australia, and some countries in the European Union).

All influenza researchers agree that we need better influenza vaccines. The current ones must be reformulated each year to match the viruses that keep changing. Some years the vaccine produced is not a good match for the circulating viruses and protection is poor. Even under the best of circumstances the vaccine usually gives only 50% to 60% protection. Most of the vaccine is made using an egg-based production system (virus is grown in eggs), which is slow and requires a huge number of eggs. The duration of protection from the vaccine is short (months), so the vaccine must be administered each year. Many scientists are seeking to develop a better influenza vaccine, a so-called universal vaccine that would protect against the multiple influenza viruses that infect humans and would give long-lasting protection. This is worthy of a massive investment given the constant, predictable threat of influenza every year and the potential risk of another pandemic, like the one that devastated the world in 1918–1919, at a time when the global population was only 1.9 billion (in contrast to 7.6 billion in 2018). In the meantime, there are strong arguments to be made for wider use of the current vaccine as multiple laboratories continue research to develop a better one. The CDC estimates that use of influenza vaccine prevented 40,000 deaths in the United States between the 2005–2006 and 2013–2014 influenza seasons.

Measles, another viral infection for which we have an excellent vaccine, has continued to cause outbreaks and occasional deaths. Its high transmissibility means it is necessary to achieve extremely high coverage (95%) of a population with the vaccine to prevent outbreaks. Measles, a systemic infection, also affects the respiratory tract and dampens immune responses generally, making those infected more susceptible to other infections. It can also cause deaths, especially in young children and those who are immunocompromised or malnourished.

It is not clear exactly how much antibiotic consumption could be decreased with optimal vaccine coverage of the global population, but it is likely to be substantial. Current research also focuses on developing vaccines to protect against many other infections that may now prompt the use of antibiotics because of bacterial infection or concern that symptoms might be caused by bacterial infection. Some of the highest priorities for vaccines against bacterial infections are for *E. coli*, nontyphoid *Salmonella*, *Shigella* and Group A *Streptococcus*. A better vaccine against tuberculosis is also needed.

Vaccines also play an important role in decreasing some vector-borne infections that cause fever, especially the mosquito-transmitted viral infections yellow fever and Japanese encephalitis. These vaccines are used widely in some endemic areas but currently do not cover all at-risk populations. Vaccines have been approved for mosquito-transmitted dengue and malaria, two more fever-causing infections, though better vaccines are needed for both. There are also vaccines in development or in trials that would protect against Ebola, Zika, *S. aureus*, Group B *Streptococcus*, and other infections.

Are vaccines used to prevent infections in animals? Can they prevent infections that could affect humans?

Vaccines are not just for people, and antibiotics are also used widely in animals (pets and work and food animals). Use of vaccines in animals potentially can also reduce antibiotic use in animals. A vaccine against *Salmonella* infections in chickens could also reduce the likelihood of *Salmonella* contamination of eggs, which can cause human illness and lead to antibiotic use for treatment. *Salmonella* vaccination of breeder chickens can lower the rates of *Salmonella* infections in broiler chickens when they enter processing plants. This can mean less contamination of chicken carcasses with *Salmonella*, which can cause illness in humans. Commercial poultry is routinely vaccinated against a whole series of bacteria and viruses that do not infect humans (and that most people have never heard of). Marek disease vaccine, fowl pox vaccine, and Newcastle disease vaccine are among some of the poultry vaccines.

Commercial swine can be vaccinated against influenza and a whole range of other pathogenic bacteria and viruses. Pigs can be a source of influenza viruses that can infect humans. *E. coli* diarrhea in piglets can be reduced by vaccinating sows. Food animals typically are raised in high-density settings and are genetically similar. An infection that enters the flock, herd, or gaggle can easily spread.

Vaccines are also used to prevent infections in fish. Increasingly fish for human consumption is being raised in a range of artificial ponds, tanks, and specially prepared bodies of water. Vaccines can be injected into fish individually, placed in the water, or mixed with the fish food. Infections in fish are treated with many of the same antibiotics that are used to treat human infections. Websites with fish antibiotics display many familiar drugs marketed for ornamental fish—ampicillin, amoxicillin, ciprofloxacin, cephalexin, penicillin, metronidazole, erythromycin, and others.

How can controlling vectors like mosquitoes and ticks reduce antibiotic use?

It may seem paradoxical, but controlling mosquitoes and other arthropod vectors (e.g., ticks, fleas, mites, and flies) could also potentially decrease use of antibiotics. Vector-borne infections are those that are transmitted from one person to another or from an animal to a person by the bite of a mosquito, tick, or other biting arthropod (includes insects and eight-legged critters like ticks and mites) that moves the bacteria, virus, or parasite from one host to another. These vector-borne infections cause more than 700,000 deaths annually (more than 17% of all infectious diseases globally). Most of these infections are caused by parasites (like malaria) or viruses (like dengue, Zika, chikungunya, or yellow fever). Fewer are caused by bacteria (e.g., Lyme disease, rickettsial infections like Rocky Mountain spotted fever, and murine typhus in the United States). However, acute infections caused by all of these pathogens cause fever in the infected individual. A typical response to the presence of fever is treatment with one or more antibiotics. Of course, someone with a fever caused by a virus or parasite like malaria will not be helped by treatment with an antibiotic. When rapid diagnostic tests are not available to define the specific cause of fever, antibiotics are usually given "just in case they might work."

An example of this comes from India. In a study of children and adults in Pune, India, hospitalized with fever in a setting where laboratory testing could be done, 94% of the children and 82% of the adults were given antibiotics. Most of them received broad-spectrum antibiotics, and most received more than one antibiotic. Those who were suspected of having dengue or malaria were less likely to be given antibiotics, but on day 5, 59% of all of the patients were still receiving antibiotics, including patients whose cultures for bacteria were negative. Before admission 22% reported they had already taken antibiotics.

Poor nutrition and micronutrient deficiencies also make people more susceptible to infections and more likely to have poor outcomes. This is especially apparent in malnourished young children in low-income countries, who also lack access to clean food and adequate sanitation. Malnourished children may also have a less vigorous immune response to vaccines, compounding their problems.

Are health care–associated infections a common reason for antibiotic treatment?

A third major area where reducing infections could reduce the need for antibiotics is in the health care setting, whether inpatient, outpatient, chronic care, or other health care facilities (Magill 2014; Magill 2014). Regrettably, health care–associated infections, also known as nosocomial infections, are far more common than they should be and lead to frequent use of antibiotics as well as disability and death. In the past, these infections were considered inevitable—the price of receiving health care—but it is now clear from multiple studies that some can be virtually eliminated, for example, the bloodstream infections related to having an intravenous catheter in place to deliver antibiotics, and others can be markedly decreased.

The CDC, based on a 2011 study, found that on any given day about 1 in 25 hospitalized patients had at least one health care–associated infection. A survey done in 2010 found that about a quarter of them are related to devices, like catheters or ventilators (for patients who need assistance with breathing). The CDC tracks health care–associated infections and has an action plan to reduce these infections. They regularly publish data reports. Among other indicators, they track central line bloodstream infections, catheter-associated urinary tract infections, surgical site infections, and ventilator-associated pneumonia. They also track two specific infections that may be acquired in the health care setting—methicillin-resistant *S. aureus* and *Clostridioides difficile*, which can cause severe diarrhea (see section on *C. difficile* in chapter 3). In a report published in 2016 they found a 50% decrease in central line–associated bloodstream infections between 2008 and 2014. Overall, the risk of having a health care–associated infection in 2015 had dropped to 3.2% (from 4% in 2011), a 16% decrease (Magill 2018). This was based on a study of 199 hospitals spread over 10 states. In 2015 the most common health care–associated infections were pneumonia, gastrointestinal infections (primarily *C. difficile*), and surgical site infections.

A landmark study published in 2006 in the *New England Journal of Medicine*, a leading medical journal, helped to change the thinking about hospital-acquired infections (Pronovost 2006). At that time in the United States an estimated 80,000

ANTIBIOTICS

central venous catheter–related bloodstream infections were
occurring each year and causing up to 28,000 deaths and costing
up to $2.3 billion. Clinicians in 104 intensive care units prima-
rily in Michigan agreed to participate in a study that involved
consistently using five simple evidence-based procedures, including handwashing, using full-barrier precautions (gloves,
gowns, masks) during the insertion of central venous catheters
(placement of a plastic catheter into a large vein), cleaning the
patient's skin with chlorhexidine (a liquid disinfectant to prepare the site of insertion), avoiding the groin site if possible,
and removing unnecessary catheters (ones that were no longer
clearly needed). They combined these five procedures with
education of the staff. They also created a cart (that could be
moved to the patient's bedside) stocked with all of the necessary supplies and used a checklist to ensure that clinicians
were following all of the appropriate procedures. The result
of the combination of these simple procedures was dramatic.
In some intensive care units catheter-associated infections
dropped to zero. The median rate of infections per 1,000
catheter-days dropped from 2.7 at baseline to 0 at 3 months.
Even after 16 to 18 months the benefit was sustained. The rate
was 66% lower than at baseline. This changed clinical practice
and the mindset about the prevention of these infections.

Catheter-related urinary tract infections are also common
in health care settings and were once considered an expected
consequence of care. However, with a clear focus on finding
ways to reduce infections, a bundle of interventions used together has been found to be successful in markedly reducing
the rates of these infections. While these infections have not
been eliminated, research has now shown, as with intravenous
line–related infections, that they can be reduced to a fraction
of past levels. It has also been learned that giving antibiotics
every time a urine culture from a person with a catheter is
positive for bacteria is not only unnecessary but also coun-
terproductive, leading to more and more resistant bacteria.
Unless a patient has signs and symptoms of an infection (or is

going to undergo a surgical or other invasive procedure), the recommended approach today is to avoid doing cultures. In fact, laboratories in some health care systems will not culture a urine specimen unless there is evidence of infection or unless the health provider specifically requests it.

In the United States more than 1.4 million people reside in nursing homes. Infections are especially common in nursing homes. Residents are frequently frail and have multiple chronic medical problems. It has been estimated that up to 3 million infections occur annually in nursing home residents and about 300,000 die from them. Urinary tract infections are among the leading causes of infections in nursing home residents, especially those who require an indwelling urinary catheter, a catheter used to drain urine from the bladder into a bag. On entry into nursing homes up to 12% to 13% of residents have an indwelling catheter (and long-term use is usually 5% to 8%). Infections occur as frequently as 1 for every 100 days that a catheter is in place. This is also an infection for which antibiotics are frequently prescribed. Good news came from a study that was published in 2017. In a large study involving more than 400 nursing homes across the United States, researchers showed that with a series of interventions they could reduce the number of urinary tract infections by more than half (54%) (Mody 2017). There was not a simple, single intervention that was introduced, but the project used a bundle of interventions: catheter removal when not needed, proper aseptic insertion when needed, training for catheter care, incontinence care planning, effective communication, and active engagement of the resident and the family. Overall use of catheters did not change, but the rate of infections decreased. In this large study 75% of the nursing homes showed at least a 40% decrease in infections. The nonprofit nursing homes had rates of catheter-associated infections that were approximately half of those of for-profit nursing homes, suggesting that overall infection rates could be reduced even more. Nursing homes included in this study agreed to participate, so results may not be representative of all nursing homes. Although the study was large, there are almost 15,000 nursing homes in the United States. A laudable goal would be to scale up the interventions and reduce infections in all (Turnipseed 2017).

This study and others since then have shown that it is possible to eliminate many infections that are associated with health care, but this requires time and attention—and resources and commitment. To reduce these infections a clinic or hospital needs personnel with knowledge and training, adequate staffing and space, and materials such as gowns, gloves, masks, sterile equipment, and disinfectants. Unfortunately, many health care settings in low- and middle-income countries lack the resources for these interventions.

Surgical site infections (infections at the body site where the surgery was done) cause pain and suffering, sometimes death, and prolong hospitalizations and increase health care costs—and typically antibiotics are part of the treatment. They are especially common in hospitals in low-income countries. A recent study that looked at surgical site infections after gastrointestinal (stomach and bowel) surgery in high-income, middle-income, and low-income countries found that the highest rates of infection were in low-income countries and the lowest rates of infection in high-income countries (GlobSurg Collaborative 2018). Bacteria causing the infections in the low-income countries were more likely to be resistant to the commonly used antibiotics than those in the high-income countries, further increasing the burden and potential consequences of these infections. The WHO has developed and published guidelines for prevention of surgical site infections in addition to an earlier WHO Surgical Safety Checklist.

All of this points to ways to reduce the need for antibiotics. Good diagnostics, by pinpointing the specific diagnosis, can often show that an illness is not caused by bacteria that will benefit from antibiotic treatment—or can identify which antibiotic is likely to work in a bacterial infection. These are other avenues to improve the appropriate use of antibiotics.

The WHO has also been active in many of the areas related to reducing the need for antibiotics. At the World Health Assembly in 2017, WHO member states adopted a resolution aimed at improving the prevention, diagnosis, and management of sepsis (severe infection). Although hospital and other health care settings are a source of many infections, the majority originate in the community. Many infection prevention and control measures can be implemented even in low-resource settings. The WHO has focused on handwashing (hand hygiene) as one of these measures. The WHO slogan in 2017 for the campaign was "It's in your hands – prevent sepsis in health care." The campaign focused on health workers but also on patients and patient advocacy groups.

May 5, 2017, was designated global hygiene day. Social media has been used to promote messages such as "fight antibiotic resistance – it's in your hands," and many health care facilities have registered support. There is also a "Clean Care Is Safer Care" website (http://www.who.int/gpsc/5 may/en/).

Health care–associated infections are a major source of antibiotic-resistant bacteria in high-income countries. A recent study analyzed deaths and disability caused by antibiotic-resistant bacteria in the European Union and the European Economic Area (Cassini 2019). Researchers found that the burden from antibiotic-resistant infections is substantial and increasing. What was especially notable in the population studied was that overall almost two-thirds (63.5%) of the infections caused by antibiotic-resistant bacteria were related to health care. They estimated, as have others, that more than half of these could be prevented. The burden from antibiotic-resistant infections was greatest in infants (younger than 1 year old) and those 65 years and older, the latter a population that is growing in Europe, the United States, and elsewhere.

Do antiseptics and alcohol-based hand sanitizers work against all microbes?

Antibiotics are used to treat infections in humans, but disinfectants and antiseptics play an important role, especially in hospitals, in preventing bacteria from being spread among patients and health care workers and in the environment and on equipment. Other interventions are also used including high heat (autoclaving instruments) and ultraviolet radiation. One approach that has become common in both hospitals and the community is the use of hand sanitizers. These have become widely used in hospitals because they are generally better tolerated than repeated scrubbing of the hands by those who must do so between dozens of patient visits or procedures— and use of alcohol-based hand sanitizers is generally faster and they are more available than a sink with running water, soap, and clean towels. The alcohol is active against most of the common microbes that cause infection, if used in high enough concentrations. It is generally recommended that hand washes should contain at least 60% to 70% ethyl alcohol. Isopropanol (isopropyl alcohol) is also used widely in hospitals to clean surfaces. It is also used in rubbing alcohol. It has the advantage of drying rapidly and not leaving much residue.

But hand sanitizers do not work well against all bacteria and viruses. Several years ago surveys found that long-term care facilities (like nursing homes) that used alcohol-based hand sanitizers had an increased risk for outbreaks of norovirus, a common virus that has caused many nasty outbreaks of diarrhea and other gastrointestinal symptoms in many settings—on cruise ships and in hospitals, schools, and other settings where people have close contact. They also found that institutions that had had multiple norovirus outbreaks were more likely to have been using hand sanitizers than soap and water. Other studies have shown that the alcohol-based sanitizers may not be effective against certain viruses (nonenveloped), like norovirus. Based on these findings, the CDC revised recommendations for the control and prevention of norovirus during an outbreak. They now recommend using soap and water instead of hand sanitizers to clean hands in the event of an outbreak. Hand sanitizers may also be suboptimal for cleaning hands contaminated with spores of *C. difficile.*

Use of hand sanitizers has made hand cleaning easier, faster, and more accessible—and adherence is higher with hand sanitizers than washing with soap and water. Any changes in recommendations for hand cleaning must be carefully assessed and based on the best available science. Alcohol has broad activity against many microbes but is also used extensively. But can bacteria adapt to alcohol? Can bacteria evolve ways to resist its activity the way they do with antibiotics?

A recent study raised questions about this. Investigators in Australia were prompted to do a study because they observed that while the incidence of infections due to most bacteria had been decreasing, infections caused by one particular type of bacteria (*Enterococcus faecium*) had increased. They had access to 139 isolates (bacteria that had been grown in the microbiology laboratory) of *E. faecium* from two hospitals. This is one of the "bad bugs"—one that has been targeted for attention and monitoring because it tends to produce serious and difficult-to-treat infections. This is because *E. faecium* tends to be resistant to most of the commonly used antibiotics. In many locations throughout the world these infections have also been observed to increase in hospitals in recent years and to become more resistant to antibiotics.

The Australian investigators tested their 139 isolates of bacteria that had been collected between 1997 and 2015 to determine if there had been any change in their response to isopropanol (isopropyl alcohol), the form of alcohol used in disinfectants to clean surfaces in hospitals and in hand sanitizers. They found that strains collected between 2010 and 2015 were more tolerant to (able to survive) exposure to alcohol than those collected earlier. They studied this in a mouse model by housing mice in cages that had been intentionally contaminated with the bacteria (early-year isolates or late-year isolates) and disinfected (cleaned) in a standard way with 70% isopropyl alcohol. They found that the mice were more likely to become colonized (pick up bacteria on their bodies) if they were kept in the cages contaminated with the bacteria collected from the later years (2010 to 2015). They did genomic analysis and found that the E. *faecium* that could survive better in the presence of alcohol had mutations in genes for carbohydrate uptake and metabolism. They concluded that these bacteria were adapting to the presence of alcohol, which is one of the mainstays of controlling the spread of bacteria in hospitals. Additional studies will be needed to confirm or refute this— and to determine how widespread this is. If the bacteria can become tolerant to (survive in the presence of) or resistant to alcohol, this would have an enormous impact on infection control procedures throughout health care systems globally. Studies should include other bacteria to assess the seriousness of these findings. This suggests, however, that there is the potential for tolerance or resistance to develop to alcohol-based hand rubs and the possible future need for alternatives to this commonly used product.

How can copper be used to reduce infections?

A totally different approach is also being tested to reduce hospital- and health care–associated infections. Copper and its alloys have broad activity against many bacteria—as well as against many viruses, algae, fungi, and other microorganisms. An ancient Egyptian text written between 2600 and 2200 BC mentions the use of copper to sterilize wounds. Bronze, formed by combining copper and tin, was also likely to have antibacterial activity. Copper was apparently used widely in medicine in 19th and early 20th centuries to treat a whole range of diseases. When antibiotics became available in the 1930s and after, the use of copper for treatment disappeared. The idea that its antimicrobial activity on surfaces might be valuable was noted at least as early as 1983, when it was shown that brass door knobs could prevent the spread of microbes in hospitals. More recently in an era of multidrug-resistant bacteria contaminating many surfaces in health care settings, there has been renewed interest in and study of copper and its alloys for their antimicrobial activity. As of 2008, the Environmental Protection Agency (EPA) had registered almost 300 copper surfaces as having antimicrobial activity. Many studies have shown that microbes are killed or inactivated when they have contact with copper-containing surfaces. The response can vary depending on the copper content of the alloy (higher content means more effective) and the temperature and humidity (higher is better for both for the elimination of microbes). Even spores that are formed by bacteria like *C. difficile* and that can survive heat, radiation, drying, and some chemicals can be killed by metallic copper in some settings. One study showed that living spores were decreased by more than 99% in 3 hours after being exposed to solid copper.

How rapidly bacteria are killed by contact with copper surfaces varies greatly depending on the microbe, the numbers, and the local conditions. The killing time at room temperature for most common bacteria ranges from minutes to hours (Grass 2011).

Today in many health care facilities many working surfaces are made of stainless steel. It looks clean; however, studies of survival of bacteria on stainless steel show that survival is not decreased—in marked contrast to what happens after contact with copper surfaces. Several trials in hospitals and clinics have shown that refitting with copper surfaces reduces bacterial counts. The copper surfaces also affect drug-resistant pathogens such as methicillin-resistant *S. aureus* and multiply drug-resistant *E. coli*.

In a hospital in Hamburg, Germany, surfaces that people would touch in patient rooms, staff rooms, and rest rooms were refitted with brass, a copper and zinc alloy (Mikolay 2010). Surfaces in control rooms were aluminum and plastic and were unchanged for the study. The investigators then studied what happened over a period of 32 weeks. They took samples from the surfaces and checked them for the presence of ciprofloxacin-resistant *S. aureus*. During the study the usual cleaning with a disinfectant was continued in all areas each morning. The researchers found that on average, the bacteria had decreased by 63% on the copper surfaces when compared to the surfaces that had not been changed. Door handles had the highest numbers of bacteria—and showed the greatest reduction with the presence of copper (brass). After the surfaces were cleaned, bacteria returned to the copper surfaces half as quickly as they returned to the aluminum and plastic surfaces.

But it is not enough to show that bacteria can be killed by copper surfaces. Do copper surfaces make a difference? Do they have any impact on infections and outcomes for patients? A systematic review and meta-analysis published in 2017 identified studies that assessed the role of copper surfaces in reducing health care–associated infections (Pineda 2017). Fourteen studies published between 2000 and 2016 compared antimicrobial copper versus regular surfaces in patients' environments. In 12 studies, antimicrobial copper alloy (mix of copper and something else) surfaces were used. Surfaces on which copper alloys were used varied, including bed rails, toilet seats, faucet handles, tray tables, poles for transporting intravenous fluids, and other surfaces. In one study, biocidal copper-impregnated linens were used, and another compared regular pens and copper-containing pens used by nurses in an intensive care unit. All but one study was done in a high- or middle-income country. In all studies usual cleaning procedures and handwashing were continued along with the copper intervention. Overall, they found that the settings using copper alloy for high-touch surfaces reduced the incidence of health care–associated infections by about a quarter. Bacterial counts were lower on copper-containing than on regular surfaces. The results did not have enough data on deaths to comment on whether deaths were reduced by use of copper. Studies were done in multiple different countries and included both pediatric and adult intensive care units and a rural clinic in South Africa. No adverse effects were observed from using refitted areas with copper-containing surfaces. An analysis of the cost required to implement the copper intervention estimated that in a 20-bed intensive care unit the cost of refitting with copper surfaces could be recovered in 2 months given the expected decrease in infections (and the high cost of treating these infections).

Others have also looked into multiple potential uses of copper in materials in the health care setting (Souli 2017). This looks like a promising avenue to explore as another intervention to reduce infections and allow a reduction in the use of conventional antibiotics.

Alloys that contain copper include bronze and brass—and many others. They will need to be studied for safety, effectiveness, durability, aesthetic appeal, and capacity to withstand repeated cleaning if used in a hospital setting. Copper alone will not solve the problem of health care–associated infections but used with other interventions may make it easier to eliminate these infections.

In low-income countries some researchers have looked into using the antimicrobial activity of copper to treat drinking water. Researchers in India filled three types of different sterilized containers with distilled water: a copper pot, a glass bottle, and a glass bottle with a copper coil device. They then inoculated each with *E. coli* and the bacteria that cause typhoid fever (*Salmonella typhi*) and cholera (*Vibrio cholerae*) and let them stand overnight. After 16 hours, the water stored in the copper pots and glass bottles with copper coils showed no growth of the bacteria, whereas the bacteria in water stored in plain sterilized bottles had increased 3- to 4-fold for the *S. typhi* and *V. cholerae* and more than 30-fold for the *E. coli* (Sudha 2009). They measured the amount of copper leached into the water stored in the copper pot and found that it was within the limits stipulated by the WHO as safe for human consumption. The authors of this study recommend more field trials of this approach as a potential low-cost way to make water safer in low-income areas.

Health care–associated infections are generally more prevalent in low- and middle-income countries than in high-income countries. This includes surgical wound infections. Improved training and staffing may help, but facilities often lack basic infrastructure and have inadequate buildings with poor ventilation, lack of handwashing facilities, and chronic shortages of essential medications. In many low- and middle-income countries rates of antibiotic-resistant bacteria are higher than in many high-income countries, partly reflecting the wide access to antibiotics without prescriptions.

In summary, many approaches are available today that could drastically reduce the need for antibiotics by reducing the occurrence of infections: improved sanitation and clean water globally; vaccination using available vaccines that have not yet reached many populations; interventions to reduce spread of infections in the health care setting, including improved training and education of health professionals for interventions known to be effective; and protecting the food supply to reduce foodborne infections. Other less direct approaches include making populations healthier and more able to resist infections. Many risk factors for infections are modifiable through behavioral changes or public health interventions. For example, one can work to eliminate malnutrition and micronutrient deficiencies that can contribute to risk of infection and poor outcome; reduce and eliminate smoking; reduce obesity; reduce illicit drug use and needle sharing; and use barrier protection to avoid sexually transmitted infections. All of these can reduce the risk of some infections. Some interventions to reduce infections are even more indirect, such as improving early diagnosis and treatment linked to contact tracing to avoid ongoing spread of infections like tuberculosis and gonorrhea—both of which continue to be global problems. Even improved vector control (like mosquitoes and ticks) can lead to decreased use of antibiotics by decreasing fever-causing illnesses.

Are there approaches to treating infections that do not involve antibiotics—treatment approaches that do not drive the development of resistance the way that use of antibiotics does?

We should be pursuing approaches to decrease the need for antibiotics and to eliminate unnecessary, inappropriate use while also looking at alternative approaches for treatment. Eliminating unnecessary or low-priority use is especially difficult because this involves multiple sectors, not just human health sectors. Other sectors and industries, including agriculture, aquaculture, veterinary, and pharmaceutical industries, have large economic interests in the use of antibiotics.

Concern remains that no matter what alternative antibiotics are developed, bacteria will find a way around them, to subvert them, or otherwise to change so that bacterial life and function can continue as usual. The most promising approaches may include teaming up with microbes and identifying the microbes or combinations of them associated with good health and allowing them to assist the host in displacing the disease-causing bacteria. Nuking bacteria with blasts of broad-spectrum antibiotics that destroy or disrupt populations of beneficial bacteria and their associated community members seems like a shortsighted approach and offers brief benefits at the cost of potential long-term harm.

Fecal microbiota transplantation is already being used to treat severe *C. difficile* colitis (see chapter 3) and is being evaluated for use for other diseases.

Bacteria inhabiting the body have generated outsized attention because we have been able to see and grow many of them for more than a century. Although the majority of them are nonculturable by traditional methods, they are now detectable through genetic sequencing and other technologies. The body also has abundant archaea, which were originally classified with bacteria. The viral communities that are a normal part of the fecal microbiota have received less attention, but the fecal virome (assemblage of viruses) is immense and diverse. Not surprisingly, the gut microbiota include abundant bacteriophages, viruses that infect bacteria but do not infect human cells. The largest reservoir of phages in humans is in the human gut, the location of most of the body's bacteria.

Recent use of fecal transplantation for treatment of *C. difficile* and other medical problems has raised concerns about exactly what is being transplanted. One study of fecal microbiota transplantation from a single donor to three different recipients found that multiple viral lineages were transferred during the transplantation. Investigators analyzed the donor fecal microbiota for viral particles and could identify up to 32 different donor viruses. Investigators used metagenomic sequencing to document that multiple viral lineages had been transferred. They were reassured to find that none of the viruses transferred were ones that replicated in animal cells or were known to cause disease—but this is one study.

Fecal microbiota transplantation is also being studied for possible use for other medical problems. There is extensive ongoing research to better understand the function of bacteria and especially communities of them and their possible role in treating infections and other medical problems. These approaches may have an important role in treatment in the future. Some have dubbed the human microbiota a treasure trove for next-generation medicine.

What other approaches to treating infections are being tried that do not involve antibiotics?

Several approaches are being tried but are not yet in wide use. In general, antibiotics are cheap, familiar, and available to use on a wide scale, so it is easy to see why and how they have become the preferred approach to treating infections.

Alternatives are often more complicated to create and to use in broad populations.

One example of approaches being tried is the use of a human monoclonal antibody (identical antibodies made in the laboratory) that binds to and neutralizes (inactivates) toxin B of *C. difficile*. It reduces recurrences of *C. difficile*, which occur in about 25% of people after first infections. Among those with a recurrence of *C. difficile*, about 40% will have a second recurrence. The monoclonal antibody named bezlotoxumab is FDA approved for use to prevent recurrences in people 18 years and older. Risk factors for recurrence of *C. difficile* that have been identified include people who are older (age >65 years), are immune compromised, have severe disease, have a history of previous episodes of *C. difficile*, and are infected with a particular strain of *C. difficile* (B/NAP1/027). Populations with multiple risk factors are likely to have the greatest reduction in recurrent infections after treatment with bezlotoxumab. A downside of using this agent is its high cost. Because of its high cost, hospitals may try to reserve it for those patients at highest risk for recurrence. However, recurrences are also expensive to treat.

Another approach to treating a different infection involves neutralizing the toxin produced by *Bacillus anthracis*, the cause of anthrax. A humanized monoclonal antibody was developed that prevents the toxin produced by the anthrax bacteria from binding to the human cell. If the toxin cannot bind to the cell, it cannot damage it. The antibody does not, however, kill the anthrax bacteria. It was approved for use by the FDA in 2012 to prevent and treat inhalation anthrax—but it is given along with an antibiotic. It must be given as an intravenous infusion and can cause itching and other allergic symptoms—so the directions for administration also include use of a drug like diphenhydramine (Benadryl). The monoclonal antibody is notable because it was the first drug that was approved on the basis of efficacy data in animals. This is not a drug expected to have wide use. It was created for use against one specific infection (that is considered a bioterrorism threat).

There is a long history of using antibodies produced in another human to treat or prevent infections—and those still have a potential role. These are used more often for viral than for bacterial infections, in instances when no other therapy is available. This requires having humans who have been infected or immunized and have developed antibodies and are willing to donate their blood so that antibodies can be extracted and used in another human. It is labor intensive and has limited use. An example of this approach used today is human rabies immune globulin that can be used along with rabies vaccine if someone is bitten by an animal infected with the rabies virus.

To overcome some of the limitations of using humans to produce antibodies, a new platform has been developed. It involves using specially designed cows whose lymphocytes (type of white blood cell that produces antibodies) are able to secrete human polyclonal immunoglobulin (antibodies). The cows have trans-chromosomal B lymphocytes and can be immunized against various bacteria and viruses. The cow lymphocytes are programmed to produce potent, antigen-specific, human antibodies (immunoglobulin). This is a biological system (special cow) that has the capacity to produce large volumes of antibodies quickly—and it can be used for a range of disease-causing microbes. The system will produce pathogen-specific, even isolate-specific, antibodies. In one study, infusions of antibodies against the Middle East respiratory syndrome virus from trans-chromosomal cattle were studied in healthy adults in a phase 1 trial and appeared safe and well tolerated. This approach could potentially be used to create antibodies to treat specific, antibiotic-resistant infections. One published report describes the use of this approach to obtain antibodies to treat a *Mycoplasma hominis* infection.

Probiotics have been used to treat periodontal disease by trying to replace disease-producing bacteria with *Streptococcus salivarius* and *Lactobacillus* species.

What is bacteriophage therapy? How does it work? Is it being used today?

Recent reports describe use of phage therapy for treating bacterial infections. Bacteriophages, often referred to as phages, are viruses that infect bacteria. They also infect archaea, microbes long lumped with bacteria in classification systems but now known to be a distinctive class of organisms, separate from bacteria. Infection of bacteria by phages can lead to lysis (breakdown and death) of the bacteria, hence the interest in them for possible use in treating infections.

Bacteriophages were first discovered more than 100 years ago and first visualized by electron microscopy in the 1940s. They are diverse, abundant—the most common organisms in the biosphere—and widespread, found in water, soil, terrestrial subsurfaces, and humans and animals. They contain a core nucleic acid (usually DNA) and a protein or lipoprotein capsid. A drop of seawater is estimated to contain a million particles. They are found wherever bacteria are found and are more plentiful than bacteria. They are found in nature and can be purified and saved. They play a critical role in biology and the evolution of microbes. They have specificity—a particular bacteriophage is capable of infecting only specific types of bacteria, sometimes only a single strain. This is one of the benefits of their potential use. They offer a precision approach to killing a specific type of bacteria. They do not affect human cells. Humans are regularly exposed to large numbers of them.

It may not be surprising to learn that bacteria and archaea have developed multiple sophisticated ways to defend against them—or antiphage defense systems. The genes encoding these are found in the genome of the bacteria. These antiphage systems can protect against invasion by foreign DNA.

Phages have two potential life cycles. Some bacteriophages have the capacity to lyse (break apart or destroy) bacteria (lytic or virulent). They can attach to receptors (like a docking station) on bacterial cell walls, inject DNA into the bacterium, and take over the bacterial host machinery to produce more phages, often releasing 10 to 100 virions (particles) per phage. They can produce enzymes (endolysins or lysins) that disrupt the function of the cell. Other bacteriophages, termed "temperate" or lysogenic phages, infect bacteria but do not kill them. They replicate with the host bacterial genome. Some phages can transfer genetic material to the bacterium. One example is the transfer of cholera toxin genes to nontoxigenic strains of cholera by means of a lysogenic phage. They can also play a role in spreading resistance genes.

Bacteriophages have long been studied at the Eliva Institute of Bacteriophage, Microbiology, and Virology in Tblisi, Georgia (former Soviet Union), and used to treat infections. Study of them in other institutions was largely discontinued because of the discovery and easy availability of sulfonamides and then antibiotics. Although some research has been conducted, the types of studies have not met those expected of rigorous clinical trials, and the potential use and benefit of phage therapy has been mostly ignored by much of the scientific community.

The looming crisis in antibiotic resistance has led to more willingness, even eagerness, to look into potential use of bacteriophage therapy. A recent highly publicized event—saving the life of a man dying from a multidrug-resistant infection by using phage therapy—by an innovative group that worked with a number of collaborators and partners has catalyzed interest in moving forward with phage research in the United States.

In 2015 a 69-year-old professor from California became ill during a holiday in Egypt. He was hospitalized with severe abdominal pain and fever and diagnosed with pancreatitis, an inflammation of the pancreas. He was later airlifted to Frankfurt, Germany, where he was found to have a complication of pancreatitis, a pancreatic pseudocyst (collection of fluid rich in pancreatic enzymes and other material). It was drained and found to be infected with a multidrug-resistant strain of *Acinetobacter baumannii*, a Gram-negative bacterium known to cause severe and deadly infections. It is often acquired in hospitals and was a problem in many US veterans who had served in the Middle East. (It has sometimes been called Iraqibacter because of its association with veterans from Iraq and Afghanistan who have become infected with it, typically after being hospitalized for injuries.) The patient was treated with multiple antibiotics, stabilized, and transferred to the intensive care unit at Thornton Hospital at the University of California San Diego (UCSD) Health. Repeat testing showed that the bacteria had become resistant to all antibiotics. After initial improvement, the patient developed life-threatening sepsis related to slippage of a drain. He fell into a coma.

His team of physicians, including Robert Schooley, who was chief of the infectious diseases division at UCSD, decided to explore possible use of phages given that no antibiotic options remained and the clinical situation was desperate. They found three other teams willing to help that had suitable phages—ones that were active against the *A. baumannii* bacteria infecting this patient. They were able to establish rapid collaboration with teams at the Biological Defense Research directorate at the Naval Medical Research Center in Frederick, Maryland; the Center for Phage Technology at Texas A&M University; and AmpliPhi, a San Diego–based biotechnology company specializing in bacteriophage-based therapies. They were able to enlist a research team at San Diego State University that was able to purify the phage samples so that they could be safely used in a human. Dr. Schooley applied for and obtained an Emergency Investigational New Drug status from the FDA to use the phages from the three other research groups in this last-ditch effort.

They administered the phage therapy, initially a cocktail of four phages introduced via catheter into the pseudocyst, and later intravenously. The bacteria developed resistance to the initial phage therapy, and the team revised the treatment with new phage strains. The patient was ultimately cured of the infection—but had lost 100 pounds and had a slow recovery.

In this setting, multiple efforts aligned to produce a successful outcome. The team was able to draw upon work already in progress by multiple other groups who were willing to share phages and work together. More important is the effect the experience with a single patient has had on catalyzing new efforts.

This case points out some of the potential benefits and hurdles to use of phage therapy. The benefits of using phage therapy include the following:

It allows treatment of a specific bacterial infection in an individual without disruption of the person's resident microbiota. It is precise and elegant. It hits only the target bacteria.

It can be used against Gram-negative and Gram-positive bacteria.

A cocktail of multiple phages can be used.

It works against antibiotic-resistant bacteria (independent of antibiotic resistance).

The viruses (phages) replicate when the target bacteria are present and disappear when the target is gone.

The viruses do not affect human host cells. Phages are not known to be toxic.

It potentially can be delivered by different routes.

It does not have known side effects.

It can act rapidly.

One could potentially engineer bacteriophages with specific properties.

Phage treatment does not seem to cause release of high levels of endotoxin from bacteria (toxins present inside some bacteria). (One recent study found that the rapid killing of bacteria by bacteriophages would release lower levels of toxins [endotoxin] than would be released by use of an antibiotic to kill bacteria.)

Phages can penetrate biofilm or can be engineered to deal with it.

Potential uses exist for products of bacteriophages (e.g., lysins, other enzymes).

Despite the possible benefits, the potential problems and unknowns are numerous. Much more research is needed to answer many practical questions about its efficacy, safety, and use. The potential hurdles to use of phage therapy include the following:

Bacteria can become resistant to phages; one might have to modify the phage or the cocktail of phages during the course of treatment.

Phage therapy needs to be individualized for the specific bacteria causing the infection.

There are questions about how to deliver phage so that it reaches the target bacteria. Phages do not move independently. Phages must reach the site of infection to be effective.

Routes of administration that are effective are not known. It has been used on surfaces (topically), intravenously, via aerosol administration, and by instillation via a catheter.

The pharmacokinetics and pharmacodynamics are unknown.

Regulatory issues would exist around testing, production, and consistency of the product.

The current regulatory model for testing and approving drugs is for chemical molecules. Phages are viruses.

It is unknown whether it is safe in the short or long-term.

Clinical trials would be complicated given the variety of bacteriophage options and types of treatments.

It is unknown whether there could be unanticipated adverse events or whether bacteriophages could infect bacteria and increase their virulence.

It would be expensive and complicated if each treatment course has to be individualized.

Data on use to date are limited. Good outcomes in individual cases have been reported, for example, phage treatment of an aortic graft infected with *Pseudomonas aeruginosa*.

Looking to the future

Phage therapy is one of many alternatives to traditional antibiotic therapy being studied as bacteria become increasingly resistant to all available drugs. It received a high-visibility boost from the aforementioned case. The team caring for the patient was able to secure approval for use of phage therapy through the FDA's emergency pathway.

This successful outcome was followed by successful outcomes in five other patients and has led to the recent announcement by this San Diego group that they are launching a clinical center to refine phage treatments. They will work with companies to bring phages to market. The new center will launch with a 3-year, $1.2 million grant from UCSD and will be called the Center for Innovative Phage Applications and Therapeutics (IPATH). It will not manufacture phage treatments but will collaborate with companies and other academic centers to do multicenter clinical trials. It will focus, at least initially, on treating patients with chronic, multiply drug-resistant infections caused by a single bacterial pathogen—patients with organ transplants, implanted devices such as pacemakers or artificial joints—and patients with cystic fibrosis.

Another example of its use includes a cocktail of six bacteriophages called Biophage-PA. This has been developed for treating *P. aeruginosa* causing chronic otitis (ear infection). It was delivered directly into the ear. In a small trial (24 patients), it was more effective than placebo in decreasing the bacterial counts of *P. aeruginosa*. It was used without antibiotics and was well tolerated.

How are phages and bacteriocins used today?

Although research on use of phages in clinical medicine is in its early stages, other interventions employing phages for other uses have been tested and are marketed. An agent named Listex P100 is a bacteriophage that has received GRAS (generally recognized as safe) status from the FDA and is approved by the US Department of Agriculture's Food Safety and Inspection Service as an antimicrobial that can be used in ready-to-eat meat and poultry products. Because its use is considered a processing aid, it does not require labeling. It is aimed specifically at control of *Listeria monocytogenes*, a bacterium that can contaminate food (including meat, cheese, milk, and other products) and has been responsible for many severe outbreaks of foodborne infections. It can be especially severe (with high mortality) in pregnant women, infants, the elderly, and individuals who are immunocompromised. Because *L. monocytogenes* has the unusual feature of being able to multiply at low temperatures—even under refrigerated storage (in contrast to most bacteria whose replication is slowed or stopped at low temperatures)—refrigerated foods, especially those stored for long periods, can become heavily contaminated with the bacteria.

Listex P100 is available as a liquid and is used in the postprocessing environment (before packaging) when cooked foods can become recontaminated. It can be sprayed on products before packaging and is also used on surfaces, such as slicing blades. It can be used on meat, fish, and cheeses. It has been approved in the United States, the European Union, Canada, Australia, New Zealand, Switzerland, and Israel.

The importance of *Listeria* as a cause of foodborne outbreaks was highlighted by an outbreak in South Africa in 2017–2018. As of June 2018 more than 1,000 cases had been reported. Of those whose outcome was known, more than a quarter had died. In the South Africa outbreak, 42% of the cases were in young infants who were infected during pregnancy or delivery. After an intensive investigation, the source of the outbreak was identified—a widely consumed ready-to-eat processed meat product called "Polony." The product was exported to 15 countries in the African region. Even after the source of the outbreak was identified, investigators expected more cases to occur because of the long incubation period of infection (usually 1 to 3 weeks but up to 70 days).

Bacteriocins

Bacteriocins are proteins or peptides produced by bacteria that can kill or inhibit the growth of bacteria (antimicrobial proteins or peptides produced by bacteria). They are used in food but have not been used to treat infections in humans. They were discovered in 1925. They are synthesized by bacterial ribosomes, tiny particles inside bacteria. They are abundant and diverse—structurally, functionally, and ecologically—and can be found in Gram-negative and Gram-positive bacteria. Virtually every species of bacteria and archaea can produce at least one bacteriocin.

Most have a narrow spectrum and inhibit growth of similar or closely related bacteria. They are part of the microbiota of the gut. Genes for them are located on chromosomes or on mobile genetic elements such as transposons or plasmids. Some have commercial use, especially in the food industry, such as use in acceleration of cheese ripening. They are categorized as GRAS and so can be used in food. They work by affecting the inner membrane, causing leakage of cellular contents; digesting DNA and RNA of the bacteria; or targeting a peptidoglycan precursor and hence blocking cell wall synthesis.

Pediocin PA-1 inhibits growth of *L. monocytogenes* and is used in a number of foods. Nisin is produced by the bacterium *Lactococcus lactis* and is used as a food preservative. In contrast to many bacteriocins that inhibit only closely related species, nisin is relatively broad spectrum and inhibits *Listeria, S. aureus, Bacillus cereus,* and *Clostridium botulinum,* all pathogens that can potentially contaminate food. It can also extend the shelf life of food and is a common food additive.

8

PRESERVING ANTIBIOTICS AND DEVELOPING NEW ANTIBACTERIAL TREATMENTS

How common is inappropriate prescribing of antibiotics?

Many studies have tried to estimate what percentage of antibiotic use in people is unnecessary or inappropriate. Most estimates come up with about a quarter to a third of all use. For some specific types of infections like upper respiratory infections, it may be 50% or higher. The Centers for Disease Control and Prevention (CDC) has concluded that 20% to 50% of antibiotics in US acute care hospitals are unnecessary or inappropriate. Repeated studies suggest that there is a lot of room for improvement in prescribing antibiotics in the United States (Fleming-Dutra 2016; Hicks 2015). Types of inappropriate prescribing include using antibiotics when no antibiotic is needed, using the wrong antibiotic or the wrong dose, giving it by the wrong route (e.g., giving an antibiotic by injection or intravenous route when an oral drug would work, or vice versa), giving it for the wrong duration (too long or too short a course of treatment), and administering an antibiotic when there are clear reasons that it should not be used in that particular patient (e.g., because of allergies, interactions with other drugs taken by the patient, or other factors). In general, in the United States most of the inappropriate use is in the direction of overuse rather than underuse. In low- and middle-income countries many patients who would benefit from antibiotics are still not receiving them, often because of lack of resources or access to them.

Many factors go into deciding whether to give an antibiotic and then choosing one that is appropriate for a specific patient with a particular type of infection. Most antibiotics used by humans are taken for respiratory tract infections, including colds, coughs, sore throats, sinus infections, bronchitis, and pneumonia. Ear infections may accompany infections of the upper respiratory tract. The majority of the infections of the respiratory tract are caused by viruses for which antibiotics will provide no benefit. Occasionally viral infections of the respiratory tract will be complicated by a secondary bacterial infection (the viral infection makes a person more susceptible to a bacterial infection), but the majority are not.

Because of the alarming increase in antibiotic-resistant infections in the United States and globally, many organizations and institutions have become engaged in tracking inappropriate use and identifying ways to eliminate unnecessary and inappropriate use of antibiotics. All antibiotic use, whether appropriate or not and whether in humans, plants, or animals, can drive the emergence of antibiotic-resistant bacteria. The goal is to use antibiotics only when the potential benefits outweigh the potential adverse consequences. Ideally the antibiotic chosen should have the narrowest spectrum of antibacterial activity needed to treat a given infection. Unfortunately, many antibiotics in wide use today have a relatively broad spectrum of antibacterial activity and can produce long-lasting effects on the microbiota.

Many factors affect decision making about prescribing antibiotics and patterns of use can be slow to change.

The US Food and Drug Administration (FDA) warned about fluoroquinolone (FQ) use in 2008 and updated these warnings in 2016 because of adverse events (including damage to tendons, muscles, joints, nerves, and the central nervous system). Researchers looked at FQ use in the United States for adults in outpatient care in 2014 to assess whether prescribing was in line with the FDA recommendations about more limited prescribing of these drugs. They found that about 5% of FQ prescriptions were for problems for which no antibiotics should be prescribed (such as upper respiratory tract infections) and almost 20% were given for infections for which FQs were not the first choice—instances in which other antibiotics would be preferred treatment. The researchers concluded that about a quarter of all quinolone prescriptions in ambulatory patients were inappropriate. The overall number of FQ prescriptions for ambulatory patients in the United States in 2014 was 31.5 million. The most common use was for genitourinary conditions (like urinary tract infections), and the second most common use was for respiratory infections. Almost 8 million prescriptions were given to patients for conditions that did not warrant an antibiotic or for which an alternative was preferred (Kabbani 2018). A follow-up study prompted by this looked at FQ outpatient prescriptions at one hospital and found that 18% of FQ prescriptions did not comply with FDA recommendations (Mercuro 2018). On further analysis they found that 75% of all FQ prescriptions were suboptimal when they took into account the dose and duration of the treatment being prescribed. The largest factor in FQ overuse was excessively long duration, found in 54% of cases. Among patients treated with FQs, 4% had serious adverse events and 3% developed recurrent infections due to quinolone-resistant organisms.

FQs have been available for decades. They are relatively inexpensive, are generally well tolerated, and can treat many kinds of infections. Clinicians became comfortable prescribing them for many kinds of infections, and many clinicians have not changed their prescribing habits or have modified them only slightly in response to FDA warnings. Warnings about new and unfamiliar drugs may be followed more explicitly.

As noted earlier, antibiotics are often given for infections that will not benefit from them, and they are also often continued longer than necessary. In treating cases of sinusitis for which antibiotics are needed, a course of 5 to 7 days is recommended based on best available data (outlined in the evidence-based Infectious Diseases Society of America guidelines), yet a recent study showed that 70% of prescriptions were for 10 days or longer (King 2018). In another type of infection, severe intra-abdominal infections, researchers found that most patients could be treated effectively with an 8-day course rather than a 15-day course.

Better guidelines about recommended duration of treatment based on high-quality studies could be useful to clinicians. A well-done study compared 5- or 10-day treatment courses of antibiotics for young children (under age 2 years) with acute otitis media (infection of the middle ear often caused by bacteria) and found that the shorter course was more likely to fail—34% versus 16% (Hoberman 2016). This suggests that unless a test can be developed to better define duration for an individual patient, in this instance a longer course should be used in children younger than 2 years.

Recent guidelines have also recommended against long-duration treatment for patients with Lyme disease.

Urinary tract infections are a relatively common reason for antibiotic treatment in ambulatory and hospitalized patients—though much less frequent than respiratory tract infections. Guidelines now recommend not treating people with bacteria found in the urine who are not having symptoms (so-called asymptomatic bacteriuria) except in special situations. Urinary tract infections are more common in older populations and are often caused by Gram-negative bacteria. There is general agreement that patients with acute symptoms and bacteria present in the urine should be treated. There is also general agreement about treating pregnant women who have bacteria in their urine even if they do not have symptoms because not treating them may affect pregnancy outcomes. Treatment is also recommended for patients with bacteriuria who will be undergoing a surgical or other procedure involving the genito-urinary tract. Urine specimens are easy to collect (in contrast to blood, cerebrospinal fluid, or some other specimens) and they are frequently sent to the laboratory for testing, especially in hospitalized patients, even in the absence of symptoms of a urinary tract infection. But treating women who have bacteria in the urine and no symptoms is more likely to lead to recurrent bacteria in the urine after 12 months than not treating them. It often does not work. After more than 3 years of follow-up, women who received antibiotics were more than four times as likely to have bacteriuria—and antibiotic resistance was significantly higher in those who had been treated (Cai 2015).

Antibiotics are generally prescribed for patients with acute diverticulitis (inflammation or infection of small pouches in the wall of the intestine), yet a recent study found that patients with a first episode of uncomplicated acute diverticulitis managed without antibiotics recovered just as rapidly as those who received antibiotics. This and other studies suggest that antibiotics can be used selectively—and not routinely for all episodes of acute uncomplicated diverticulitis (Daniels 2017). Patients hospitalized with severe and complicated diverticulitis do require antibiotics. In severe diverticulitis bacteria may leak out of the bowel.

What approaches have been effective in increasing the appropriate use of antibiotics and decreasing inappropriate prescribing by clinicians?

Some approaches target individual clinicians, and others are done at the institutional level—at the clinic or hospital. It turns out that extra educational sessions alone do not work very well. Guidelines are useful but are not always followed. Automatic stop orders for antibiotics are used in some settings.

Professional societies like the Infectious Diseases Society of America, some hospital and health care systems, and other groups have developed guidelines for clinicians. These describe, sometimes in great detail, when antibiotics should be used and in what dose and duration. Practice algorithms— roadmaps for clinical decisions—have also been developed for health care providers to follow. With support from the CDC, a group has put together the "MITIGATE Antimicrobial Stewardship Toolkit," a guide for health care providers and administrators that outlines how facilities can implement effective programs in acute care settings, such as emergency department and urgent care settings.

In the end, the clinician typically decides whether to prescribe a drug, but these guidelines may influence choice. Some health systems, as part of a review of quality of care, track whether clinicians are following the recommended guidelines. They can provide rewards and favorable feedback to those who follow guidelines and penalties for those who do not.

The American College of Physicians and the CDC issued guidelines in 2016 for appropriate use of antibiotics in adults with acute respiratory tract infections (Harris 2016). They were published in a major medical journal and CDC patient information sheets were also made available online (http://www.cdc.gov/getsmart/community/materials-references/print-materials/hcp/index.html). They describe the instances when patients with bronchitis (>90% viral cause), pharyngitis, and acute sinusitis should receive antibiotics.

In the United Kingdom Chief Medical Officer Dame Sally Davis has been active and outspoken about the dangers of antibiotic resistance (and antibiotic overuse) and has helped to mobilize a number of efforts in the United Kingdom and globally. One approach that was studied in the United Kingdom involved identifying about 1,500 general practitioner (GP) practices whose prescribing rates were in the top 20% for their National Health Service local team area (Hallsworth 2016; Gould 2016). Half were randomly assigned to receive a letter from England's chief medical officer stating that their GP practice was prescribing antibiotics at a rate higher than 80% of practices in that area. The other half received no communication. The researchers then assessed whether those who received the letter with feedback changed their rates of prescribing antibiotics. They found that the group that received the intervention letter with feedback about use actually reduced the prescribing by about 3.3%. Now 3.3% may seem like a trivial decrease, but given the size of the population participating, it meant that 73,406 fewer antibiotic prescriptions were dispensed. Does providing information to patients work? In another part of the study researchers sent patient-focused information that promoted reduced use of antibiotics. Unfortunately, in this setting the intervention did not have an impact on antibiotic prescribing. This study and others suggest that feedback about social norms could be effective and could be inexpensive to deliver in electronically connected systems.

In Europe, as among states in the United States, there is great variation in antibiotic use by country and over time. In the United Kingdom 80% to 90% of human antibiotic use occurs in the community, most often prescribed by general practitioners. It is notable that between 2000 and 2014, antibiotic use in primary care increased 46% (from 14.3 to 20.9 defined daily doses [DDDs] per 1,000 residents), but between 2014 and 2017, there was a 13.2% drop in antibiotic prescriptions in the primary health care setting. Within Europe in 2014, there was almost a threefold difference in total consumption of antibiotics for systemic use (defined as DDDs) between the lowest- and highest-using countries. Use was lowest in the Netherlands at about 10 DDDs and highest in Greece at about 30 DDDs per 1,000 inhabitants (Gould 2016).

Some interventions seem to make a difference. In the United Kingdom, where there has been strong government support for improved antibiotic prescribing, total antibiotic consumption decreased by 6.1% between 2014 and 2017. More sobering is the report that while antibiotic prescribing in clinical care was decreasing in the United Kingdom, resistant bacteria persisted and the percentage of infections of the bloodstream (serious infections when bacteria enter the blood) caused by resistant bacteria increased by a third.

Another approach was tried in Spain in a randomized trial. In 23 primary care centers, researchers tested different approaches in patients with acute uncomplicated respiratory infections, usually caused by viral infections not benefiting from antibiotics. Some patients were given antibiotic prescriptions but told to take antibiotics only if they were not better in 5 days. Others were told that antibiotic prescriptions were available for pickup at the primary care center if they were not better but only after 3 days passed. Others received an antibiotic prescription and instructions to start antibiotics that same day. The last group received no antibiotic prescription but had the option of returning to see their doctors if not improved. Not surprisingly, overall antibiotic use was lower in those with delayed antibiotics or a return visit if not improved than in the group who received immediate antibiotics (de la Poza 2016). Burden of symptoms was similar in all groups.

Other approaches to reduce inappropriate prescribing have been studied. Two were done with an electronic medical record (EMR) system. In one study health providers were prompted in the EMR to consider nonantibiotic alternatives when a diagnosis of acute respiratory infection was made, and another required the health provider to enter a justification in free text if he or she prescribed an antibiotic. A third intervention involved sending monthly emails to clinicians in which their prescribing performance was compared with the "best performers" with respect to antibiotic use. Two interventions were effective in reducing inappropriate antibiotic prescribing: requiring justification for using an antibiotic and giving peer comparison (Meeker 2016).

In a Cochrane Review of trials about use of antibiotics for acute respiratory infections in primary care practices, the investigators assessed more than 10 different interventions to reduce inappropriate antibiotic prescribing. These included educational materials for the clinicians, educational meetings, audits and feedbacks, financial interventions (including penalties for inappropriate prescribing), delayed prescribing as described in one of the aforementioned studies (prescription that patient could use later if symptoms did not improve), communication strategies, and point-of-care tests (Tonkin-Crine 2017). The reviewers found moderate-quality evidence that three types of strategies probably are useful in helping to reduce antibiotic prescribing for acute respiratory infections in primary care practices. These were shared decision making between doctors and patients and the use of two point-of-care tests: testing for C-reactive protein (CRP) and procalcitonin. These tests measure the amount of specific substances in the blood. Levels are higher in bacterial infections than in viral infections. Use of procalcitonin results could also guide management of patients with acute respiratory infections in the emergency room.

Yet another approach using laboratory reporting was tried by researchers in Canada in a large community teaching hospital where there was concern about the overuse of ciprofloxacin and its contribution to *Clostridiodes difficile* infections (Landford 2016). Microbiology laboratories typically test bacteria that they recover from a clinical specimen (like urine, sputum, blood, or cerebrospinal fluid) against antibiotics to determine whether the bacteria are sensitive or resistant (and in some instances how sensitive or how resistant). They typically test a large number of antibiotics and make all of this information available to the clinician. The clinician can review this information and revise the treatment course as needed to make certain the patient is receiving an antibiotic that is likely to work for that patient's specific bacteria. In this study the Canadian researchers instructed the laboratory not to report the results of ciprofloxacin susceptibility for *Enterobacteriaceae* (group of bacteria including common Gram-negative bacteria like *Escherichia coli* and *Klebsiella*) if the bacteria were sensitive to (likely to be killed by) other commonly used antibiotics. Clinicians could still learn the ciprofloxacin sensitivity results, but they had to call the laboratory and request them. After this policy was put in place, ciprofloxacin use plummeted—dropping from 87 to

39 daily doses per 1,000 patient-days. Use of older antibiotics, like ampicillin-clavulanate, increased. The investigators also found that 12 and 24 months after starting this policy of selective reporting, *E. coli* isolates were more likely to be sensitive to ciprofloxacin than when the study started. Some have suggested that selective antimicrobial reporting should be used more widely as a way to guide prescribing practices and reduce overuse of certain antibiotics.

What can individuals do to reduce the inappropriate use of antibiotics?

Patient expectations and requests for antibiotics affect the prescribing behavior of clinicians. Greater awareness of the lack of benefit from antibiotics (and lack of need for them) for upper respiratory tract infections among the general public might help. The CDC and other organizations have targeted the general public with messages (on websites and available as posters for clinics) reinforcing the lack of benefit from antibiotics in treating upper respiratory infections.

In the United States, in contrast to many countries, most antibiotics require a prescription from a health provider. Exceptions are some topical agents, like bacitracin and neomycin ointments. A large percentage of antibiotic treatments are given outside of a hospital setting. Targets for education about proper use have generally been health providers, but there is an increasing realization that patients also influence the decision about whether they receive an antibiotic. They decide whether or when to call the health provider for various symptoms. They may request an antibiotic or put subtle or not-so-subtle pressure on the health provider to give them a prescription for an antibiotic—because it "always works." Health providers are not immune to pressure from patients. One study found that physicians were more likely to write prescriptions for upper respiratory infections, those that typically do not warrant an antibiotic, later in the day. They wrote more antibiotic prescriptions for upper respiratory infections late in the morning than early and more in the late afternoon than in the early afternoon. The authors called it "decision fatigue." It takes more energy and time to convince a patient why an antibiotic is not likely to help than to just write a prescription. In a study of telemedicine encounters for respiratory tract infections (that usually do not require antibiotics), patients were asked to complete a patient satisfaction survey at the end of the encounter. Patients who had been prescribed an antibiotic were the happiest with their encounters and gave top scores to their physicians. Those who received a nonantibiotic prescription were less satisfied, and those who received no prescription were the least satisfied (Martinez 2018). Appointments also take longer when patients are not given an antibiotic.

Recent efforts have also included providing information to the general public through publications like *Consumer Reports*. The American Board of Internal Medicine (ABIM) Foundation worked together with multiple medical professional societies (like those for primary care, pediatrics, and surgery) to develop and publicize practical recommendations about antibiotics called "Choosing Wisely." They identified some of the most common reasons for inappropriate use of antibiotics and are making them available to the public so that patients will not expect to receive antibiotics for these conditions. These include asymptomatic bacteriuria (bacteria in the urine causing no symptoms of infection), suspected viral upper respiratory tract infection (colds, stuffy and runny noses), and others. The CDC has also developed educational programs and resources for health providers but also for the public through the "Get Smart: Know When Antibiotics Work" program. They also collaborate with international partners during annual observance of US Antibiotic Awareness week. The CDC website covers multiple topics aimed at the general public. They also offer resources such as posters, fact sheets, brochures, videos, and graphics.

What are antibiotic stewardship programs?

The Infectious Diseases Society of America has defined antimicrobial stewardship as "coordinated interventions designed to improve and measure the appropriate use of antimicrobials by promoting the selection of the optimal antimicrobial drug regimen, dose, duration of therapy, and route of administration" (Fishman 2012). The goals are to achieve the best possible clinical outcomes, minimize toxicity and adverse events, reduce costs, and limit the emergence of resistance. The Joint Commission (an independent not-for-profit organization that certifies health care organizations; many states recognize Joint Commission accreditation as a condition for licensure for receipt of Medicaid and Medicare reimbursement) announced a new standard for hospitals, critical access hospitals, and nursing care centers effective January 1, 2017, that addresses antimicrobial stewardship. They have published elements of performance. This will have wide influence on hospitals because Joint Commission accreditation is sought by a large number of hospitals in the United States.

The CDC has defined the core elements of an effective antimicrobial stewardship program (ASP): leadership commitment (adequate personnel, financial, and information technology resources available), accountability (a single leader is responsible for program outcomes), drug expertise (ASP-dedicated pharmacists are responsible for assisting with the implementation of ASP goals and initiatives), action (recommendations are implemented that are supported by scientific evidence and endorsed by professional societies), monitoring (antimicrobial prescribing and local resistance patterns are tracked), feedback (data on antimicrobial use and resistance are reported to physician and nonphysician prescribers), and education (physicians and nonphysician prescribers receive education regarding rational antimicrobial prescribing and local resistance patterns).

An international group (15 experts from 12 countries) recently reviewed hospital antibiotic stewardship programs from published literature, websites, and other sources (Pulcini 2018). Their goal was to develop a set of core elements and a related checklist that would be used for antibiotic stewardship programs that would be relevant globally, including in hospitals and settings with limited resources and staffing. There have already been many efforts in Europe, North America, and Australia to define and develop programs, such as the one described previously by the CDC.

The group reached consensus in identifying 7 core elements and a checklist of 29 items that would be relevant for antibiotic stewardship in low- to high-income countries. These provide a baseline of key elements to start a hospital antibiotic stewardship program and could facilitate the development of national stewardship guidelines in countries that currently lack them. The seven core elements are leadership commitment, accountability, drug expertise, action, tracking, reporting, and education. These are similar to ones outlined by the CDC but the checklist can be used for any country.

While improving the appropriate use of antibiotics, it is also essential for hospitals to maintain surveillance for multidrug-resistant bacteria and prevent their spread within the institution and outside of it when patients are transferred to other facilities. Meticulous infection control can reduce hospital-acquired infections and provide another way to reduce the need for antibiotics.

Do antibiotic stewardship programs work?

Several studies have shown that antibiotic stewardship programs reduce antibiotic use and reduce hospital costs. An analysis of 32 studies published between 1960 and 2016 found that antibiotic stewardship programs reduced infections and colonization (carrying bacteria without having symptoms) with antibiotic-resistant bacteria, including multidrug-resistant Gram-negative bacteria, extended-spectrum beta-lactamase (ESBL) bacteria, and methicillin-resistant *Staphylococcus aureus*. The programs could also be shown to decrease *C. difficile* infections in hospitalized patients (Baur 2017). They were more effective when combined with infection control measures, like programs to improve hand hygiene (handwashing and use of other hand cleaning methods like hand sanitizers).

In South Africa one barrier to implementation of antibiotic stewardship programs has been inadequate numbers of clinicians with infectious disease expertise. In an area with limited infectious disease expertise, an alliance implemented a pharmacist-driven system that included audits of antibiotic use with a focus on reducing prolonged duration, multiple antibiotics, and redundant coverage across 47 hospitals. They were able to show a reduction in antibiotic use (Brink 2016).

In the United Kingdom a national antibiotic stewardship program was started in 2015 to improve antibiotic prescribing in primary care. The National Health Service established what was called Quality Premium that included financial rewards for the groups that plan and commission health care services for their local population—if they met defined goals for improvement. Among the measures of improvement in antibiotic prescribing was a reduction in antibiotic prescribing of at least 1% and a decrease of at least 10% in the proportion of broad-spectrum antibiotics as a percentage of antibiotics prescribed in primary care. When researchers compared antibiotic use for the period of 2 years before and about 2 years after the financial incentives were introduced, they found that antibiotic items prescribed decreased by 8.2% (Balinskaite 2018). They also found an almost 19% reduction in the prescribing of broad-spectrum antibiotics. During the same period they did not find adverse outcomes related to reduced antibiotic use.

Currently many approaches are being tried to improve antibiotic use in multiple settings (Doernberg 2018) and targeting different populations. There is no single silver bullet that will improve antibiotic use. As with programs to reduce health care–associated infections, a bundle of interventions may be needed to make substantial and sustainable improvements in antibiotic use.

Why do stewardship programs include focus on reported allergies to antibiotics?

In January 2017, the Joint Commission (formerly the Joint Commission on Accreditation of Healthcare Organizations) mandated that all hospitals have antibiotic stewardship programs and defined elements of performance. The Infectious Diseases Society of America also has developed antibiotic stewardship guidelines, and these state that penicillin allergy assessment and testing could aid in appropriate use of first-line antibiotic treatment. Many hospitals already have programs to reduce antibiotic use and some include allergy assessment.

Many patients are labeled allergic to antibiotics when they are not truly allergic (Blumenthal 2017). It is estimated that as many as 18% to 25% of hospitalized patients are labeled as allergic to an antibiotic. Labels of penicillin allergy are especially common, reported by about 10% of the general public. Once a label of allergy is placed on a medical record it is typically carried forward on medical records for years or for life. Although labeling and documenting an allergy is critically important when someone is truly allergic, being classified as antibiotic allergic when one is not truly allergic has a downside. It influences decisions about treatment and prevention. Patients labeled as allergic often receive a second-line antibiotic, often inferior, to treat an infection (or for prevention) rather than the first-choice and most effective drug. The alternative drug may be less effective, more toxic, broader in spectrum (having greater effect on the person's microbiota), and more expensive. A large study in the United Kingdom found that patients labeled as penicillin allergic were more likely to develop complications, like *C. difficile* infection, related to alternative antibiotics. In

Massachusetts, patients labeled penicillin allergic and given an alternative antibiotic to prevent an infection related to a surgical procedure had a 50% increase in the risk of developing a surgical site infection postoperatively (Blumenthal 2017). In that setting 11% of all patients had been labeled penicillin allergic. Patients labeled as penicillin allergic also have greater risk for prolonged hospital stays and readmissions. So correct labeling of allergy becomes really important. The outcomes with second-line antibiotics often are not as good as with the first-choice treatment (MacFadden 2016).

Why would someone be labeled as allergic when he or she is not? Often patients receive multiple drugs simultaneously, so it may be unclear which one is causing a skin rash or other finding that suggests an allergy. So sometimes a patient is labeled as possibly allergic to multiple medications, including antibiotics. A patient may have a predictable side effect related to taking a drug, such as nausea, vomiting, or diarrhea, that may be interpreted as an allergy when it is not—and therefore should not be listed as an allergy. This may reflect miscommunication or ignorance about the nature of allergies. A person may have had an adverse event, such as a yeast infection, following use of an antibiotic. That is not an allergic reaction and would not preclude future use. True allergies to penicillin occur in only about 1% of the population, but often medical records list penicillin allergies in 10% or more of patients.

Some approaches have been tried to improve the accuracy of labeling of patients. Clinicians in Australia developed an integrated program to delabel (remove the "allergy" label) from many patients who were labeled allergic and thereby improve antibiotic usage and appropriateness of treatment. Through careful review of histories, plus testing for allergy in some instances, they were able to remove penicillin allergy labels in 85% of the cases that were labeled allergic (Trubiano 2017). In Toronto a program in three hospitals that involved having allergists train teams available to do point-of-care skin testing for allergies to beta-lactam antibiotics (a group of antibiotics that includes all penicillins and cephalosporins) allowed them to increase the use of beta-lactam antibiotics by 81% in the patients for whom a penicillin or other beta-lactam was the preferred antibiotic.

A few types of adverse reactions to penicillin can be severe or life-threatening. Patients with these types of reactions should not have further sensitivity testing or consideration of repeat use. These include a severe skin reaction called Stevens-Johnson syndrome or toxic epidermal necrolysis and anaphylaxis. In a study in Boston only 5 of 922 patients with a history of allergy had one of the severe types of reactions. Taken together, several studies suggest that more than 95% of patients evaluated for possible penicillin allergy can be found to be able to tolerate penicillins and cephalosporins—two valuable, highly effective, and frequently used groups of antibiotics.

Another approach that has been tried in assessing allergy labeling is a computerized guideline application with decision support that is available to clinicians in a hospital setting. One study compared skin testing and use of a computerized guideline (with standard care) and found that skin testing increased penicillin or cephalosporin use almost sixfold; use of the computerized app increased it nearly twofold (Blumenthal 2017).

When a patient is labeled penicillin allergic, health providers are often reluctant to give any beta-lactam antibiotics. Given that many first-line drugs (both treatment and prevention) for many infections are cephalosporins, which are also beta-lactam antibiotics, this can markedly narrow choices available for treatment. But studies have shown that when penicillin-allergic patients are given cephalosporins, less than 5% show allergy. With the so-called third-generation cephalosporins, only about 2% will show cross-reactivity.

Penicillin allergy management needs to be incorporated into antibiotic stewardship programs because labels of allergy are common and consequences are expensive and serious. Many health systems are now implementing inpatient and outpatient penicillin-testing programs to increase appropriate prescribing of penicillin. Guidelines from the Infectious Diseases Society of America and the Society for Healthcare Epidemiology of America (SHEA) now recommend penicillin allergy skin testing (PAST) as part of antibiotic stewardship protocols. In many centers this involves a version of PAST that uses penicilloyl-polylysine (PRE-PEN) and penicillin G combined with an amoxicillin challenge, which rules out virtually all immediate-type hypersensitivity (the ones that are serious) reactions.

Correctly identifying those who are not truly penicillin allergic can allow treatment with beta-lactam antibiotics and lead to improved outcomes, and can reduce health care expenditures.

What is the role of better diagnostic testing in reducing use of antibiotics?

Many patients are given antibiotics because the clinician is uncertain of the diagnosis and does not want to miss treating a treatable infectious disease—the "just in case" approach. Often the antibiotic given has a broader spectrum (active against more bacteria) than needed because the clinician does not know the specific bacterial cause or the antibiotic sensitivity profile of the bacteria involved. Even if the clinician suspects a staphylococcal infection, for example, it is usually not known at the outset whether it is methicillin-resistant *S. aureus* (MRSA) or methicillin-susceptible *S. aureus* (MSSA). Better diagnostic tests could clearly help in allowing more accurate and precise treatment of patients.

Several types of diagnostic tests could be helpful. These fall into the big categories: Is illness caused by infection? Is the infection treatable (with antibiotics, antivirals, antimalarials, antifungal, or other drugs)? If it is a bacterial infection, which bacteria are involved? Where is the infection (in what part of the body)? What antibiotics are most active against the patient's strain of bacteria? Later in the course it is useful to know when the infection has been cleared so that it is safe to stop the antibiotic.

One would like to have tests that are accurate (sensitive and specific), fast, available wherever patients are treated, easy to do (do not require trained personnel and fancy laboratory equipment), and inexpensive. It would also be useful to have rapid tests that would indicate whether a patient is likely to have an unusual allergic or other adverse reaction to an antibiotic (based on genetics) and whether the person's metabolism might lead to usually high or low levels of the drug. These are currently not available in most instances.

These kinds of data could allow more narrowly targeted treatment and help avoid an excess spectrum of antibiotic activity and days of antibiotic treatment.

Much of the inappropriate use of antibiotics is for treating acute respiratory infections. It may be difficult to distinguish between a bacterial infection that might benefit from antibiotics and a viral infection that would not. We do not have rapid diagnostic tests available in most instances to rapidly distinguish between a viral and bacterial infection.

What is procalcitonin and can it help guide antibiotic treatment?

The body often mobilizes different immune responses for viral and bacterial infections, and researchers have tested whether there are simple tests that would better distinguish between bacterial and viral infections. This has received increased attention because of wider recognition of the downside of using antibiotics, especially when they provide no benefit.

One approach being tested is to measure levels of something called procalcitonin. Procalcitonin (peptide precursor to the hormone calcitonin) is a substance expressed by human cells in response to bacterial infections and is released into the blood. Measuring the level of procalcitonin will not identify the specific bacteria causing an infection but may help answer the question about a viral versus bacterial cause of an infection and aid in the decision whether or not to give an antibiotic. Levels can be measured in a clinical laboratory. Decreasing levels over time in a person with a bacterial infection can also indicate a good response to treatment and may help in deciding when treatment can be stopped. Procalcitonin is thought to increase within 6 to 12 hours of the start of a bacterial infection; levels drop by half daily when an infection is being effectively treated. Cutoff ranges may be different for adults and children because children have a more reactive immune system. Many studies have been done and more are in progress to assess how measuring these levels might aid decisions about antibiotics.

Because acute respiratory tract infections are the most frequent reason for the inappropriate use of antibiotics, multiple studies have been done to assess whether and under what circumstances this test might be useful. A Cochrane Review in 2017 that assessed all of the published studies concluded that using procalcitonin (PCT) levels to guide decisions about starting and stopping antibiotics in acute respiratory infections reduced mortality and reduced antibiotic usage (Schuetz 2017). The number who had died within 30 days were lower and antibiotic-related adverse events were 25% lower in patients whose clinical care was managed using procalcitonin levels to guide decisions. Studies came from 12 different countries and included patients with acute upper and lower respiratory tract infections. Most of the studies looked at adults and did not include immunocompromised patients. When they used PCT to guide treatment, 71.5% received antibiotics. In those managed without PCT testing, 86.3% were given antibiotics. Duration of antibiotic treatment was also shorter in patients whose care was guided by PCT results.

In February 2017 the FDA approved the use of procalcitonin to guide decisions about use of antibiotics in patients with acute respiratory tract infections—but only in patients who are hospitalized or treated in the emergency department (Schuetz 2018).

A recent study that involved 1,656 patients from 14 US hospitals assessed whether using procalcitonin to guide use of antibiotics would decrease antibiotic use in patients with lower respiratory tract infections (primarily pneumonia). In half of the patients decisions about antibiotic use were guided by using procalcitonin levels; the other half received usual care. All hospitals included in the study had high levels of adherence to quality measures for treating pneumonia. In this study looking only at lower respiratory tract infections, the researchers could not show that using procalcitonin levels made a difference in duration of antibiotic treatment or the proportion of patients with adverse outcomes. They did show, however, that in patients with acute bronchitis, antibiotic prescriptions in the emergency department decreased by 50% (Huang 2018).

The results of this study contrast those in many other studies. Critics of the study have noted that the use of procalcitonin levels was not combined with an antibiotic stewardship program. Despite the laboratory results suggesting antibiotics were not necessary, they were still prescribed in many instances (Pulia 2018). The desire for a simple test that can guide treatment remains, but tools and perhaps the implementation are still imperfect.

Studies using PCT in managing patients with other types of infections, like urinary tract infections, are more limited. A study published in 2017 that assessed patients admitted to intensive care units with the diagnosis of sepsis found no benefit—but it was a retrospective study. An analysis of patients with bloodstream infections (serious infection manifested by finding bacteria in the bloodstream) found that the duration of antibiotic treatment was shorter when patients were managed by following PCT levels. Mortality was the same in groups managed with and without use of PCT levels (Meier 2018).

Are procalcitonin levels useful in diagnosing infections in infants?

Young infants are vulnerable to infections. Neonatal sepsis (serious infection of a neonate, especially a newborn younger than 1 month of age) is a leading cause of death. As many as 30% to 60% can die if they do not receive appropriate treatment. Prompt treatment is crucial—but diagnosis is often challenging because the signs and symptoms of sepsis are often subtle and nonspecific. Because physicians do not want to miss treating an infection that could be fatal, in high-income countries up to 7% (or more) of young infants are given intravenous antibiotics within the first 3 days of life. In reality fewer than 1 in 1,000 newborns has sepsis but many more are treated "just in case."

This is another setting where using procalcitonin levels has been studied (Stocker 2017). In a large study from 2009 to early 2015, investigators conducted a controlled trial in hospitals in four countries (the Netherlands, Switzerland, Canada, and Czechoslovakia). Neonates with suspected infection whose parents consented were randomly assigned to a procalcitonin-testing or a control group (treatment as usual). In the procalcitonin-testing group the procalcitonin levels were used to determine how soon to stop antibiotics in infants in whom infection was not documented with cultures or other tests. They found the PCT-tested babies ended up receiving less antibiotic therapy. This study did not look at preterm neonates ("preemies"), another group with high risk of sepsis, but this is likely to be studied in the future.

In a study on the use of antibiotics in 127 neonatal intensive care units (NICUs) across the state of California in 2013, researchers found that there was a 40-fold variation in antibiotic use (meaning that the top users of antibiotics used 40 times more antibiotics than the lowest users), a dramatic difference (Schulman 2015). In NICUs that used more antibiotics, babies had a longer length of stay. On average babies were on antibiotics about a quarter of the days they were in the NICUs, but this varied from 2.4% to 97.1% of baby patient-days—also a remarkable difference. When researchers analyzed other data about the units, they found levels of infection were similar across the units, suggesting that antibiotics were severely overused in some of the NICUs. The study was large, involving data on more than 52,000 infants.

In a different study in 40 children's hospitals, antibiotic-days ranged from 37% to 60% of patient-days, though there were no obvious reasons for this in the clinical mix of diagnoses and type of care (Gerber 2010). Much of antibiotic use is "empiric," and large differences exist in different health care settings with respect to the threshold and "tradition" for giving antibiotics. Stewardship and other programs aim to reduce the excessive use in many hospital and outpatient settings through guidelines and feedback.

Antibiotics in early life may have a profound effect on the assembly and development of the infant's microbiota with potentially long-lasting consequences, so decisions about using antibiotic treatment should be made carefully.

Why did use of rapid diagnostic tests lead to increased use of antibiotics in some settings?

Use of diagnostic tests can also have unexpected consequences. Rapid diagnostic tests (RDTs) for malaria were developed to provide rapid specific diagnosis and to reduce unnecessary and excessive use of antimalarial drugs, which could contribute to development of drug-resistant malaria parasites. However, increased use of RDTs for malaria has led to an increase in use of antibiotics in some areas. Before these tests were available, every child with fever living in a malarious area was assumed to have malaria and treated with antimalarial drugs because most local health facilities did not have the equipment, materials, and experience to do malaria smears and make a specific diagnosis of malaria. Two factors have changed. Malaria has decreased in many parts of the world because of investments in malaria control programs, including use of long-lasting insecticide-treated bednets, residual spraying of insecticide in some areas, availability of better drug treatment, and intermittent preventive therapy for certain high-risk groups. Second, rapid diagnostic tests for malaria have become available that do not require expensive equipment or extensive training. These tests can be done in local clinics without sophisticated laboratory support. Many patients with fever who in the past would have been treated for malaria are now diagnosed as "not malaria." So what can local health providers do when faced with a sick child with fever and negative RDT for malaria? They typically give what they do have, which is an antibiotic.

Several studies have shown that antibiotic use has increased in areas where RDTs for malaria are being used. In some places almost all patients who test negative for malaria are given antibiotics, even though in areas like Thailand and Tanzania, where studies have looked carefully for alternative, specific causes of fever, only 5% to 10% of patients with fever actually have bacterial infections that are likely to respond to antibiotic treatment. Most fevers in children are caused by viral and other nonbacterial infections that will not benefit from antibiotics.

The proportion of fevers caused by malaria varies widely even within Africa from 0% to close to 80%. Other approaches are being tested. Measuring a substance in the blood called C-reactive protein (CRP) to help distinguish between a bacterial and viral infection has been helpful in some settings. Like procalcitonin, the level is elevated in bacterial infections and not in viral infections, allowing one to decide when an antibiotic might be helpful, even if it does not identify the specific bacteria causing an infection. It has been useful in some settings in Europe. The problem with relying on it in many low-income countries is that many children are malnourished, a condition that suppresses the production of CRP, making levels falsely low in a bacterial infection. In addition, some parasitic infections can cause it to be elevated, giving a signal that makes clinicians suspect bacterial infection when none is present.

Other approaches to managing fever have involved developing an application that can be used on a smartphone or tablet and can incorporate results from a few simple diagnostic tests (that can be done in a local lab), like hemoglobin (found in red blood cells; levels are low in anemia), glucose (blood sugar level), and oxygen saturation (oxygen in blood can be checked with a simple device that snaps onto a finger). The app can also incorporate pulse, breathing rate, and arm circumference. The latter is a quick, inexpensive way to identify malnourished patients. Use of breathing rate can help to distinguish an upper respiratory tract infection from pneumonia (lower respiratory tract infection), which might require antibiotic therapy. Studies have shown that use of some apps and simple diagnostic tests can help to reduce the number of children given antibiotics. Other research teams are developing tests to identify the most common fever-causing infections. One problem is that some infections vary by geographic area, so one needs an area-specific panel of tests—or a panel with a large number of infections that can be identified.

There are few reliable rapid diagnostic tests for infections other than for malaria, tuberculosis, and HIV, and these are still often found in limited areas or in specialized clinics. Rapid tests for influenza and strep infections are also available in some settings. More unusual infections and fungal and parasitic infections other than malaria often go undiagnosed. A primary challenge remains to improve fever diagnosis and management in malaria-risk and other areas.

Are there other approaches that use urine, saliva, breath, or other specimens to diagnose infection?

Some new diagnostics potentially can use saliva, urine, and other materials that are easier to collect than blood samples. One example is use of serotype-specific urinary antigen detection for diagnosing pneumococcal pneumonia (Wunderink 2018). Samples of sputum are often difficult to obtain, especially in children, who often do not cough and spit out sputum. A test using urine would be easier to use. An early version of the test only identifies 13 of the serotypes (types of pneumococcal bacteria that cause pneumonia), but it is a start. Some innovative approaches are being explored, including some that take advantage of smartphones.

Other avenues are being explored (Fidock 2018). It has been observed that malaria-infected red blood cells produce tiny amounts of gases—volatile organic compounds (VOCs). VOCs are chemicals emitted as gases from solids or liquids. Some have odor or scent. Some are toxic, for example, some of those found in cigarette smoke. Some are attractants for mosquitoes and may influence a mosquito's host preference. Skin bacteria can also affect VOCs and may influence mosquito preferences in choosing a host for taking a blood meal.

These gases, VOCs, can also be expelled in breath. Starting with the observation that malaria-infected red blood cells in humans produce VOCs, investigators analyzed the composition of the breath of people infected with malaria. They found six VOCs in patients with malaria. In a preliminary study, they found that by analyzing the composition of breath (breathprint), they were able to diagnose malaria in more than 80% of children who were infected (Schaber 2018).

Using this feature of parasite biology—production of VOCs—it may be possible to make a malaria diagnosis without taking blood samples. It would be useful to have a noninvasive test that does not rely on the presence of a specific protein (histidine-rich protein, HRP2) in the parasite. This is used by the current RDTs. Because of changes in the malaria parasite, the RDTs are already showing negative results in some patients with malaria. Parasites that lack the specific protein (HRP2 antigen) used by the RDT have spread in India, Peru, and parts of Africa. It is projected that current RDTs may miss up to 20% of cases of malaria in Africa by 2030. The prospect of a "malaria breathalyzer" or breathprint for diagnosis is appealing but needs more work to translate the concept into practice.

It is interesting evolutionarily that infection of human red blood cells by the malaria parasite can release substances that are exhaled by the human and make the infected human host more attractive to mosquitoes. The mosquito is seeking a blood meal to survive and reproduce (needs blood to nourish eggs); finding human hosts with parasites in their blood is of no extra benefit to the mosquito—but if a mosquito bites a person infected with malaria parasites, this improves the likelihood that the malaria parasites may survive and be passed on to more and more human hosts. The malaria parasites are ancient and have been remarkably successful survivors throughout history.

There has already been use of a breath-based test for diagnosing infection with *Helicobacter pylori*, a bacterium that can infect the stomach lining and cause ulcers and other problems. In this instance the test takes advantage of the presence of urease (an enzyme) in *H. pylori*. Patients drink a liquid containing urea that is labeled with a marker. Their breath is collected before and after drinking the solution. In persons with *H. pylori* infection, the urea is decomposed by the bacteria, releasing carbon dioxide. The difference between the values in exhaled air before and after the drink can indicate whether the person is infected with *H. pylori*. Infection can also be diagnosed with blood tests (antibody), cultures (to grow the bacteria), and tissue biopsies.

Other diagnostic tests are being studied for tuberculosis (TB). HIV-infected patients with latent TB have a 20 to 30 times greater risk of developing active TB than TB-infected, HIV-negative individuals. Good sputum samples are often difficult to obtain, so there is continuing need for better diagnostic approaches. There is now a urine test called the urine lipoarabinomannan assay (TB-LAM) that the World Health Organization (WHO) endorsed in 2015 to try to improve diagnosis of TB in HIV-infected individuals. It is inexpensive and easy to perform.

It is recommended under specific circumstances: adults with HIV who are hospitalized with signs and symptoms of tuberculosis and who have a low CD4 count (<100 cells/µL) or who are seriously ill. In a multicenter study in southern Africa investigators showed that using the urine test for TB on all HIV-infected hospitalized patients, regardless of symptoms, increased the number of patients diagnosed with tuberculosis. Although using the test did not reduce overall deaths among HIV-infected individuals, it did decrease deaths among those with CD4 counts less than 100 cells/µL, severe anemia, or clinically suspected TB.

Other studies have looked at the possibility of using stool (feces) samples to diagnose TB. Given that it is difficult to collect sputum samples from some adults and most young children, and that most sputum is swallowed, researchers have assessed the feasibility of looking for *Mycobacterium tuberculosis* DNA in stool specimens. They adapted DNA extraction and concentration techniques developed for use on soil samples. They applied these to stool samples and then used polymerase chain reaction (PCR) to detect *M. tuberculosis*. This could be used to diagnose TB and to monitor response to treatment. Cultures (to grow the bacteria) are still needed because PCR and traditional microscopy do not distinguish between live and dead tuberculosis bacteria. Cultures are slow and require specialized laboratory support. These newer approaches may allow earlier diagnosis—and thus earlier treatment of TB. Treating TB is good for the patient and reduces onward transmission.

There are compelling reasons for eliminating unnecessary use of antibiotics. Whether reducing use of antibiotics in some parts of the world can reverse the inexorable increase in resistance that is seen globally in multiple pathogens—in humans, animals, and the environment—is less certain. We will not (in the foreseeable future) return to a world where most bacteria are sensitive to most antibiotics, but we may be able to slow the emergence and spread of multiply resistant bacteria, the so-called superbugs. At the same time, it is essential to assess and control other uses of antibiotics (in animals, in fish, on plants) and the contamination of the environment with antibiotics and their residues.

What is the role of national and international agencies in reducing inappropriate use of antibiotics?

These agencies provide essential leadership. All embrace a One Health perspective. In the United States, the CDC has an active program to improve antibiotic use. They have identified actions to be taken by various groups: health care providers; patients and families; health systems, hospitals, clinics, and nursing homes; health care quality organizations; health insurance companies; health care provider professional organizations; and federal, state, and local health agencies. The FDA in September 2018 released a 5-year plan for supporting antimicrobial stewardship in veterinary settings. The Presidential Advisory Council on Combating Antbiotic-Resistant Bacteria (PACCARB) has been meeting since September 2015. It issued its last report in Septermber 2018 with recommendations for human and animal health (PACCARB 2018).

In the United Kingdom an expert panel chaired by Jim O'Neill delivered "Tackling Drug-Resistant Infections Globally: Final Report and Recommendations" in May 2016 after publishing eight thematic papers from 2014 to 2016. They identified 10 fronts for tackling antimicrobial resistance: public awareness; sanitation and hygiene; antibiotics in agriculture and the environment; vaccines and alternatives; surveillance; rapid diagnostics; human capital; drugs; global innovation fund; and international coalition for action.

In the United Kingdom the Responsible Use of Medicines in Agriculture Alliances set up sector-specific targets. Antibiotic use in the United Kingdom in agricultural animals dropped by 27% between 2014 and 2016, with levels dropping to 45 mg of antibiotic use per kilogram of livestock, better than the government target of 50 mg/kg by 2018. The United Kingdom has achieved agricultural use of antibiotics that is more than 50% below the EU average.

The United Nations has also taken an active role. In 2016 the UN General Assembly recognized the global problem of antimicrobial resistance, including use of antimicrobials in food animals as a leading cause of rising antimicrobial resistance (United Nations 2016). Other groups, including the World Bank (World Bank 2017), have released reports about the global problem of antimicrobial resistance and have proposed a range of interventions to slow antimicrobial resistance.

The WHO has also been active in the area of antibiotics. Starting in 1977, the WHO has published a model list of essential medicines, defined as those that "satisfy the priority health care needs of the population." The list is revised every 2 years in consultation with an expert committee (World Health Organization 2017).

For the first time in 2017, to improve stewardship of antibiotics and reduce antibiotic resistance, the WHO committee developed three categories for antibiotics: ACCESS, WATCH, and RESERVE groups. Antibiotics in the ACCESS group are those used to treat many common infections and should be widely available. The WATCH group includes antibiotics with higher resistance potential and that are recommended as first- or second-line treatment for a limited number of specific indications. This includes seven classes of drugs: the quinolones and fluoroquinolones, third-generation cephalosporins, macrolides, glycopeptides (like vancomycin), antipseudomonal penicillins with beta-lactam inhibitors, carbapenems, and penems. The WHO suggests monitoring to ensure their use is in line with recommended indications.

The RESERVE group includes drugs that should be considered "last resort" antibiotics and used for selected specific indications or in settings where other options are unavailable or have failed. These drugs should be protected and their use monitored by stewardship programs. These include aztreonam, fourth-generation cephalosporins, fifth-generation cephalosporins, polymyxins (like colistin), fosfomycin IV, oxazolidinones (linezolid), tigecycline, and daptomycin.

Why aren't pharmaceutical companies developing more new antibiotics? Why don't we have more antibiotics in the pipeline?

From an economic perspective it is easy to understand why pharmaceutical companies are not investing in developing new antibiotics. Antibiotics are typically used for short periods by patients with an episode of infection, in contrast to drugs used for chronic problems like high blood pressure, diabetes, and heart disease. Antibiotics may be taken for a few days or a week or two. In contrast, drugs for chronic diseases are taken every day for years or for life and by large numbers of people in the population. The market for antibiotics is much smaller and less predictable. Another characteristic of antibiotics makes them unique among drugs: their targets become resistant to them. The more they are used, the more likely it is that bacteria will become resistant to them and they will become less effective or even stop working for some infections. Drugs for chronic diseases like hypertension continue to work the same way and with the same effectiveness year after year. Many remain in wide use decades after they were developed. New and improved drugs for chronic diseases are developed, but it is not because the old ones stop working. For these reasons most large pharmaceutical companies have stopping investing in research and development of antibiotics. The traditional economic incentives do not work well for antibiotics. They provide poor return on investment.

In 2018 Novartis announced that it would discontinue antibacterial and antiviral research. It joins other companies that have made this choice and highlights the challenges for pharmaceutical companies. Relative to other drugs, such as cancer drugs, biologics, and agents for treating chronic diseases, antibiotics do not sell in large quantities and are generally not profitable. They are costly to develop and may become ineffective after a few years. The public would benefit from the development of new antibiotics, but pharmaceutical companies are acting rationally (in their own best economic interests) when they decide not to pursue antibiotic research.

Which bacteria are the highest priority for development of new antibiotics?

In 2017 the WHO released a list of antibiotic-resistant bacteria that are a priority for research and development (World Health Organization 2017). *M. tuberculosis* is among the most important given its continued high burden globally. It was not included in this list because it is covered in a separate program, but the WHO reiterated the need for new approaches to treat and prevent tuberculosis, including multidrug-resistant (MDR) and extensively drug-resistant (XDR) TB.

The list was developed using multiple criteria to rank priority pathogens in a transparent process. Experts applied a multicriteria decision analysis technique, a method that incorporates expert opinion and evidence-based data. The expert committee selected 10 assessment criteria for each pathogen evaluated: all-cause mortality, health care burden, community burden, prevalence of resistance, 10-year trend of resistance, transmissibility, preventability in the hospital setting, preventability in community settings, treatability, and current pipeline.

Taking into account these criteria, they developed a list of pathogens that they stratified into three groups in terms of priority for research and development of new antibiotics.

Priority 1 group, which they termed "critical," included *Acinetobacter baumannii*, carbapenem resistant; *Pseudomonas aeruginosa*, carbapenem resistant; and *Enterobacteriaceae*, carbapenem resistant, third-generation cephalosporin resistant. These Gram-negative infections are typically treated in hospitals, are often seen in patients with chronic diseases, and are often lethal.

Priority 2 group, which they termed "high priority," included *Enterococcus faecium*, vancomycin resistant; *S. aureus*, methicillin resistant, vancomycin intermediate and resistant; *H. pylori*, clarithromycin resistant; *Campylobacter*, fluoroquinolone resistant; *Salmonella* spp., fluoroquinolone resistant; and *Neisseria gonorrhoeae*, third-generation cephalosporin resistant, fluoroquinolone resistant. Many of these infections are usually community acquired and often treated in the community.

The Priority 3 group, listed as "medium priority," includes *Streptococcus pneumoniae*, penicillin nonsusceptible; *Haemophilus influenzae*, ampicillin resistant; *Shigella* spp., fluoroquinolone resistant.

What antibiotics or antibacterial products are currently in the pipeline?

A recent review of the global clinical antibiotic pipeline found that as of July 1, 2018, there were only 30 new antibacterial drugs that were considered new chemical entities (Theuretzbacher 2019). Only 11 out of the 30 were expected to be active against a critical bacterial pathogen that is carbapenem resistant. Ten have activity against *M. tuberculosis*, and four are active against *C. difficile*. Most of the new drugs are derivatives from classes of antibiotics already used. Of the 11 with activity against Gram-negative bacteria, 10 are beta-lactams or tetracyclines. In a few instances, a new chemical entity was combined with a well-known approved drug to extend its spectrum of antibacterial activity. In addition to antibiotics, there are 10 antibacterial agents that fall into the category of "biologics." These include six monoclonal and two polyclonal antibodies and two phage endolysin products. All of these are directed against one of three problem (hard-to-treat) bacteria: *S. aureus* (six), *C. difficile* (two), and *P. aeruginosa* (two). All except one must be given intravenously. This review summarized only products that have reached at least a phase 1 trial or beyond. It also included three agents approved by the FDA in 2017/2018. Products that are still in the early stages of development were not included. The general conclusion is that much more investment is needed to develop a broader array of safe and effective antibacterial products.

Whose responsibility is it to develop new antibiotics? Who pays for their development? What incentives or other approaches might increase the development of new antibiotics?

Usual incentives for developing new drugs involve creating a large market for them. With antibiotics, the incentives are different. To keep them working, we need to limit their use. We want new antibiotics but need to use them sparingly. The low return on investment makes them unattractive for pharmaceutical companies.

Recognizing the global crisis caused by antibiotic resistance and the limited supply of effective antibiotics, a number of organizations and institutions working with government and industry are trying to find ways to increase investment in antibiotic research and development. Some have called for the development of an intergovernmental panel on antimicrobial resistance (Woolhouse 2014) or more recently a One Health Global Leadership Group on Antimicrobial Resistance. The WHO, the CDC, the United Nations, the World Bank, the Interagency Coordination Group on Antimicrobial Resistance (in consultation with the FAO, OIE, and WHO), the Wellcome Trust, Pew Charitable Trusts, and many governments and organizations have issued reports, guidelines, roadmaps, and recommendations. CARB-X, a nonprofit public-private partnership dedicated to accelerating antibacterial research, is investing in the early development pipeline for new antibiotics, vaccines, and rapid diagnostics. The research project DRIVE-AB (driving re-investment in R&D and responsible antibiotic use) includes a consortium of public sector partners and pharmaceutical companies. The Duke Margolis Center for Health Policy has laid out value-based strategies for encouraging new development of antimicrobial drugs.

There is general agreement about the need to preserve and improve use of current antibiotics, reduce the need for antibiotics, and develop and employ better diagnostics in all sectors. Dr. John Rex, who has decades of development and policy experience with antimicrobial agents, along with others have suggested that we should reframe our thinking about antibiotics. Instead of seeing antibiotics like other drugs, we should view them as part of the infrastructure or like fire extinguishers. As such, they are fundamental to the health of society. We need to have them available, but we hope to use them infrequently. To encourage research and development of drugs that we want to stay on the shelf most of the time, we need different pathways and incentives. Strategies that have been proposed to increase research, development, and testing of new antibiotics include what have been called "push" and "pull" approaches. Push incentives include giving grants, funds, and other financial rewards to groups to find and develop new products. These funds or investments could reward a focus on the products of highest priority. In the United Kingdom a report and discussion took place at the House of Commons in October 2018. The report called for investment in the United Kingdom by government and industry. They and others have called for other approaches to make the landscape more favorable for antibiotic development, including changes in patent laws for antibiotics. Options for "pull" incentives have been more limited and largely focus on increased payment for antibiotics—and payments even if antibiotics are not used. Today the financial rewards favor increased prescribing, a behavior that we do not want to incentivize.

What are priority areas in looking for other ways to treat bacterial infections?

A blue-ribbon panel of 24 scientists from academia and industry was commissioned by the Wellcome Trust and jointly funded by the Department of Health England to consider the prospects for alternatives to antibiotics. They came up with 19 alternatives to be considered and published their report in 2016 (Czaplewski 2016). They focused on treatments for systemic and invasive infections and not superficial ones and on products that would be used by injection, by mouth, or inhaled and not on products that would be used topically.

Ten approaches were prioritized. Most of the approaches have been known for a long time, but specific products would need to be developed and tested. They considered all possible approaches, including those that would target the bacteria as well as those that target the host. Many are specific to the particular bacterial pathogen or even specific strain of bacteria, in contrast to many of the currently used antibiotics, which are broad spectrum and active against multiple bacteria. Many would be used only as an adjunct to traditional antibiotics, at least initially. They will likely be more expensive than current antibiotics, many of which are cheap. They will take time and money to develop and move through clinical trials and will likely be only a partial replacement to antibiotics. Most of them target some of the most problematic bacteria: *S. aureus, P. aeruginosa,* or *C. difficile.* There are gaps in the key pathogens that are being targeted—as they do not include many of the priority pathogens highlighted by the WHO and others. The targeted nature of these treatments will make diagnostics more important than ever. Their use may require innovative regulatory approaches because they do not fall into the usual categories of drugs. Some experts have speculated that some newer agents might require different delivery systems, more like a blood transfusion service or stem cell harvesting, in contrast to the global manufacturing system for antibiotics.

Will there be a role for point-of-care development for some products? All would have potential uses in animal health, whether in food animals, work animals, or pets, but costs might be prohibitive for animal use.

The commission report concluded that a bigger investment is needed to develop these approaches and gave as examples the Large Hadron Collider project, which cost approximately 6 billion pounds, and the International Space Station, which cost about 96 billion pounds. They estimate that the investment needed to develop alternatives to antibiotic treatment would lie somewhere between the two. The report is sobering.

A quick tour of the approaches that made the top 10 list is worthwhile to get some sense of the range of interventions that might work. They also included a list of another nine that have lower priority because they were less well developed or there was insufficient information about them to assess their potential impact.

The priority approaches for investment are as follows:

Use of antibodies. Some versions of antibodies have been used for a long time, but new technologies make it possible to engineer specific antibodies for a range of activities. They can bind to a specific strain or pathogen or interrupt virulence factors or neutralize toxins. Development of antivirulence products is complicated because bacteria often have multiple and redundant pathways for producing toxin, damaging cells, or otherwise injuring the host. If one pathway is blocked, they may use an alternative path, a detour around the barrier.

Use of probiotics. This involves giving live microorganisms to a person. The microbes chosen are those that can confer a health benefit. A mix of microbes may be used. This may also be used in combination with other approaches. Many studies of probiotics to treat and prevent a range of problems have already been published, including use to prevent or treat *C. difficile* infections. Results have been mixed.

Use of lysins. These are enzymes used by bacteriophages (phages) to destroy the cell walls of the target bacteria. They act directly on the bacteria and can also weaken biofilms.

Use of wild-type bacteriophages. These are the viruses, widespread in nature, that can infect bacteria. They target specific bacteria. They can replicate as long as their target bacteria are present but do not affect other resident bacteria. One can also develop cocktails of phages to target specific infections.

Use of engineered bacteriophages. There is potential to genetically engineer phages with specific properties to counter specific infections. They might be mixed with wild-type bacteriophages.

Stimulate host immunity. This would be an adjunct to antibiotic therapy. Agents that might enhance expression of innate resistance could be identified and studied.

Use of vaccines. New targets for vaccines can be developed; expanded knowledge of potential vaccination in elderly and immune-compromised individuals is also needed.

Use of antimicrobial peptides. These have a broad spectrum, rapid killing, and low resistance. Studies to date, however, have not yielded any breakthroughs for treatment of systemic infections. Some of these are bacteriocins and are used in the food industry; some are used in food animals.

Use of host defense peptides and innate defense peptides. These have indirect effects on bacteria and act by increasing expression of anti-inflammatory cytokines and reducing expression of proinflammatory cytokines.

Use of antibiofilm peptides. Peptides have been identified that specifically inhibit bacterial biofilm. These would be used along with antibiotics. Creation of biofilms is a mechanism that allows bacteria to survive despite the presence of antibiotics. Survival of bacteria in biofilms is important in clinical medicine (as well as in industry and manufacturing) in infections that involve catheters, prosthetic joints, heart valves, and other sites.

Now that scientists better understand the factors that contribute to the creation and persistence of biofilms, they are working on approaches to prevent the development of biofilms and on ways to disrupt biofilms. These include coatings of catheters and other devices with materials that prevent bacteria from adhering to the surface—the first step in creating a biofilm. Other approaches involve trying to interrupt the communication among the bacteria, called quorum sensing. Bacteria respond to environmental signals from the host and from other bacteria.

Confronting the challenges created by antibiotic resistance will require creative and innovative approaches and input from multiple disciplines. We have underestimated the contributions of microbes to human life and the adverse consequences of antibiotic use. The genetic capabilities of bacteria are protean. Can human wit harness microbial communities to our benefit instead of trying only to disrupt or destroy them? Our future health and the health of the planet depend on it.

GLOSSARY

Institutions, Organizations, Documents, Policies, Acts

Acronyms and Abbreviations

ACIP: Advisory Committee on Immunization Practices (CDC)
AMR: antimicrobial resistance
APUA: Alliance for the Prudent Use of Antibiotics
AR: antibiotic resistance
AR Isolate Bank: antibiotic-resistant isolate bank (CDC-FDA)
ARSI: Antibiotic Resistance Solutions Initiative (CDC)
ASM: American Society of Microbiology
ASP: Antimicrobial Stewardship Program
AST: antimicrobial susceptibility testing
BARDA: Biomedical Advanced Research and Development Authority
BCG: bacillus Calmette-Guerin (vaccine to protect against tuberculosis)
CARE: Collective Antimicrobial Resistance Ecosystem
CBRN: Chemical Biological Radiological and Nuclear threats
CDC: Centers for Disease Control and Prevention
Antibiotic Resistance Laboratory Network (ARLN)
Antibiotic Resistance Solutions Initiative (ARSI)
CDDEP: Center for Disease Dynamics, Economics and Policy
CMS: Centers for Medicare and Medicaid Services
CRE: carbapenem-resistant *Enterobacteriaceae*
CRP: C-reactive protein
CTX-M ESBL: cefotaxime extended-spectrum beta-lactamase
DDD: defined daily doses
DEA: Drug Enforcement Administration

DNA: deoxyribonucleic acid

DRI: drug-resistant infection

ECCMID: European Congress of Clinical Microbiology and Infectious Diseases

ECDC: European Centre for Disease Control

EPA: Environmental Protection Agency

ESBL: extended-spectrum beta-lactamase

ESCMID: European Society of Clinical Microbiology and Infectious Diseases

ESKAPE: *Enterococcus faecium, Staphylococcus aureus, Klebsiella pneumoniae, Acinetobacter baumannii, Pseudomonas aeruginosa, Enterobacter* spp.

EU: European Union

EU-JAMRAI: European Union Joint Action on Antimicrobial Resistance and Healthcare-Associated Infections

FAO: Food and Agriculture Organization of the United Nations

FDA: Food and Drug Administration

Center for Biologics Evaluation and Research (CBER)

Center for Devices and Radiological Health (CDRH)

Center for Drug Evaluation and Research (CDER)

Center for Veterinary Medicine (CVM)

National Center for Toxicological Research (NCTR)

FQ: fluoroquinolone

GAP: Global Action Plan

GARDP: Global Antibiotic Research and Development Partnership

GFSI: Global Food Safety Initiative

GLASS: Global Antimicrobial Surveillance System

GMP: good manufacturing practices (CGMF: current good manufacturing practices).

GRAS: generally recognized as safe

Hib vaccine: *Haemophilus influenzae* B vaccine

IACG: Inter-Agency Coordination Group on Antimicrobial Resistance

ICU: intensive care unit

IDSA: Infectious Diseases Society of America

IHR: International Health Regulations

IM: intramuscular (injected directly into muscle)

IMI: Innovative Medicines Initiative

IV: intravenous (injected into a vein)

JCAHO: Joint Commission on Accreditation of Healthcare Organizations; replaced by Joint Commission

LPAD: Limited Population Pathway for Antibacterial and Antifungal Drugs (legislation enacted by Congress in 2016; aims to advance development and approval of drugs to treat serious infections in limited populations)

MDR: multidrug resistant

MDR-TB: multidrug-resistant tuberculosis

MI: microbiome index

MRL: maximum residue limit (level)

MRSA: methicillin-resistant *Staphylococcus aureus*

MSSA: methicillin-susceptible *Staphylococcus aureus*

MTB: *Mycobacterium tuberculosis*

NAM: National Academy of Medicine

NAP: National Action Plan

NARMS: National Antimicrobial Resistance Monitoring System (comanaged by the FDA, USDA, CDC; monitors resistance in foodborne and other enteric bacteria)

NASEM: National Academies of Sciences, Engineering, and Medicine

NDA: New Drug Application

NDARO: National Database of Antibiotic Resistant Organisms (NIH)

NHSN: CDC's National Healthcare Safety Network

NICU: neonatal intensive care unit

NIFA: National Institute of Food and Agriculture

NIH: National Institutes of Health

OIE: World Organization for Animal Health

PAST: penicillin allergy skin testing

PCR: polymerase chain reaction

PCT: procalcitonin

PCV: pneumococcal conjugate vaccine

RDT: rapid diagnostic test, often used to describe RDTs for malaria

RIF: rifampin

RNA: ribonucleic acid

SDG: Sustainable Development Goals

SHEA: Society for Health Care Epidemiology of America

SHIELD: Systemic Harmonization and Interoperability Enhancement for Lab Data

Staph: *Staphylococcus*

Strep: *Streptococcus*

TB: tuberculosis

UN: United Nations

UNGA: United Nations General Assembly

USDA: United States Department of Agriculture

UV: ultraviolet

VFD: veterinary feed directive (includes guidelines about antibiotic use in feed for animals)

VOCs: volatile organic compounds

VRE: vancomycin-resistant *Enterococcus*

WHO: World Health Organization

XDR-TB: extensively drug-resistant tuberculosis

Definitions of Terms

Acquired resistance: capacity of bacteria to develop ways to resist antibiotics. Can be acquired through mutation of the bacteria or through acquiring new genetic material from other microbes.

Acronize: describes the coating of chicken (and other kinds of meat and fish) with a solution containing the tetracycline antibiotic aureomycin (accomplished by dipping killed, cleaned chickens into bucket with solution of aureomycin); term used in 1950s, now obsolete.

Adverse drug event: harmful effects as a result of using a drug, like an antibiotic.

Aminoglycosides: class of antibiotics active against many Gram-negative bacteria; includes streptomycin, gentamicin, and tobramycin. Toxic side effects can affect kidney function and hearing.

Antiseptics: substances active against microbes; often applied to tissues or skin to prevent infection; examples are alcohol, iodine, hydrogen peroxide, and chlorhexidine.

Archaea: unicellular organisms that differ from bacteria in genetics and biochemistry. Their membranes are made of ether lipids. Often found in extreme environments. Part of the microbiota.

Azithromycin: a macrolide antibiotic active against many common respiratory, diarrheal, and other infections.

Bacteria: single-celled organisms. Widespread, varied, abundant, old. Live in, on, and all around us. Some are essential for human health; a few cause disease.

Bactericidal: capacity of antibiotic or other substance to kill bacteria.

Bactericide: term often used to describe antibiotics used to treat or prevent infections in plants.

Bacteriocins: proteins or peptides produced by bacteria that kill or inhibit bacteria.

Bacteriophage: viruses that can infect bacteria or archaea.

Bacteriostatic: antibiotic or other substance that slows the growth of bacteria but does not kill them.

BCG: vaccine to prevent tuberculosis; used in most countries globally.

Beta-lactam ring: key chemical structure that is present in penicillin and cephalosporin antibiotics.

Beta-lactamase: enzyme produced by bacteria that can break the beta-lactam ring, making these antibiotics ineffective; many different beta-lactamases have been identified, including penicillinase, extended-spectrum beta-lactamases (ESBLs), and carbapenemase.

Biofilms: collection or aggregation of bacteria that stick to a surface; may produce sticky substance (slime) that helps to protect the bacteria from being killed.

Broad-spectrum antibiotic: active against many different bacteria.

C-reactive protein: produced by the body in response to inflammation, injury, certain diseases, and some infections, especially bacterial; released into the bloodstream; can be measured with laboratory test.

Carbapenem: broad-spectrum, beta-lactam antibiotics developed to evade the action of most beta-lactamases.

Carbapenem-resistant *Enterobacteriaceae*: bacteria that resist the action of carbapenem antibiotics, usually via production of carbapenemase.

Carbapenemase: enzyme produced by bacteria that can inactivate carbapenem antibiotics.

Cephalosporins: type of beta-lactam antibiotic, including many commonly used antibiotics, such as cefixime and ceftriaxone; multiple generations of these antibiotics have been developed.

Chromosomes: strings of genes; made of DNA; usually found in nucleus of cell.

Ciprofloxacin: a commonly used broad-spectrum fluoroquinolone antibiotic.

Clindamycin: antibiotic active against many Gram-positive bacteria and anaerobes; associated with *Clostridioides difficile* colitis.

Codex Alimentarius or "Food Code": collection of guidelines, standards, and codes of practice.

Colonization: bacteria living on tissues, like in the throat or gut, without invading or causing symptoms.

Colonization resistance: capacity of a normal community of bacteria to resist the colonization or invasion by other microbes that do not normally inhabit that body site, such as the gut, vagina, or mouth.

Conjugate vaccine: type of vaccine made from attaching an antigen to a carrier protein; examples include Hib, pneumococcal, meningococcal, and typhoid vaccines.

Disinfectants: substances/chemicals that are active against microbes and are used to clean or treat surfaces.

DNA: deoxyribonucleic acid; made up of adenine, guanine, thymine, and cytosine; instructions for genes.

Dysbiosis: disruption of the normal balance of microbiota.

E. coli: *Escherichia coli*, Gram-negative bacteria; rod shaped; commonly found in the gastrointestinal tract.

Enterobacter **spp**.: genus of bacteria within the family of *Enterobacteriaceae*; some are multidrug resistant

Enterobacteriaceae: large family of Gram-negative bacteria that includes *E. coli*, *Klebsiella*, *Salmonella*, and *Shigella*. Many are found in gastrointestinal tracts of humans and animals.

Enzymes: proteins (substances) that cause specific chemical reactions; can speed up or catalyze reactions.

Erythromycin: macrolide antibiotic.

ESKAPE: collection of hard-to-treat bacteria that escape action of most antibiotics. Common cause of health care–associated infections. Includes *Enterococcus faecium*, *Staphylococcus aureus*, *Klebsiella pneumoniae*, *Acinetobacter baumanii*, *Pseudomonas aeruginosa*, and *Enterobacter* species.

Eukaryotes: includes unicellular (many are microscopic) and many multicellular organisms, like plants and animals. Their cells have a nucleus and other internal components, like mitochondria and Golgi apparatus.

Extended spectrum beta-lactamases (ESBLs): enzymes produced by bacteria that make them resist antibiotics that were created to resist beta-lactamases.

Extensively drug resistant (XDR): resistant to most drugs that would normally be used to treat that infection.

Fluoroquinolones: class of broad-spectrum antibiotics; includes ciprofloxacin and moxifloxacin.

Genes: instructions for making proteins; arranged on chromosomes. Usually found in nucleus of cells.

Genome: an organism's complete set of DNA including all genes (humans have >3 billion DNA base pairs).

Gram-negative: bacteria that have an outer membrane, a thin peptidoglycan cell wall plus an inner (cytoplasmic) cell wall; stain pinkish-red with Gram's stain.

Gram-positive: bacteria with thick peptidoglycan cell wall and inner membrane. Stain purple with Gram's stain.

Gram stain: developed in 1800s by Danish scientist Hans Christian Gram to stain bacteria; allows classification based on appearance under microscope; bacteria appear pinkish-red (Gram negative) or purple (Gram positive).

GRAS: generally recognized as safe; substance can be used without obtaining FDA approval.

Growth promotion: giving food animals, like chickens and pigs, low doses of antibiotics to make them gain weight faster.

HAI: health care–associated infection; includes hospital-acquired infections; sometimes called nosocomial infections.

Hand hygiene: cleaning hands; includes handwashing with soap and water and use of hand sanitizers.

Horizontal gene transfer: bacteria acquire foreign DNA (via transformation, transduction, conjugation); can confer resistance to antibiotics.

Integrons: assembly platforms in bacteria; gene acquisition systems found in bacteria.

Invasive bacteria: bacteria that can invade and damage body tissues or organs.

Isolate/bacterial isolate: growth of bacteria in the laboratory after incubating a clinical or other specimen; can be studied for resistance to antibiotics and other characteristics.

Isoniazid (INH): one of the key drugs used to treat tuberculosis and prevent reactivation of latent tuberculosis.

Klebsiella pneumoniae: Gram-negative bacterium that is common cause of severe infections; some are multidrug resistant.

Macrolides: class of antibiotic; includes erythromycin and azithromycin.

MDR-TB: *Mycobacterium tuberculosis* bacteria resistant to INH (isoniazid) and rifampin, two of the first-line drugs for the treatment of tuberculosis.

Metagenomics: study of genetic material recovered directly from samples; can study communities of organisms; analysis of microbial DNA from environmental samples.

Metallo-beta-lactamases: type of enzyme produced by bacteria; can break the beta-lactam ring of most antibiotics.

Methicillin: type of penicillin developed to work against penicillin-resistant *Staphylococcus aureus*; most staphylococci are now resistant to it.

Microbes (microorganisms): organisms too small to be seen with naked eye; need microscope to see them; includes bacteria, archaea, viruses, fungi, and some parasites; may be harmful (pathogenic), neutral, or beneficial.

Microbiome: collection of all genomes of microorganisms in a shared environment.

Microbiota: collection of all microorganisms in a defined environment or that inhabit a particular ecosystem, such as the gut, throat, or skin.

Mobile genetic elements: genetic material that can move within the genome or can be transferred from one species to another; examples include plasmids and transposons.

Monoclonal antibodies: proteins made in the laboratory that bind to a specific target (antigen) in body; made by identical immune cells.

Mortality: Deaths.

Multidrug resistant (MDR): bacteria that are resistant to multiple antibiotics that usually are effective against that bacterial species.

Mycobacterium tuberculosis: bacteria that cause tuberculosis (TB).

Mycobiome: collection of all fungi in a defined environment.

Narrow-spectrum antibiotic: antibiotic active against a limited number of bacteria.

Natural resistance: bacteria that resist the action of antibiotics even though they have never been exposed to them.

One Health: transdisciplinary approach among human, animal, plant, and environmental health disciplines; health of people, animals, plants, and their shared environment are interconnected.

Pan-drug resistant: resistant to all drugs.

Pathogen: Microbe or other organism capable of causing disease.

Penicillinase: enzyme produced by some bacteria; breaks the beta-lactam ring of penicillin, making it inactive.

Penicillins: Class of beta-lactam antibiotics including ampicillin, amoxicillin, methicillin, piperacillin, ticarcillin, and others.

Phage (bacteriophage): viruses that infect bacteria or archaea.

Plasmids: circular strand of DNA in the bacterial cell, outside of the chromosome; can carry antibiotic resistance genes.

Pneumococcal or pneumococcus: *Streptococcus pneumoniae.* Common cause of pneumonia, ear, sinus, and other respiratory infections.

Pneumonia: infection of the lungs.

Polymerase chain reaction (PCR): method used to make many copies of a specific region of DNA from a sample in the laboratory; it can then be tested; used frequently to diagnose infections; does not distinguish between live and dead microbes; can identify microbes when present in small numbers.

Polymyxins: old drugs; use in past was limited because of toxicity; now used as last-resort antibiotics to treat some multidrug-resistant infections.

Prebiotics: nutritional substrate (nutrients or substances) that can promote growth of microbes that are beneficial to health.

Probiotics: live microbes that confer health benefits.

Procalcitonin: peptide precursor to the hormone calcitonin; blood levels increase in bacterial infections but not usually in viral infections.

Prokaryotes: bacteria and archaea; unicellular microbes; lack nucleus.

Prophylaxis: prevention; chemoprophylaxis; common reason for use of antibiotics in humans and animals.

Proteins: molecules made up of one or more long chains of amino acids; perform many functions within the body (and in biological systems).

Pseudomonas aeruginosa: Gram-negative bacteria, typically resistant to multiple drugs; causes serious infections, especially in immunocompromised individuals.

Quinolones (fluoroquinolones): class of synthetic antibiotics; includes ciprofloxacin.

Quorum sensing: capacity of bacteria to sense the size of the bacterial population and communicate about it with other bacteria through chemical signals.

Resistance: describes the capacity of bacteria to resist the effect of an antibiotic or other substances; can be natural or acquired and pertain to a few or multiple antibiotics.

Resistome: collection of all antimicrobial resistance genomes derived from microbes in a defined environment.

Ribosome: particles found in cells involved in protein building (synthesis).

Rifampin: one of the first-line drugs for treating tuberculosis.

Sepsis (septicemia): the body's response to severe infection; can damage tissues and lead to organ failure and death; can progress to septic shock.

Staph: short term commonly referring to *Staphylococcus aureus* (or occasionally other staphylococci, like *Staphylococcus epidermidis*, commonly found on skin.

Strains, serotypes, group, serogroup, lineages, ribotype: terms commonly used to identify specific strains or types within a species of bacteria (or other microbes).

Strep: Commonly used to refer to *Streptococcus* sp., sometimes a specific strep, Group A *Streptococcus*, the cause of strep throat infections, rheumatic fever, and other serious infections. Many other types of streptococci cause infections in humans.

Superbugs: casual term used to describe bacteria (or other microbes) that resist treatment, cause severe disease, spread rapidly, or have some combination of these characteristics.

Susceptible (or sensitive) bacteria: ones that can be killed or inhibited by specific antibiotics.

Synbiotics: combination of prebiotics and probiotics.

Systemic antibiotic: antibiotic that enters the bloodstream and can reach many tissues throughout the body.

Tetracyclines: class of antibiotics that includes tetracycline, doxycycline, and minocycline.

Transposons (transposable elements): DNA sequences or segments that can change position within the genome; can replicate.

Triclosan: chemical active against many microbes added to many products including toothpaste, cosmetics, and cleaning supplies.

Trimethoprim-sulfamethoxazole (TMP-SMX): antibiotic that combines two different agents.

Vaccine: substance that causes the body to produce immunity to it; immunity may be partial or complete.

Virome: collection of all viruses in a defined environment.

Virulent: capacity to cause severe disease or damage tissues; bacteria use many virulence factors, including production of toxins.

VRE: vancomycin-resistant *Enterococcus*.

XDR: extensively drug resistant. Refers to bacteria that are resistant to all or almost all of the drugs commonly used to treat them.

XDR-TB: TB isolates that are resistant to INH and rifampin, the fluoroquinolones (such as levofloxacin or moxifloxacin), and at least one of the three injectable second-line drugs (amikacin, capreomycin, or kanamycin).

BIBLIOGRAPHY

Books and reports

AMR Industry Alliance. Tracking progress to address AMR. 2018. https://www.amrindustryalliance.org/.

Blaser M. Missing microbes: how the overuse of antibiotics is fueling our modern plagues. Henry Holt & Co., 2014.

British Society for Antimicrobial Chemotherapy. Antimicrobial stewardship: from principles to practice. 2018. Available as ebook. In collaboration with ESGAP (ESCMID—European Society of Clinical Microbiology and Infectious Diseases, Study Group for Antimicrobial Stewardship) and ESCMID (Managing Infections Promoting Science).

Bud R. Penicillin: triumph and tragedy. Oxford University Press, 2007. ISBN 0-19-925406-0.

CDC. National Antimicrobial Resistance Monitoring System (NARMS). Centers for Disease Control and Prevention, 2018.

CDC. Outpatient Antibiotic Prescriptions – United States, 2015. Centers for Disease Control and Prevention.

CDC. Patient information sheets. http://www.cdc.gov/getsmart/community/materials-references/print-materials/hcp/index.html.

Center for Disease Dynamics, Economics & Policy (CDDEP). 2015. State of the world's antibiotics, 2015. Washington, DC: CDDEP. http://www.cddep.org/ publications/state_worlds_antibiotics_2015#sthash.XhiMCKG6.dpbs (accessed July14, 2016).

Douglas AE. Fundamentals of microbiome science: how microbes shape animal biology. Princeton University Press, 2018.

Dubos RJ. Mirage of health. George Allen & Unwin, 1959.

Hall W, McDonnell A, O'Neill J. Superbugs. An arms race against bacteria. Harvard University Press, 2018.

House of Commons Health and Social Care Committee. Antimicrobial resistance. Eleventh report of a session 2017–2019. Report, together with formal minutes relating to the report. Ordered by the House of Commons to be printed October 18, 2018. Published October 22, 2018.

How top restaurants rate on use of antibiotics in their meat. September 2017. Chain Reaction III.

Initiatives for addressing antimicrobial resistance in the environment: Current situation and challenges. 2018. https://wellcome.ac.uk/sites/default/files/antimicrobial-resistance-environment-report.pdf

Institute of Medicine. Antibiotic resistance: implications for global health and novel intervention strategies: Workshop summary. Washington, DC: National Academies Press, 2010.

Kahn LH. One health and the politics of antimicrobial resistance. Baltimore: Johns Hopkins University Press, 2016.

Levy SB. The antibiotic paradox. How the misuse of antibiotics destroys their curative powers. 2nd edition. Perseus Books, 2002.

McKenna M. Big chicken: the incredible story of how antibiotics created modern agriculture and changed the way the world eats. National Geographic, 2017.

National Academies of Sciences, Engineering, and Medicine. Combating antimicrobial resistance: a One Health approach to a global threat: proceedings of a workshop. Washington, DC: National Academies Press, 2017. https://doi.org/10.1722/24914

National Academies of Sciences, Engineering, and Medicine. Understanding the economics of microbial threats: proceedings of a workshop. Washington, DC: National Academies Press, 2018. https://doi.org/10.17226/25224

O'Neill J. Tackling drug-resistant infections globally: final report and recommendations. The review on antimicrobial resistance. May 2016 (Independent review on antimicrobial resistance, UK). https://amr-review.org/sites/default/files/160518_Final%20paper_with%20cover.pdf

Pew Charitable Trusts. A scientific roadmap for antibiotic discovery. A sustained and robust pipeline of new antibacterial drugs and therapies is critical to preserve public health. Available online.

Pikkemaat MG, Yassin H, van der Fels-Klerx, et al. Antibiotic residues and resistance in the environment. 2016. Wageniingen, RIKILT Wageningen UR (University & Research Centre).

Pew Commission. Putting meat on the table: industrial farm animal production in America. A Report of the Pew Commission on Industrial Farm Animal Production. 2008.

Quammen D. The tangled tree. A radical new history of life. Simon and Schuster, 2018.

OIE. Annual report on antimicrobial agents intended for use in animals: better understanding of the global situation. Second report. Paris. World Organization for Animal Health: 2017.

Re-vitalizing the antibiotic pipeline. DRIVE-AB (driving re-investment in R & D and responsible antibiotic use). http://drive-ab-eu/. www.imi.europa.eu/projects-results/project-factsheets/drive-ab.

Rosen W. Miracle cure: the creation of antibiotics and the birth of modern medicine. Viking, 2017.

United Nations. Political Declaration of the High-level Meeting on Antimicrobial Resistance (Resolution A/Res/71/3). New York: United Nations; 2016.

Walsh C, Wencewicz T. Antibiotics. Challenges, mechanisms, opportunities. ASM Press, 2016.

World Bank. Drug-resistant infections: a threat to our economic future. Washington, DC: World Bank, 2017. License: creative commons Attribution CC BY 3.0 IGO.

World Health Organization (WHO). Antibiotic agents in clinical development: an analysis of the antibiotic clinical development pipeline, including tuberculosis. Geneva: World Health Organization; 2017.

World Health Organization (WHO). Antimicrobial resistance (WHO fact sheet). Geneva: World Health Organization; February 2018.

World Health Organization (WHO). Global antimicrobial resistance surveillance system (GLASS) report: early implementation 2106–2017. Geneva: World Health Organization; 2017.

World Health Organization (WHO). Global tuberculosis report 2018. Geneva: World Health Organization; 2018.

World Health Organization (WHO). WHO model list of essential medicines. 20th list (March 2017). Geneva: World Health Organization; 2017.

World Health Organization (WHO). Prioritization of pathogens to guide discovery, research and development of new antibiotics for drug-resistant bacterial infections including tuberculosis. Geneva: World Health Organization, 2017.

World Health Organization (WHO). WHO Regional office for Europe. Antimicrobial medicines consumption (AMC) network. AMC data 2011–2014. Copenhagen; World Health Organization Regional Office for Europe; 2017.

World Health Organization (WHO). World report on surveillance of antibiotic consumption 2016–2018. Early independent. Geneva: World Health Organization; 2018.

World Health Organization (WHO). Top 10 causes of death, 2015. Global Health Observatory data repository. Geneva: World Health Organization; 2018

World Health Organization (WHO), FAO, OIE. Global framework for development & stewardship to combat antimicrobial resistance. Daft roadmap. WHO, Food and Agriculture Organization of the United Nations and World Organization for Animal Health; 2017.

Yong E. I contain multitudes: the microbes within us and a grander view of life. Ecco/HarperCollins, 2016.

Chapter 1

Abraham EP, Chain E, Fletcher CM, et al. Further observations on penicillin. Lancet 1941;Aug 16:177–88.

Auta A, Hadi A, Oga E. Global access to antibiotics without prescription in community pharmacies: a systematic review and meta-analysis. J Infect 2018. https://doi.org/10.1016/j.jinf.2018.07.001

Chain E, Florey HW, Gardner AD, et al. Penicillin as a chemotherapeutic agent. Lancet 1940;Aug 24:226–28.

Chikowe I, Bliese SL, Lucas S, et al. Amoxicillin quality and selling practices in urban pharmacies and drug stores of Blantyre, Malawi. Am J Trop Med Hyg 2018;99:233–38.

FDA drug safety communication: FDA updates warnings for oral and injectable fluoroquinolone antibiotics due to disabling side effects. May 16, 2016. https://www.fda.gov/Drugs/DrugSafety/ucm511530.htm

Fleming A. On the antibacterial action of cultures of penicillium, with special reference to their use in the isolation of B. influenza. Br J Exper Pathol 1929;10:226–36.

Fleming A. Aseptics in war-time surgery. Pharm J (London) 1940;145:172.

Fleming A. An address to the Alumni Association. Harvard Alumni
    Bulletin 1945;47:580–81.
Gaynes R. The discovery of penicillin—new insights after more than
    75 years of clinical use. Emerg Infect Dis 2017;23(5):849–53.
National Academies of Science, Engineering, and Medicine (NASEM).
    Committee on Understanding the Global Public Health
    Implications of Substandard, Falsified and Counterfeit Medical
    Products. Buckley GJ, Gostin LO, eds. Countering the problems of
    falsified and substandard drugs. Institute of Medicine. Washington,
    DC: National Academies Press, 2013.
Ozawa S, et al. Prevalence and estimated economic burden of
    substandard and falsified medicines in low- and middle-income
    countries. A systematic review and meta-analysis. JAMA Network
    Open 2018;1(4):e181662.
Waksman SA, Woodruff HB. The soil as a source of microorganisms
    antagonistic to disease-producing bacteria. J Bacteriol
    1940;40:581–600.
World Health Organization (WHO). Substandard and falsified (SF)
    medical products. 2017. http://www.who.int/medicines/
    regulation/ssffc/en/ (accessed June 22, 2017).

Chapter 2
Auta A, Hadi A, Oga E. Global access to antibiotics without
    prescription in community pharmacies: a systematic review
    and meta-analysis. J Infect 2018. https://doi.org/10.1016/
    j.jinf.2018.07.001
Baggs J, Fridkin SK, Pollack LA, et al. Estimating national trends in
    inpatient antibiotic use among US hospitals from 2006 to 2012.
    JAMA Intern Med 2016;176:1639–48.
Bcheraoui EC, Mokdad AH, Dwyer-Lindgren L, et al. Trends and
    patterns of differences in infectious diseases mortality among US
    counties, 1980–2014. JAMA 2018;319(12):1248–60.
Berrios-Torres SI, Umscheid CA, Bratzler DW, et al. Centers for Disease
    Control and Prevention guideline for the prevention of surgical site
    infection, 2017. JAMA 2017;152(8):784–91.
Chow AW, Benninger MS, Brook I, et al. Infectious Diseases
    Society of America. IDSA clinical practice guideline for acute
    bacterial rhinosinusitis in children and adults. Clin Infect Dis
    2012;54(8):e72-e112.
Diven DG, Barenetein DW, Carroll DR. Extending shelf life just makes
    sense. Mayo Clin Proc 2015;90(11):1471–74.

Doan T, Hinterwirth A, Arzika AM, et al. Mass azithromycin
distribution and community microbiome: a cluster-randomized
trial. Open Forum Infect Dis 2018. doi:10.1093/ofid/ofy182

Durkin MJ, Jafarzadah SR, Hsueh K, et al. Outpatient antibiotic
prescription trends in the United States: a national cohort study.
Infect Control Hosp Epidemiol 2018;39:584–89.

Fleming-Dutra KE, Hersh AL, Shairo DJ, et al. Prevalence of
inappropriate antibiotic prescriptions among US ambulatory care
visits, 2010–2011. JAMA 2016;315(17):1864–73.

Hicks LA, Bartoces MG, Roberts RM, et al. US outpatient prescribing
variation according to geography, patient population, and provider
specialty in 2011. Clin Infect Dis 2015;60(9):1308–16.

Hoberman A, Paradise JL, Rockette HE, et al. Shortened antimicrobial
treatment for acute otitis media in young children. N Engl J Med
2016;375:2446–56.

Keenan JD, Bailey RL, West SK, et al. Azithromycin to reduce
childhood mortality in sub-Saharan Africa. N Engl J Med
2018;378(17):1583–92.

Keenan JD, Chin SA, Amza A, et al. The effect of antibiotic selection
pressure on the nasopharyngeal macrolide resistome: a cluster-
randomized trial. Clin Infect Dis 2018;67(11):1736–42.

Klein EY, Van Boeckel TP, Martinez EM, et al. Global increase and
geographic convergence in antibiotic consumption between 2000
and 2015. Proc Natl Acad Sci USA 2018;15:E3463–E3470.

LaPara TM, Burch TR, McNamara PJ, et al. Tertiary-treated municipal
wastewater is a significant point source of antibiotic resistance genes
into Duluth-Superior Harbor. Environ Sci & Tech 2011;45(22):9543–49.

Laxminarayan R, Matsoso P, Pant S, et al. Access to effective
antimicrobials: a worldwide challenge. Lancet 2016;387:168–75.

Leach AJ, Shelby-James TM, Mayo M, et al. A prospective study of the
impact of community-based azithromycin treatment of trachoma
on carriage and resistance of Streptococcus pneumoniae. Clin Infect
Dis 1997;24:356–62.

Lyon RC, Taylor JS, Porter DA, et al. Stability profiles of drug
products extended beyond labeled expiration dates. J Pharm Sci
2006;95(7):1549–60.

Martinez KA, Rood M, Jhangiani, et al. Association between
antibiotic prescribing for respiratory tract infections and patient
satisfaction in direct-to-consumer telemedicine. JAMA Intern Med
2018;178:1558–60.

Mendelson M, Rottingen JA, Goinathan U, et al. Antimicrobials: access and sustainable effectiveness 3. Maximising access to achieve appropriate human antimicrobial use in low-income and middle-income countries. Lancet 2016;387:188–98.

Mitja O, Godornes C, Houinei W, et al. Re-emergence of yaws after single mass azithromycin treatment followed by targeted treatment: a longitudinal study. Lancet 2018;391:1599–1607.

Mosites E, Frick A, Gounder P, et al. Outbreak of invasive infections from subtype emm26.3 Group A Streptococcus among homeless adults—Anchorage, Alaska, 2017–2017. Clin Infect Dis 2018;66(7):1068–74.

Palms DL, Hicks LA, Bortoces M, et al. Comparison of antibiotic prescribing in retail clinics, urgent care centers, emergency departments, and traditional ambulatory care settings in the United States. JAMA Intern Med 2018;178(9):1267–69.

Peal A, Evans B, Blackett I, et al. A review of fecal sludge management in 12 cities. World Bank – Water and Sanitation Program. 2015.

Skalet AH, Cevallos V, Ayele B, et al. Antibiotic selection pressure and macrolide resistance in nasopharyngeal Streptococcus pneumoniae: a cluster-randomized clinical trial. PLoS Med 2010;7(12):e1000377.

Steffen R, Jiang Z-D, Garcia MLG, et al. Rifamycin SF-MMX for treatment of travellers' diarrhea: equally effective as ciprofloxacin and not associated with the acquisition of multi-drug-resistant bacteria. J Travel Med 2018; doi:10.1093/jtm/tay116.

Suda KJ, Hicks LA, Roberts RM, et al. Antibiotic expenditures by medication, class, and healthcare setting in the United States, 2010–2015. Clin Infect Dis 2018;66:185–90.

Tita ATN, Szychewski JM, Boggess K, et al. Adjunctive azithromycin prophylaxis for cesarean delivery. N Engl J Med 2016;375:1231–34.

US Burden of Disease Collaborators. The state of US health, 1990–2016. Burden of diseases, injuries, and risk factors among US states. JAMA 2018;319(14):1444–72.

Wiese AD, Griffin MR, Schaffner W, et al. Opioid analgesic use and risk for invasive pneumococcal diseases. Ann Intern Med 2018;169(5):355.

Zhu Y-G, Zhao Y, Li B, et al. Continental-scale pollution of estuaries with antibiotic resistance genes. Nature Microbiol 2017;Jan 30. doi: 10.1038/microbiol.2016.270

Chapter 3

Andremont A. Too early to recommend early fecal microbiota transplantation in patients with severe Clostridium difficile, or not too early? Clin Infect Dis 2018;66:651–52.

Bartlett JG. Bezlotoxumab—a new agent for Clostridium difficile infection. N Engl J Med 2017;376:381–82.

Bartlett JG, Chang T-W, Gurwith M, et al. Antibiotic-associated pseudomembranous colitis due to toxin-producing clostridia. N Engl J Med 1978;298:531–34.

Bilinski J, Grzesiowski P, Sorensen N, et al. Fecal microbiota transplantation in patients with blood disorders inhibits gut colonization with antibiotic-resistant bacteria: results of a prospective single-center study. Clin Infect Dis 2017;65(3):364–70.

Blaser MJ. Missing microbes: how the overuse of antibiotics is fueling our modern plagues. Henry Holt & Co., 2014.

Blaser MJ, Falkow S. What are the consequences of the disappearing human microbiota? Nat Rev Microbiol 2009;7:887–94.

Blumenthal KG, Ryan EE, Li Y, et al. The impact of reported penicillin allergy on surgical site infection risk. Clin Infect Dis 2018;66:329–36.

Brown KA, Jones M, Daneman N, et al. Importation, antibiotics, and Clostridium difficile infection in veteran long-term care. Ann Intern Med 2016;164:787–94.

Clemente JC, et al. The microbiome of uncontacted Amerindians. Sci Adv 2015;1. Pii:e1500183.

Collins J, Robinson C, Hanhof H, et al. Dietary trehalose enhances virulence of epidemic Clostridium difficile. Nature 2018;553:292–94.

de Gunzburg J, Ghozlane A, Ducher A, et al. Protection of the human gut microbiome from antibiotics. J Infect Dis 2018;217:628–36.

Dethlefsen L, Huse S, Sogin ML, et al. The pervasive effects of an antibiotic on the human gut microbiota, as revealed by deep 16S rRNA sequencing. PLoS Biol 2008;6(11):e280.

Doan T, Arzika AM, Ray KJ, et al. Gut microbial diversity in antibiotic-naïve children after systemic antibiotic exposure: a randomized controlled trial. Clin Infect Dis 2017;64:1147–53.

Dominguez-Bello MG, Knight R, Gilbert JA, Blaser MJ. Preserving microbial diversity. Science 2018;362:33–34.

Dubberke ER, Mullane KM, Gerding DN, et al. Clearance of vancomycin-resistant enterococcus concomitant with administration of a microbiota-based drug targeted at recurrent

Clostridium difficile infection. Open Forum Infect Dis
2016:3(3):ofw133.

Eyre DW, Fawley WN, Rajgopal A, et al. Comparison of control of
Clostridium difficile infection in six English hospitals using whole-
genome sequencing. Clin Infect Dis 2017;65:433–41.

Faith JJ, Guruge JL, Charbonneau M et al. The long-term stability of the
human gut microbiota. Science 2013;341:1237439.

Goldenberg JZ, et al. Probiotics for the prevention of Clostridium
difficile-associated diarrhea in adults and children. Cochrane
Database Syst Rev 2017;12:CD006095.

Hocquart M, Lagier M-D, Cassir N, et al. Early fecal microbiota
transplantation improves survival in severe Clostridium difficile
infections. Clin Infect Dis 2018;66:645–50.

Hoffmann D, Palumbo F, Ravel J, et al. Improving regulation of
microbiota transplants. Science 2017;358:1390–91.

Juul FE, Garborg K, Bretthauer M, et al. Fecal microbiota
transplantation for primary Clostridium difficile infection. N Engl J
Med 2018;378:2535–36.

Kao D, Roach B, Silva M, et al. Effect of oral capsule vs colonoscopy-
delivered fecal microbiota transplantation on recurrent
Clostridium difficile infection: a randomized clinical trial. JAMA
2017;318(20):1985–93.

Lessa FC, Mu Y, Bamberg WM, et al. Burden of Clostridium difficile
infection in the United States. N Engl J Med 2015;372:825–34.

Lynch SV, Pedersen O. The human intestinal microbiome in health and
disease. N Engl J Med 2016;375:2369–79.

Ma GK, Brensinger CM, Wu Q, et al. Increasing incidence of multiply
recurrent Clostridium difficile infection in the United States. Ann
Intern Med 2017;167:152–58.

Magill SS, O'Leary SJ, Janelle DL, et al. Changes in prevalence of
health care-associated infections in U.S. hospitals. N Engl J Med
2018;379:1732–44.

Maier L, et al. Extensive impact of non-antibiotic drugs on human gut
bacteria. Nature 2018;555:623–28. doi:10.1038/nature25979

Moeller AH, Suzuki TA, Pifer-Rixey M, et al. Transmission modes of the
mammalian gut microbiota. Science 2018;262:453–57.

Motta EVS, Raymann K, Moran NA. Glyphosate perturbs the
gut microbiota of honey bees. Proc Natl Acad Sci USA
2018;115:10305–10.

Pasternak B, Inghammar M, Svanstrom H. Fluoroquinolone use and risk of aortic aneurysm and dissection: nationwide cohort study. BMJ 2018;360:678.

Prabhu VS, Dubberke ER, Dorr MB, et al. Cost-effectiveness of bezlotoxumab compared with placebo for the prevention of recurrent Clostridium difficile infection. Clin Infect Dis 2018;66(3):355–62.

Raguideau R, Lamaitre M Day-Spira R, et al. Association between fluoroquinolone use and retinal detachment. JAMA Ophthalmol 2016;134:415–21.

Rothschild D, Weissbrod, Barkan E, et al. Environment dominates over host genetics in shaping human gut microbiota. Nature 2018;555:210–15.

Smits SA, Leach J, Sonnenburg ED, et al. Seasonal cycling in the gut microbiome of the Hadza hunter-gatherers of Tanzania. Science 2017;357:802–6.

Tamma PD, Avdic E, Li DX, et al. Association of adverse events with antibiotic use in hospitalized patients. JAMA Intern Med 2017;177:1308–15.

Tariq R, Pardi DS, Tosh PK, et al. Fecal microbiota transplantation for recurrent Clostridium difficile infection reduces recurrent urinary tract infection frequency. Clin Infect Dis 2017;65(10):1745–47.

Vangay P, Johnson AJ, Ward TL, et al. US immigration westernizes the human gut microbiome. Cell 2018;175:962–72.

Winkel P, Hilden J, Hansen JF, et al. Clarithromycin for stable coronary heart disease increases all-cause and cardiovascular mortality and cerebrovascular morbidity over 10 years in the CLARICOR randomized, blinded clinical trial. Int J Cardiol 2015;182:459–65.

Zeidler S, Hubloher J, Schabacker K, et al. Trehalose, a temperature- and salt-induced solute with implications in pathobiology of Acinetobacter baumannii. Environ Microbiol 2017;19(12):5088–99.

Zhang D, Prabhu VS, Marcella SW. Attributable healthcare resource utilization and costs for patients with primary and recurrent Clostridium difficile infection in the United States. Clin Infect Dis 2018;66:1326–32.

Zitvogel L, Ma Y, Raoult D, et al. The microbiome in cancer immunotherapy: diagnostic tools and therapeutic strategies. Science 2018;359:1366–70.

Chapter 4

Bar-On YM, Phillips R, Milo R. The biomass distribution on Earth. Proc Natl Acad Sci USA 2018;115(25):6506–11.

Berendes DM, Yang PJ, Lai A, et al. Estimation of global recoverable human and animal faecal biomass. Nature Sustainability 2018:1:679–85.

Cabello FC, Godfrey HP, Buschmann AH, et al. Aquaculture as yet another environmental gateway to development and globalisation of antimicrobial resistance. Lancet Infect Dis 2016;16(7):e127–e133.

Collignon PC, Conly JM, Andremont A, et al. World Health Organization ranking of antimicrobials according to their importance in human medicine: a critical step for developing risk management strategies to control antimicrobial resistance from food animal production. Clin Infect Dis 2016;63:1087–93.

Federal Register. Environmental Protection Agency. Aureobasidium pullulans strains DSM 14940 and DSM 14941: exemption from the requirement of a tolerance. 2015;80(227):73661–62.

Food and Agriculture Organization of the United Nations (FAO). The state of the world fisheries and aquaculture (FAO). 2016.

Graham DW, Knapp CW, Christensen BT, et al. Appearance of β-lactamase resistance genes in agricultural soils and clinical isolates over the 20th century. Sci Rep 2016;6:21550.

Islam MA, Hasan R, Hossain MI, et al. Environmental spread of New Delhi metallo-β-lactamase-1-producing bacteria in Dhaka, Bangladesh. Appl Environ Microbiol 2017;83:e00793–17.

Jukes TH, Stokstad ELR, Taylor RR, et al. Growth promoting effect of aureomycin on pigs. Arch Biochem 1950;26(2):324–25.

Klein EY, Van Boeckel TP, Marinez EM, et al. Global increase and geographic convergence in antibiotic consumption between 2000 and 2015. Proc Natl Acad Sci USA 2018;15:E3463–70.

Kosgey A, Shitandi A, Marion JW. Antibiotic residues in milk from three popular Kenyan milk vending machines. Am J Trop Med Hyg 2018;98:1520–22.

Lubbert C, Baars C, Lippmann N, et al. Environmental pollution with antimicrobial agents from bulk drug manufacturing industries in Hyderabad, South India, is associated with dissemination of extended-spectrum beta lactamase and carbapenemase producing pathogens. Infection 2017;45:479–91.

Marshall BM, Levy SB. Food animals and antimicrobials: impacts on human health. Clin Microbiol Rev 2011;24(4):718–33.

McGhee GC, Sundin GW. Evaluation of kasugamycin for fire blight
    management, effect on nontarget bacteria, and assessment
    of kasugamycin resistance potential in Erwinia amylovora.
    Phytopathology 2011;101(2):192–204.

McKenna M. Big chicken: the incredible story of how antibiotics created
    modern agriculture and changed the way the world eats. National
    Geographic; 2017.

Nguyen Dang Giang C, Sebesvari Z, Renaud F, et al. Occurrence and
    dissipation of the antibiotics sulfamethoxazole, sulfadiazine,
    trimethoprim, and enrofloxacin in the Mekong Delta, Vietnam.
    PLoS One 2015;10(7);e0131855.

Nigra AE, Nachman KE, Love DC, et al. Poultry consumption and
    arsenic exposure in the U.S. population. Environ Health Perspect
    2017;125(3):370–77.

Osterholm M. Preparing for the next pandemic. N Engl J Med
    2005;352(18):1839–42.

Speedy AW. Global production and consumption of animal source
    foods. J Nutr 2003;133:4048S–53S.

Stockwell VO, Duffy B. Use of antibiotics in plant agriculture. Rev Sci
    Tech 2012;31(1):199–210.

Teillant A, Laxminarayan R. Economics of antibiotic use in U.S. swine
    and poultry production. Choices, Publication of the Agricultural &
    Applied Economics Association 2015;30(1).

Van Boeckel TP, Brower C, Gilbert M, et al. Global trends in
    antimicrobial use in food animals. Proc Natl Acad Sci
    2015;112:5649–54.

Van Boeckel TP, Glennon EE, Chen D, et al. Reducing antimicrobial use
    in food animals. Science 2017;357:1350–52.

Zhang T, Li B. Occurrence, transformation, and fate of antibiotics in
    municipal wastewater treatment plants. Crit Rev Environ Sci Techol
    2011;41(11)951–98.

Zhang M, Powell CA, Zhou L, et al. Chemical compounds effective
    against the citrus Huanglongbing bacterium "Candidatus
    Liberibacter asiaticus" in plants. Phytopathology 2011;101:1097–103.

Chapter 5

Arcilla MS, van Hattem JM, Haverkate MR, et al. Import and spread of
    extended-spectrum β-lactamase-producing Enterobacteriaceae by
    international travelers (COMBAT study): a prospective, multicenter
    cohort study. Lancet Infect Dis 2017;17:78–85.

Bar-On YM, Phillips R, Milo R. The biomass distribution on Earth. Proc Natl Acad Sci USA 2018;115(25):6506–11.

Chen L, Todd R, Kiehlbauch J, et al. Pan-resistant New Delhi metallo-beta-lactamase-producing Klebsiella pneumonia—Washoe County, Nevada, 2016. MMWR Morb Mortal Wkly Rep 2017;66:33.

Chen LH, Wilson ME. The globalization of healthcare: implications of medical tourism for the infectious disease clinician. Clin Infect Dis 2013;57:1752–59.

Collaborative Group for the Meta-Analysis of Individual Patient Data in MDR-TB treatment 2017. Lancet 2018;392:821–34.

Fifer H, Cole M, Hughes G, et al. Sustained transmission of high-level azithromycin-resistant Neisseria gonorrhoeae in England: an observational study. Lancet Infect Dis 2018;18(5):573–81.

Gillespie SH. Evolution of drug resistance in Mycobacterium tuberculosis: clinical and molecular perspective. Antimicrobiol Agents Chemother 2002;46(2):267–74.

Holt M, Lea T, Mao L, et al. Community-level changes in condom use and uptake of HIV pre-exposure prophylaxis by gay and bisexual men in Melbourne and Sydney, Australia: results of repeated behavioural surveillance in 2013–2017. Lancet HIV 2018;5:e448–56.

Houk VN. Spread of tuberculosis via recirculated air in a naval vessel. Ann N Y Acad Sci 1980;353:10–24.

Houk V, Kent D, Baker J, et al. The epidemiology of tuberculosis transmission in a closed environment. Arch Environ Health 1968;16:26–35.

Kantele A, Laaveri T, Mero S, et al. Antimicrobials increase travelers risk of colonization by extended-spectrum betalactamase-producing Enterobacteriaceae. Clin Infect Dis 2015;60:837–46.

Kantele A, Mero S, Kirveskari J, et al. Increased risk for ESBL-producing bacteria from co-administration of loperamide and antimicrobial drugs for travelers' diarrhea. Emerg Infect Dis 2016;22(1):117–20.

Kumarasamy KK, Tolman MA, Walsh TR, et al. Emergence of a new antibiotic resistance mechanism in India, Pakistan, and the UK: a molecular, biological, and epidemiological study. Lancet Infect Dis 2010;10:597–602.

Leder K, Torresi J, Libman MD, et al. for the GeoSentinel Surveillance Network. GeoSentinel surveillance of illness in returned travelers, 2007–2011. Ann Intern Med 2013;158(6):456–68.

Luo Y, Yang F, Mathieu J, et al. Proliferation and multidrug-resistant New Delhi metallo-β-lactamase genes in municipal wastewater treatment plants in northern China. Environ Sci Technol Lett 2014;1(1):26–30.

MacFadden DR, McGough SF, Fisman D, et al. Antibiotic resistance increases with local temperature. Nature Climate Change 2018;8:510–14.

Mantilla-Calderon D, Jumat MR, Wang T, et al. Isolation and characterization of NDM-positive Escherichia coli from municipal wastewater in Jeddah, Saudi Arabia. Antimicrob Agents Chemother 2016;60(9):5223–31.

Montgomery MP, Robertson S, Koski L, et al. Multidrug-resistant Campylobacter jejuni outbreak linked to puppy exposure—United States, 2016–2018. MMWR Morb Mortal Wkly Rep 2018;67(37):1032–35.

Pawlowski AC, Wang W, Koteva K, et al. A diverse intrinsic antibiotic resistome from a cave bacterium. Nature Commun 2016;7:13803.

Petersen TN, Rasmussen S, Hasman H, et al. Meta-genomic analysis of toilet waste from long distance flights: a step towards global surveillance of infectious diseases and antimicrobial resistance. Sci Rep 2015;5:11444. doi:10.1038/strp11444

Pieterman ED, te Brake LHM, de Knegt GJ, et al. Assessment of the additional value of verapamil to a moxifloxacin and linezolid combination regimen in a murine tuberculosis model. Antimicrob Agents Chemother 2018;62:9.

Ray MJ, Lin MY, Weinstein RA, et al. Spread of carbapenem-resistant Enterobacteriaceae among Illinois healthcare facilities: the role of patient sharing. Clin Infect Dis 2016;63(7):889–93.

Riley R. Ariel dissemination of pulmonary tuberculosis—the Burns Amberson Lecture. Am Rev Tuber Pulmon Dis 1957;76:931–41.

Stewart RJ, Tsang CA, Pratt RH, et al. Tuberculosis—United States, 2017. MMWR Morb Mortal Wkly Rep 2018;67(11):319–23.

Taylor SN, Marrazzo J, Batteiger BE, et al. Single-dose zoliflodacin (ETX0914) for treatment of urogenital gonorrhea. N Engl J Med 2018;379:1835–45.

Toth DJA, Khader K, Slayton RB, et al. The potential for interventions in a long-term acute care hospital to reduce transmission of carbapenem-resistant Enterobacteriaceae in affiliated healthcare facilities. Clin Infect Dis 2017;65(4):581–87.

Unemo M, Shafer WM. Antimicrobial resistance in Neisseria gonorrhoeae in the 21st century: past, evolution, future. Clin Microbiol Rev 2014;27(3):587–613.

Walsh TR, Weeks J, Livermore DM, et al. Dissemination of NDM-1-
    positive bacteria in the New Delhi environment and its implications
    for human health: an environmental point prevalence study. Lancet
    Infect Dis 2011;11:355–62.
Wilson ME. Travel and the emergence of infectious diseases. Emerg
    Infect Dis 1995;1:39–46.
Wilson ME. The traveler and emerging infections: sentinel, courier,
    transmitter. J Appl Microbiol 2003;94:1S-11S.
World Health Organization. Global TB report. Geneva: World Health
    Organization, 2017.
Zhu Y-G, Zhao Y, Li B, et al. Continental-scale pollution of estuaries
    with antibiotic resistance genes. Nature Microbiol 2017;
    doi: 10.1038/nmicrobiol.2016.270.

Chapter 6

Alexander S, Fisher BT, Gaur AH, et al. Effect of levofloxacin
    prophylaxis on bacteremia in children with acute leukemia or
    undergoing hematopoietic stem cell transplantation. A randomized
    clinical trial. JAMA 2018;320(10):995–1004.
Andrews JR, Qamar FN, Charles RC, et al. Extensively drug-resistant
    typhoid—are conjugate vaccines arriving just in time? N Engl J
    Med 2018;379:1493–95.
Cassini A, Hogberg LD, Plachouras D, et al. Attributable deaths and
    disability-adjusted life-years caused by infections with antibiotic-
    resistant bacteria in the EU and the European Economic Area in
    2015: a population-level modelling analysis. Lancet Infect Dis
    2019;19:56–66.
Chatham- Stephens K, Medalla F, Hughes M, et al. Emergence of
    extensively drug-resistant *Salmonella* Typhi infections among
    travelers to or from Pakistan – United States, 2016–2018. MMWR
    Morb Mortal Wkly Report 2019;68(1):11–13. doi: http://dx.doi.org/
    10.15585/mmwr.mm6801a
D'Agata EMC, Varu A, et al. Acquisition of multidrug-resistant
    organisms in the absence of antimicrobials. Clin Infect Dis
    2018;67(9):1437–40.
Dubinsky-Pertzov B, Temkin E, Harbarth S, et al. Carriage of extended-
    spectrum beta-lactamase-producing Enterobacteriaceae and the
    risk of surgical site infection after colorectal surgery: a prospective
    cohort study. Clin Infect Dis 2018. Published online September
    10, 2018. doi: 10.1093/cid/ciy768

Gandra S, Tseng KK, Arora A, et al. The mortality burden of multidrug-resistant pathogens in India: a retrospective observational study. Clin Infect Dis 2018. Published Nov 2018. https://doi.org/10.1093/cid/ciy955

Hall W, McDonnell A, O'Neill J. Superbugs. An arms race against bacteria. Harvard University Press, 2018.

Kaliberg C, Ardal C, Bliix HS, et al. Introduction and geographic availability of new antibiotics approved between 1999 and 2014. PLoS One 2018;Oct 16.

Klemm EJ, Shakoor S, Page AJ, et al. Emergence of an extensively drug-resistant Salmonella enterica serovar Typhi clone harboring a promiscuous plasmid encoding resistance to fluoroquinolones and third-generation cephalosporins. mBio 2018;9(1):e00105–18.

O'Neill J. Tackling drug-resistant infections globally: final report and recommendations. The review on antimicrobial resistance. May 2016 (Independent review on antimicrobial resistance, UK). https://amr-review.org/sites/default/files/160518_Final%20 paper_with%20cover.pdf

Tamma PD, Goodman KE, Harris AD, et al. Comparing the outcomes of patients with carbapenemase-producing and non-carbapenemase-producing carbapenem-resistant Enterobacteriaceae bacteremia. Clin Infect Dis 2017;64(3):257–64.

Teillant A, Gandra S, Barter D, et al. Potential burden of antibiotic resistance on surgery and cancer chemotherapy antibiotic chemoprophylaxis in the USA: a literature review and modelling study. Lancet Infect Dis 2015;15(12):1429–37.

Theuretzbacher U, Gottwalt S, Beyer P, et al. Analysis of the clinical and antituberculosis pipeline. Lancet Infect Dis 2019;19:e40–50.

Chapter 7

Boston Consulting Group. Vaccines to tackle drug resistant infections: an evaluation of R and D opportunities. Supported by the Wellcome Trust, 2018. http://www.Vaccinesforamr.org.

Cassini A, Hogberg LD, Plachouras D, et al. Attributable deaths and disability-adjusted life-years caused by infections with antibiotic-resistant bacteria in the EU and the European Economic Area in 2015: a population-level modelling analysis. Lancet Infect Dis 2019;19:56–66.

De Muri G, Gern JE, Eickhoff JC, et al. Dynamics of bacterial colonization with Streptococcus pneumoniae, Haemophilus influenzae, and Moraxella catarrhalis during symptomatic and asymptomatic viral upper respiratory tract infection. Clin Infect Dis 2018;66(7):1045–53.

GlobalSurg Collaborative. Surgical site infection after gastrointestinal surgery in high-income, middle-income, and low-income countries: a prospective, international, multicenter cohort study. Lancet Infect Dis 2018;18(5):516–25.

Grass G, Rensing C, Solioz M. Metallic copper as an antimicrobial surface. Appl Environ Microbiol 2011;77(5):1541–47.

Grayson ML, et al. Effects of the Australian National Hand Hygiene Initiative after 8 years on infection control practices, health worker education, and clinical outcomes: a longitudinal study. Lancet Infect Dis 2018;18:1269–77.

Hooton TM, Vecchio M, Oroz A, et al. Effect of increased daily water intake in premenopausal women with recurrent urinary tract infections. A randomized clinical trial. JAMA Intern Med 2018;178(11):1509–15.

Iuliano AD, Roguski KM, Change HH, et al. Estimates of global seasonal influenza-associated respiratory mortality: a modelling study. Lancet 2017;391:1285–1300.

Little P, et al. An internet-delivered handwashing intervention to modify influenza-like illness and respiratory infection transmission (PRMIT): a primary care randomized trial. Lancet 2015;386:1631–39.

Liu W-C, Lin C-S, Yeh C-C, et al. Effect of influenza vaccination against postoperative pneumonia and mortality for geriatric patients receiving major surgery: a nationwide matched study. J Infect Dis 2018;217:816–26.

Magill SS, Edwards JR, Bamberg W, et al. Multistate point-prevalence survey of health care-associated infections. N Engl J Med 2014;370(13):1198–208.

Magill SS, Edwards JR, Beldavs ZG, et al. Emerging Infections Program Healthcare-Associated Infections and Antimicrobial Use Survey Team. Prevalence of antimicrobial use in US acute care hospitals, May–September 2011. JAMA 2014;312(14):1438–1446.

Magill SS, O'Leary SJ, Janelle DL, et al. Changes in prevalence of health care-associated infections in U.S. hospitals. N Engl J Med 2018;379:1732–44.

Mikolay A, Huggett S, Takana L, et al. Survival of bacteria on metallic copper surfaces in a hospital trial. Appl Environ Biotechnol 2010;87:1875–79.

Mody L, Greene MT, Meddings J, et al. A national implementation project to prevent catheter-associated urinary tract infection in nursing home residents. JAMA Intern Med 2017;177(8):1154–62. doi:10.1001/jamainternmed.2017.1689

Pineda I, Hubbard R, Rodriguez F. The role of copper surfaces in reducing the incidence of healthcare-associated infections: a systematic review and meta-analysis. Can J Infect Dis 2017;32:13–24.

Pronovost P, Needham D, Berenholtz S, et al. An intervention to decrease catheter-related bloodstream infections in the ICU. N Engl J Med 2006;355:2725–32.

Sigurdsson S, Eythersson E, Hrafnkelsson B, et al. Reduction in all-cause acute otitis media in children <3 years of age in primary care following vaccination with 10-valent pneumococcal Haemophilus influenzae protein-D conjugate vaccine: a whole-population study. Clin Infect Dis 2018;67(8):1213–19.

Souli M, Antoniadou A, Kaatsarois I, et al. Reduction of environmental contamination with multidrug-resistant bacteria by copper-alloy coating of surfaces in a highly endemic setting. Infect Control Hosp Epidemiol 2017;38(7):765–71.

Sudha VBP, Singh KO, Prasad SR, et al. Killing of enteric bacteria in drinking water by a copper device for use in the home: laboratory evidence. Trans R Soc Trop Med Hyg 2009;103:819–22.

Taksler GB, Rothberg MB, Cutler DM. Association of influenza vaccination coverage in younger adults with influenza-related illness in the elderly. Clin Infect Dis 2015;61(10):1495–503.

Troeger C, Colombara DV, Rao PC, et al. Global disability-adjusted life-year estimates of long-term health burden and undernutrition attributable to diarrhoeal diseases in children younger than five years. Lancet Glob Health 2018;6:e255–69.

Turnipseed EG, Landefield CS. A triumph for the Agency for Healthcare Research and Quality Safety Program for Long-term Care. JAMA Intern Med 2017;177(6):1163–64.

van Weel C. Handwashing and community management of infections. Lancet. 2015;386:1603–4.

Wierzba TF, Muhib F. Exploring the broader consequences of diarrhoeal diseases on child health. Lancet Global Health 2018;6:e230–32.

Chapter 8

Balinskaite V, Johnson AP, Holmes A, et al. The impact of a national antimicrobial stewardship programme on antibiotic prescribing in primary care. An interrupted time series analysis. Clin Infect Dis 2018. Published online October 2018. doi: https://doi.org/10.1093/cid/ciy902

Baur D, Gladstone BP, Burkert F, et al. Effect of antibiotic stewardship on the incidence of infection and colonisation with antibiotic-resistant bacteria and Clostridium difficile infection: a systematic review and meta-analysis. Lancet Infect Dis 2017;17:990–1001.

Blumenthal KG, Wickner PG, Hurwitz S, et al. Tackling inpatient penicillin allergies: tools for antimicrobial stewardship. J Allerg Clin Immunol 2017;140(1):154–61. doi:10.1016/j.jaci.2017.02.005.

Brink AJ, Messina AP, Feldman C, et al. Antibiotic stewardship across 47 South African hospitals: an implementation study. Lancet Infect Dis 2016;16:1017–25.

Cai T, Nesi G, Mazzoli S, et al. Asymptomatic bacteriuria treatment is associated with a higher prevalence of antibiotic resistant strains in women with urinary tract infections. Clin Infect Dis 2015;61(11):1655–61.

Czaplewski L, Bax R, Clokie M, et al. Alternatives to antibiotics—a pipeline portfolio review. Lancet Infect Dis 2016;16(2):239–51.

Daniels S, Unlu C, de Korte N, et al. Dutch diverticular disease (3D) collaborative study group. Randomized clinical trial of observation versus antibiotic treatment for a first episode of CT-proven uncomplicated acute diverticulitis. Br J Surg 2017;104:52–61.

de la Poza M, Dalmau GM, Bakedano MM, et al. Prescription strategies in acute uncomplicated respiratory infections. A randomized clinical trial. JAMA Intern Med 2016;176(1):21–29.

Doernberg SB, Abbo LM, Burdette SD, et al. Essential resources and strategies for antibiotic stewardship programs in the acute care setting. Clin Infect Dis 2018;67(8):1168–74.

Fidock D. A breathprint for malaria: new opportunities for noninterventional diagnostics and malaria traps? J Infect Dis 2018;217:1512–13.

Fishman N. Policy statement on antimicrobial stewardship by the Society of Healthcare Epidemiology of America (SHEA), the Infectious Diseases Society of America (IDSA), and the Pediatric Infectious Diseases Society (PIDS). Infect Control Hosp Epidemiol 2012;33:322–27.

Fleming-Dutra KE, Hersh AL, Shapiro DJ, et al. Prevalence of inappropriate antibiotic prescriptions among US ambulatory care visits, 2010–2011. JAMA 2016;315(17):1864–73.

Gerber JS, Newland JG, Coffin SE, et al. Variability in antibiotic use at children's hospitals. Pediatrics 2010;126(6):1067–73.

Gould IM, Lawes T. Editorial. Antibiotic stewardship: prescribing social norms. Lancet 2016;387:1699–701.

Hallsworth M, Chadborn T, Sallis A, et al. Provision of social norm feedback to high prescribers of antibiotics in general practice: a pragmatic national randomised controlled trial. Lancet 2016;387:1743–51.

Harris AM, Hicks LA, Qaseem A, et al. Appropriate antibiotic use for acute respiratory tract infection in adults: advice for high-value care from the American College of Physicians and the Centers for Disease Control and Prevention. Ann Intern Med 2016;164:425–34.

Hicks LA, Bartoces MG, Roberts RM, et al. US outpatient antibiotic prescribing variation according to geography, patient population, and provider specialty in 2011. Clin Infect Dis 2015;60:1308–16.

Hoberman A, Paradise JL, Rockette HE, et al. Shortened antimicrobial treatment for acute otitis media in young children. N Engl J Med 2016;375:2446–56.

Huang DT, Yealy DM, Filbin MR, et al. Procalcitonin-guided use of antibiotics for lower respiratory tract infection. N Engl J Med 2018;379:236–49.

IACG (Interagency Coordination Group). Ad hoc interagency coordination group on antimicrobial resistance (IACG). New York: United Nations.

Kabbani S, Hirsh AL, Shapiro DJ, et al. Opportunities to improve fluoroquinolone prescribing in the US for adult ambulatory care visits. Clin Infect Dis 2018;67:134–36.

King LM, Sanchez G, Bartoces M, et al. Antibiotic therapy duration in US adults with sinusitis. JAMA Intern Med 2018;178(7):992–94.

Langford BJ, et al. Antimicrobial stewardship in the microbiology laboratory: impact of selective susceptibility reporting on ciprofloxacin utilization and susceptibility of gram-negative isolates to ciprofloxacin in a hospital setting. J Clin Microbiol 2016;54:2343.

MacFadden DR, LaDelfa A, Leen J, et al. Impact of reported beta-lactam allergy on inpatient outcomes: a multicenter prospective cohort study. Clin Infect Dis 2016;63(7):904–10.

Martinez KA, Rood M, Jhangiani N, et al. Association between antibiotic prescribing for respiratory tract infections and patient satisfaction in direct-to-consumer telemedicine. JAMA Intern Med 2018;178(11):1558–60.

Meeker D, et al. Effect of behavioral interventions on in appropriate antibiotic prescribing among primary care practices: a randomized clinical trial. JAMA 2016;315(6):562–70.

Meier MA, Branche A, Neeser OL, et al. Procalcitonin-guided treatment in patients with positive blood cultures: a patient-level meta-analysis of randomized trials. Clin Infect Dis 2018. https://doi.org/10.1093/cid/ciy917

Mercuro NJ, Kenney RM, Lanfranco O-A, et al. Ambulatory quinolone prescribing: moving from opportunity to implementation. Clin Infect Dis 2018;67(8):1306–7.

PACCARB (Presidents's Advisory Council on Combating Antibiotic Resistant Bacteria). Key strategies to enhance infection prevention and antibiotic stewardship. Report with recommendations for human and animal health. September 2018. Washington, DC: U.S. Department of Health and Human Services.

Pulcini C, Binda F, Lamkang AS, et al. Developing core elements and checklist items for global hospital antimicrobial stewardship programmes: a consensus approach, Clin Microbiol Infect 2018. doi:10.1016/j.cmi.2018.03.033

Pulia MS, Schulz L, Fox BC. Procalcitonin-guided antibiotic use. N Engl J Med 2018;379(20):1971–72.

Schaber CLL, Katta N, Bollinger LB, et al. Breathprinting reveals malaria-associated biomarkers and mosquito attractants. J Infect Dis 2018;217:1553–60.

Schuetz P, Wirz Y, Sager R, et al. Procalcitonin to initiate or discontinue antibiotics in acute respiratory tract infections. Cochrane Database Syst Rev 2017;10:CD007498.

Schuetz P, Wirtz Y, Mueller B. Procalcitonin testing to guide antibiotic therapy in acute upper and lower respiratory tract infections. JAMA 2018;319:925–26.

Schulman J, Dimand RJ, Lee HC, et al. Neonatal intensive care unit antibiotic use. Pediatrics 2015;135:826–33.

Stocker M, van Herk W, el Helou S, et al. Procalcitonin-guided decision making for duration of antibiotic therapy in neonates with suspected early-onset sepsis: a multicentre, randomised controlled trial (NeoPIns). Lancet 2017;390:871–81.

Theuretzbacher U, Gottwalt S, Beyer P, et al. Analysis of the clinical antibacterial and antituberculosis pipeline. Lancet Infect Dis 2019;19:e40–50.

Tonkin-Crine SKG, Tan PS, van Hecke O, et al. Clinician-targeted interventions to influence antibiotic prescribing behavior for acute

respiratory infections in primary care: an overview of systematic
reviews (Review). Cochrane Database of Systematic Reviews
2017;9:DC012252. http://www.cochranelibrary.com.

Trubiano JA, Adkinson NF, Phillips EJ. Penicillin allergy is not
necessarily forever. JAMA 2017;318:82–83.

United Nations. Draft political declaration of the high-level
meeting of the General Assembly on antimicrobial resistance.
New York: United Nations; 2016.

Woolhouse M, Farrar J. An intergovernmental panel on antimicrobial
resistance. Nature 2014;509:555–57.

World Bank. Drug-resistant infections: a threat to our economic future.
Washington, DC: World Bank, 2017. License: creative commons
Attribution CC BY 3.0 IGO.

World Health Organization (WHO). WHO model list of essential
medicines. 20th list (March 2017). Geneva: World Health
Organization; 2017.

World Health Organization (WHO). Prioritization of pathogens to
guide discovery, research and development of new antibiotics
for drug-resistant bacterial infections including tuberculosis.
Geneva: World Health Organization, 2017.

Wunderink RG, et al. Pneumococcal community-acquired pneumonia
detected by serotype-specific urinary antigen detection assays. Clin
Infect Dis 2018;66:1504–10.

INDEX